The Piercing Bible

The **Piercing** Bible

The Definitive Guide to Safe Body Piercing

ELAYNE ANGEL

CROSSING PRESS
Berkeley

Copyright © 2009 by Elayne Angel
Illustrations copyright © 2009 by Jennifer Klepacki
Front cover photo copyright © 2009 Jupiterimages Corporation
Back cover author photo copyright © ASHLEY, www.savageskin.co.uk

All rights reserved. Published in the United States by Crossing Press, an imprint of the Crown Publishing Group, a division of Random House, Inc., New York.
www.crownpublishing.com
www.tenspeed.com

Crossing Press and the Crossing Press colophon are registered trademarks of Random House, Inc.

Photos of jewelry on pages 5, 19, 43, 67, 72, 73, 81, 179, 217, 228, 240, 241, and 261 reprinted by permission of J.D. Lorenz of Industrial Strength Body Jewelry, www.isbodyjewelry.com.

Photos of jewelry and tools on the spine and pages 57, 59, 60, 66, 68, 70, 79, 94, 97, 99, 131, 222, and 223 reprinted by permission of Paul King of Cold Steel, www.coldsteelamerica.net.

Photos of jewelry on pages 97, 100, and 113 reprinted by permission of Gale Shub of Body Circle Designs, www.bodycircle.com.

Photos of tapers on pages 63 and threadless snap-together jewelry on page 73 reprinted by permission of Mark Siekierski of NeoMetal, www.neometal.com.

Library of Congress Cataloging-in-Publication Data

Angel, Elayne.
    The piercing bible : the definitive guide to safe body piercing / Elayne Angel.
        p.   cm.
Includes bibliographical references and index.
    Summary: "A manual that covers everything piercers and piercees need to know about the process, from the woman who brought tongue-piercing into the mainstream and has performed over 40,000 piercings"—Provided by publisher.
    1. Body piercing—Safety measures. 2. Body piercing—Health aspects. I. Title.

RD119.5.B82.A54 2009
617'.024—dc22   2008037558

ISBN 978-1-58091-193-1

Printed in the United States of America

Cover design by Toni Tajima
Interior design by Jeff Brandenburg

11 10 9 8 7 6 5

First Edition

To Lee Bass, with gratitude, for providing
the foundation and impetus for this book

Contents

Preface

Body piercing is not only my profession; it is my profound and lasting passion. I am still intrigued and delighted by piercing after devoting decades to the industry, performing over forty thousand piercings on other people, and receiving more than forty of my own.

Way back in 1972, I shocked my poor mother when she opened the bathroom door and caught me in the act of poking another hole through my already-pierced ear. I assured her, "Mom, other people are going to do this, too. I just *know* it!" Naturally she didn't believe me at the time; she and my father thought I was an inexplicably unusual girl.

Being a piercer wasn't a common vocation when I started working at a small business called Gauntlet in the 1980s. There was only one piercing specialty studio in the United States, and I was its manager. At the time, only ear piercing was commonly practiced elsewhere, and combination tattoo-and-piercing studios had yet to crop up. My dismayed parents visibly blanched when they learned about my career move.

More than thirty years after that first incident in the bathroom, my parents were amazed to find that the "freaky piercing stuff" I'd experimented with in my youth has actually become a part of our contemporary culture. Ultimately my folks have come to appreciate my role in professionalizing and promoting piercing. Now when my mom runs into someone who is visibly pierced, she hands out one of my business cards and proudly explains, "My daughter is a piercing pioneer! She is responsible for the popularity of tongue piercings."

One of the hardest parts of my job is seeing botched piercings and hearing horrible accounts from people who have suffered unnecessary pain, infection, and frustration at the hands of unqualified piercers. Sometimes they receive an ugly scar for their efforts instead of attractive jewelry in a healed piercing, as they wanted. There is the potential for disease transmission if piercings are improperly performed or treated; the risks are real. People have so many questions: Which jewelry is best? How do I find a good piercer? What should I use to clean my piercing?

I've written thousands of letters and emails to answer these and other piercing-related questions for individuals from around the world. I am a "career volunteer" for the Association of Professional Piercers and have served three terms on their board of directors. I've contributed to their educational materials and spoken about piercing to audiences of piercers, students, educators, and medical professionals. For years I have penned a monthly column about piercing for the body art industry publication, *Pain Magazine*. Yet still it wasn't enough. I realized I needed to disseminate more information than I could share in these ways. The solution was to write this book.

Now, the knowledge required to avoid unskilled piercers, junk jewelry, and a host of piercing pitfalls is available to everyone who is interested. Read, learn, and go forth to be pierced in safety.

—ELAYNE ANGEL, MÉRIDA, MEXICO

Acknowledgments

Tremendous thanks to my husband, Jake, for his strength, love, and perpetual belief in me; to Carolyn Ward for true friendship, moral support, and editing advice; and to Mark McDiarmid for taking me under his wing and seeing to it that *The Piercing Bible* got its chance to fly.

Much gratitude to Ten Speed Press and the whole wonderful team there for all of their expertise and hard work. Thanks to my tireless editor, Lisa Westmoreland, and my agent, Jim Donovan, for answering more questions than anybody should ever be asked.

Thank you to my esteemed colleagues for invaluable input: Paul King, David Vidra, Bethrah Szumski, Didier Suarez, Dominic Klumpe, Eric "Sque3z" Anderson, Jason Pfohl, and Erica Skadsen. Likewise to my respected supporters from the health-care professions: Dr. Stanley Steinberg (my dad), Betsy Reynolds, Scott DeBoer, and Dr. Myrna Armstrong.

Credit where credit is due: to J.D. Lorenz of Industrial Strength Body Jewelry, Paul King of Cold Steel, Gale Shub of Body Circle Designs, and Mark Siekierski of NeoMetal for the use of photos of jewelry, tapers, and tools. I deeply appreciate your generosity and assistance.

My apologies and thanks to Caitlin McDiarmid and the Association of Professional Piercers board of directors for allowing me to put my book ahead of my board duties.

Todo mi aprecio a mi ángel Yucateca, Lulu, y todo su familia, por su cuidado sobre mi familia, dándome la libertad para hacer mi trabajo. (All my appreciation to my Yucatecan angel, Lulu, and her whole family, for taking care of me and mine, which gave me the freedom to work.)

A thousand thanks to Jennifer Klepacki for doing a stunning job on the illustrations, and for unwavering dedication and patience.

I am grateful to each and every individual I've pierced, for trusting me with their skin—for without them I couldn't have gained the knowledge and experience that enabled me to create *The Piercing Bible*.

And, finally, kudos to the many people who contributed to this project but are not mentioned by name.

Introduction: Piercing 101

Whether it fascinates or repels, there is something captivating about hard metal worn through tender flesh. Piercing is thrilling. Literally. The word *thrill* originates from the Middle English word *thrillen*, "To perforate by a pointed instrument. Hence, to cause a shivering, throbbing, tingling, or exquisite sensation; to pierce; to penetrate."[1] By that account, piercing sounds quite exciting. And so it is! Body piercing is among the most ancient *and* the most contemporary of practices for ornamenting and customizing the human form.

The Art of Modern Body Piercing

In recent times, body piercing has exploded as a form of personal expression nearly anyone may use to enhance their appearance, self-image, and quality of life. The phenomenon is so pervasive that housewives, police officers, and schoolteachers wear tongue, navel, nipple, and other piercings (although you might never know if they don't tell you). Millions of people are already pierced, and countless more are considering body piercings or have pierced family members, students, or patients. Nowadays, piercing involves much more than a ring through an earlobe. Wherever there is a natural fold or flap of skin, there is a piercing waiting to happen. Multiple piercings all over the body are pervasive, and people are taking the art to an extreme never seen before.

The practice of body piercing is part of a group of activities that include tattooing, scarification, branding, and other body art. These practices are often grouped under the term *body modification*. The number of possible placements on the body; the array of jewelry styles, sizes, and materials; and the necessary aftercare all distinguish piercing from other types of body modification. Piercing breaks the protective barrier of the skin and leaves a foreign object in the body, so there are risks of infection and other potential dangers. If every aspect is not handled appropriately, complications are more likely.

The rise in the popularity of body piercing has resulted in a proliferation of piercers and jewelry. Some of the products and services are good, but unfortunately many are of very poor quality. Piercing establishments range from inexpensive jewelry kiosks at shopping malls to high-end specialty studios staffed with professional piercers, the latest equipment, and top-quality jewelry. There is a big difference between them! Choosing the right piercer and jewelry dramatically increases your chances for uneventful healing. The relative newness of professional body piercing—it has been widely practiced only since the 1990s—has many ramifications for consumers. There are still no standardized regulations, piercer training, or competency requirements in the United States. At most, local laws mandate hygiene requirements or restrict the piercing of minors. In many cities, however, even these simple regulations do not exist; in others, local laws are not enforced.

The art of body piercing is still evolving, and its practitioners continue to experiment with its limits and possibilities. Debates persist among professional piercers themselves about basic aspects of the craft, such as the use of tools and regimens for aftercare. The information in this book is intended to distill the most sensible piercing advice available. By educating yourself, you can get a great first—or twentieth—piercing or find the information you need to deal with a bungled job.

How to Use This Book

The Piercing Bible is primarily directed toward piercees, but it also contains a wealth of information for the parents of children who want to get pierced or are already pierced, teachers who work with pierced students, health-care professionals who deal with pierced patients (whether treating problem piercings or performing unrelated medical procedures), and piercers who want an authoritative reference work or an educational tool for clients.

Part 1 touches on the ancient and modern history of this art form and contains general information about who is getting pierced and what commonly motivates them. The novice piercee should carefully read parts 2 and 3, which provide a rundown on everything that should be taken into consideration when making a decision to get pierced. Part 4 describes each of the most common piercings in detail. Piercees can use it as a reference, and piercers will also find pointers here. This part includes information about jewelry sizes, styles, and piercing placements as well as the techniques I normally use to perform each piercing. Next, part 5 describes basic and alternative aftercare and provides information on troubleshooting healing complications. Part 6 explains the maintenance of healed piercings, describes special situations encountered when living with piercings, and explores advanced practices for healed piercings, including stretching. Finally, part 7 takes a look at the future of body piercing and includes a section on becoming a piercer.

The appendices include "A Piercee's Bill of Rights," a chart of minimum healing times for popular piercings, and a chart for jewelry size conversions (gauge and millimeter). There's also a handy fill-in chart to help you to keep track of your own piercings and jewelry, and a glossary of piercing-related terms.

Why This Book?

Piercing can be dangerous, and it is far more complicated than most people realize. The hazards range from tearing, scarring, migration, and rejection to localized bacterial infections and, though rare, serious infections. Consumers need facts about the risks, choices, and best practices involved. People who interact with piercees also need to be informed about various aspects of piercing. Many myths have persisted, even in academic and medical literature; they are finally dispelled here, too.

Body piercings are often associated with tattoos, and they are frequently performed in the same establishments. However, tattoos are comparatively straightforward; healing is rapid, and there are seldom complications. The same is not true of body piercings. Piercings require special attention during a prolonged period of healing plus regular maintenance once they are healed. There is a baffling array of options for where to pierce, what jewelry to put in the perforation, and how to care for the wound. Many people get the bulk of their "facts" about piercing from the Internet; unfortunately, the Web can be unreliable, offering contradictory information from questionable sources. Countless piercees have experienced needless pain, healing problems, and undesirable outcomes from a lack of sound information.

Will your pierced body part turn green and fall off if you don't follow every rule and guideline in the book? Probably not, but by educating yourself and being conscientious, you will have a much greater chance of having a healthy piercing that heals well, gives you a minimum of trouble, and provides the greatest enjoyment. Admittedly, not every piercee who fails to adhere to sound practices has a terrible catastrophe—but some of them do. This book takes a cautionary tone because the risks are real.

Disclaimers and Sound Advice

The Piercing Bible is deliberately limited in scope to provide detailed, useful information about the most common body piercings. Related subjects such as "play" (temporary) piercings, implants, and suspensions, which are all part of the broader piercing scene, will be touched on only in passing. Tattoos and more extreme forms of body modification, such as scarification, branding, tongue splitting, and so on, will not be addressed.

This book is *not* an instructional manual on how to perform body piercings on yourself or others. Visit a competent professional piercer for all permanent piercings. If you are interested in becoming a piercer, I urge you to seek out appropriate training under the guidance of an experienced mentor before attempting to do any piercings.

Some piercers exercise poor judgment and lack ethics, so you must maintain your own: never request that a piercing be performed on an animal, anyone who is intoxicated, or any other unsuitable candidate. Read more about the ethics of piercing in "Infant and Child Ear Piercing," page 251.

The Piercing Bible does not cover every possible situation, but it deals with all the areas I'm most frequently asked about. Popular terminology and names for piercings vary by region and change over time. The modern piercing industry is a new and growing field: changes are fast, frequent, and sometimes drastic. I can only present information that is current at the time of publication.

Substantive research studies, statistical analyses, and other definitive resource materials related to modern piercing are in short supply; therefore, the information, practices, and procedures described in this book are largely based on my own extensive, clinical experience. I've integrated industry standards where they exist, but there is still precious little that is truly standard, so my opinions are a primary component of many chapters.

There are few absolutes when it comes to body piercing since each individual is unique. For the sake of accuracy, words such as "frequently," "commonly," "generally," and so on are used throughout.

Finally, and importantly, I am a professional in the field of piercing, not medicine; this book is not intended to provide medical advice, diagnosis, or treatment. There is no substitute for a hands-on consultation with an experienced piercer or, when needed, the counsel of a health-care provider. This book is intended to support—not replace— the relationships that exist between piercee and piercer or doctor.

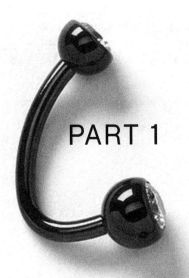

PART 1

The New Piercing

Motivations

Piercing Past and Present

1

Motivations

The urge to decorate the body and control one's appearance is a universal human trait. Each of us uses clothing, hairstyle, and so on to express our individuality and to make the most of the gifts or curses—perceived or real—bestowed by nature. Nowadays we have more choices than ever to manipulate our looks. The options range from minor adjustments such as hair dye and teeth whitener to more extreme but still socially acceptable practices such as liposuction and breast implants. Although body modification is still less conventional than, say, getting a nose job, it has become prevalent in today's world.

Piercing and other types of body modification are methods of changing the actual physical form, which is empowering in a way that may not be fully understood by those who have never participated in it. Women, in particular, are bombarded by the media's unrealistic notions of beauty, which deeply affect self-esteem and body image. They may turn to piercing or other forms of body art to help them embrace a positive attitude about themselves. While there is no unanimous consensus about whether body jewelry enhances appearance, aesthetics is a widespread motivating factor for piercing.

Who Gets Pierced and Why?

A casual observer sitting at a sidewalk café in any college town in the United States or Europe might conclude that every college student in the world has a few extra holes in the head. However, piercing is *not* exclusively a youth phenomenon nor is it always a statement of rebellion. No one should assume that their doctor or banker doesn't sport a little metal secret. I have pierced people from all professions and socioeconomic backgrounds—rocket scientists, clergy, and retired grandparents among them.

What motivates these diverse people to face their deep-seated fear of needles and pain, withstand discomfort, brave embarrassment, and endure the scorn of strangers, families, or employers and willfully undergo the needle? For piercees, the impetus to do such a thing must be very strong indeed. From the superficial to the profound, there are a multitude of reasons for getting pierced. It might be about attracting attention, the sensation of metal through flesh, or the opportunity to wear some extra "bling." For others, piercing is a response to deep internal triggers.

There is often a marked difference in age between those who are visibly pierced above the neck and those more discreetly pierced in intimate locations below the neck. Younger people are frequently motivated by a desire to fit in with their peers or the need to establish their independence from their parents. Visible piercings offer a perfect vehicle for fulfilling these desires. Young piercees tend to be more heavily influenced by popular music, media, and fashion, and they are frequently limited in their piercing options by regulations for those under the age of majority.

Older people are obviously not subject to these prohibitions nor are they typically motivated by the same impulses. Many adults endure trauma or other life experiences that lead them to turn to body modification for self-realization and healing purposes. For working adults whose employers frown on visible piercings, torso and genital piercings are popular because they are concealed under everyday clothing.

> "I have a somewhat flat face, and I feel the piercings give it the outline I would otherwise have to achieve through makeup every single morning. Also, people have a certain image of an Asian girl: the ever-smiling submissive and fragile cherry blossom princess. I think I had to do something to destroy that image, to make it visible that that isn't me." M.

> "After birthing two girls (who weighed over eight pounds each) and passing forty, I needed something to make me feel like 'me' again, not just a mom, and a wife, and a nurse, etc. I chose a navel piercing 'cause I've always thought they were sexy. I knew there was a sexy part of me somewhere inside, and my piercings helped bring that out again." J.

Group Identification

Piercing and body modification can be used to indicate and solidify one's cultural identity. There is a sense among many of my pierced and tattooed contemporaries that we belong to an intrinsically interconnected group. One popular piercing website calls itself "Tribalectic," suggesting that its members feel connected to others as part of a contemporary tribe. Many Western piercees describe themselves as "Modern Primitives" and proudly wear ethnic and tribal jewelry made of horn, wood, and stone. Conversely, some tribal people make use of modern materials. The herdsmen of northern Kenya, for example, sometimes use the metals found in telephone wires to make lip and ear ornaments.[1]

Today, many young people use piercings to visibly align themselves with rave, goth, skater, and other subcultures. It may seem contradictory, but piercing is sometimes a statement of rebellion and conformity at the same time.

Magical and Symbolic Healing

Piercing can be used as a way to restore physical and spiritual health after a trauma or to exercise some control while struggling with chronic illness or feelings of vulnerability. Many people get pierced with the intention of exchanging bad for good. This type of symbolic healing is used today when women reclaim their bodies by getting a genital piercing after childbearing or sexual assault. Through the conscious act of breaking skin and shedding blood, these people feel whole, connected with their bodies, and in control of their lives again.

> "I was drugged and raped at a party. . . . For nearly two years I let that one event get to me. I didn't like to be touched, and sex was out of the question. My husband helped with a lot of those issues, but the final touch was that ring. It was a tangible reminder that I was in control of what happened there. Those parts were mine, and even if someone else had violated that, they were for my enjoyment. Oddly, the nightmarish memories stopped shortly after having it done. I suppose it is a therapy all to its own." B.

> "Personally, I made the choice to take control of the needles. Because of my blood disorder, I am a human pincushion. . . . So, my piercings are a way for me to dictate when, where, and why I am being poked with a sharp needle! For me it is a reclaiming of me; my body is not just a pincushion for medical uses . . . . It is a piece of artwork!" S.

Rites of Passage

Ceremonial practices have provided structure and meaning to our lives throughout the ages. Unfortunately, modern society retains few of these practices, so people often struggle to create their own rites to mark the changes in their lives. Piercing accomplishes this when it is used to commemorate a milestone. Many visit a piercing or tattoo studio soon after or even on the very date of their eighteenth birthday to celebrate finally having legal possession of their own skin. Whether or not the piercing experience is consciously approached in a ritual manner, getting a piercing does effect a physical—and possibly an emotional or spiritual—transformation.

I have performed piercings to mark births, deaths, graduations, divorces, clean-and-sober time, relationship commitments, anniversaries of all kinds, and other special occasions in people's lives. One young woman memorialized the death of her peers with a piercing:

> "I wanted to get a piercing done to remember my senior year because a lot happened that I don't want to forget—most importantly, the passing of three members of my senior class. . . . I also wanted to get either a piercing or tattoo to show that—hey, I'm eighteen, I can do it now!" M.

Erotic Inspirations

Many adults are motivated to be pierced for sexual gratification. The presence of piercings and jewelry in certain locations results in increased physical stimulation for piercees or their partners. Couples sometimes use piercings to revitalize their sensual focus and reignite the flames in relationships that have lost some of their spark. Intimate piercings can bolster confidence in the bedroom and in oneself as a sexual being.

Many people do not find their private parts attractive or appealing. A large proportion of men from Western nations have had their genitals altered through nonconsensual circumcision during infancy. When an individual makes a choice about the appearance of his or her own genitals by piercing and adorning them with jewelry, it can be highly liberating, and for many it inspires a harmony with their bodies that could not be achieved through any other means.

"One of the main reasons [I got a piercing] was that I've always had confidence issues, and I felt that if I could drop my pants in front of a stranger and get a needle shoved through it, I could do damn near anything and everything else." J.

"I saw a picture of a guy with a genital piercing on the Internet . . . and it intrigued me. I wondered, like most guys would, *why* would a sensible guy go and have a piece of metal stuck through a sensitive part of his body. Well, at the time I was still coming to terms with my sexuality, and I wondered how anyone could like me if even I wasn't sure about myself. . . . I now feel more self-confident about who I am and am more comfortable with myself and the identity I present to the public." C.

A Special Connection

A piercing client and close friend of mine named Cliff willed his body jewelry to his friends when he knew the end of his life was imminent. After he passed away, I sterilized his jewelry and inserted it into the piercings of the people who loved him. Cliff's friends maintain a connection with him by wearing his jewelry. A part of him carries on, literally inside of them.

Contemporary Considerations

By getting pierced, people make bold statements about personal freedom and combat the impersonality and pressures of modern life. Piercing the body can be an effective way to exert control over one's existence. Even if their modifications are not visible to the public, people working in conservative environments often use piercings to remind themselves that they are individuals despite the conventionality of their outward appearance. One man living in the Midwest told me, "I was about fifty when I got my first. I live in a place where ignorance and poverty are a career choice. Almost everyone is religious, conservative, and tends to believe that everyone else shares that viewpoint. Bigotry is rampant. I needed to make a statement that said, in effect, I might be one of you, but I'm not one with you. Piercing was, and is, that statement."

Which Ear Is the Gay Ear?

This commonly asked question reflects an uncertainty about piercings and what they may suggest about the sexual orientation of the wearer. Some people fear that being pierced may cause others to mistakenly believe they are homosexual or participate in the BDSM (consensual bondage and discipline and sadomasochism) lifestyle. Piercing, however, has evolved a great deal since a pierced right ear was used as a coded message by gay men in the 1970s, and it's now a practice embraced by all types of people. In other words, it doesn't matter whether your ear or some other body part is pierced, or which side you choose; it doesn't mean you're gay.

While many people who engage in unconventional forms of sexual expression *do* have piercings, being pierced does not signify anything in particular—except for any meaning *you* wish to ascribe to it. Nor, of course, does getting pierced turn you gay, as was the misguided concern of one client from Atlanta. He stormed back into the piercing studio the day after he received an ear piercing and angrily reported, "You pierced the wrong ear, and now I've caught the gay!"

Well, Why Not?

Many people don't spend a lot of time considering why they choose this form of self-expression. Doing it simply because you like it and it makes you feel good about yourself are some of the best reasons for getting pierced. Upon reflection, sometimes a deeper reason will become apparent, but this isn't required for piercing to be gratifying.

"A hurricane destroyed everything my family knew. We lost our pet, who was part of the family. My kids are scarred. . . . Our bodies are our own. And, for good or bad, what happens to our bodies is generally left up to us as individuals. . . . It doesn't belong to the professional world, it doesn't belong to the government, it sure as hell doesn't belong to FEMA. It's *your* body. Treat it with respect, but don't be afraid to explore it. I fumbled around the concept of fear regarding social acceptance or even pain due to piercing. In retrospect, those fears are trivial beyond belief." C.

2

Piercing Past to Present

From the prehistoric era to the present, piercing has been an important part of the tradition of permanent body decoration. Museums are full of ear ornaments from every part of the world; the jewelry is made from the most mundane materials to the truly precious. We can better appreciate the uniqueness and diversity of modern body piercing by acknowledging the ways humans have pierced themselves in the past.

Historical Inaccuracy

Unfortunately, records about the history of body piercing are scant, often sensationalized, and filled with inaccuracies. Archaeological relics reveal little, since pierced flesh has usually long since vanished into dust. Only durable jewelry and a few rare finds of preserved human remains tell the tale. References to body piercing in written records are scarce, and scholarly interpretations are often contradictory. One source, for example, says that traditional nostril piercings worn by Indian women are a sign of beauty and status, while another claims that they are meant to induce submissiveness in women.[1] These inconsistencies may demonstrate that motivations for piercing are multifaceted, and that they change over time. Further, no researcher or historian is capable of recording anything without personal bias affecting his or her work.

Anthropologists have only recently begun to treat body decoration with any seriousness. Clarifying the history of body piercing has been made even more difficult because many of the colorful stories about its origins were entirely fabricated by an influential early modern enthusiast, Doug Malloy (see page 16). His myths were widely circulated and repeated until they were considered facts. Almost every account of piercing history—even the most scholarly—reiterates some of his fictitious tales.

Since the focus of *The Piercing Bible* is on helping the consumer with day-to-day piercing questions and concerns, it is beyond the scope of this book to provide a detailed historical study of body piercing. The emphasis of this chapter is on the development of the modern piercing industry in the late twentieth century. Therefore, only a brief overview of what is reliably known about piercing in the ancient world and in modern tribal societies is presented.

The Ancient World

Here are some of the oldest documented references to piercing:

- India's ancient religious texts, the Vedas, dating from about 1500 B.C.E., describe the goddess Lakshmi wearing earlobe and nose piercings.[2]

- Ötzi the Iceman, the 5,300-year-old mummy preserved in the Austrian Alps, had stretched earlobe piercings as well as numerous tattoos.
- The Tomb of the Ukok Princess was unearthed on the border of China and Russia in the 1990s. Artifacts there include sophisticated gold jewelry for pierced ears dating from 400 to 300 B.C.E.[3]
- Earrings and other ear ornaments for pierced ears originating from ancient Greece, Cyprus, and China have been found.
- *Infibulation* (the restriction of sexual activity through mechanical means) was extensively practiced on men in antiquity. It was usually accomplished by passing a *fibula* (fastening device) through two sides of the foreskin. This procedure was often performed on slaves in ancient Rome to assure their chastity, and on gladiators, to guard against the loss of their strength due to "sexual excesses."[4] Actors and singers would also undergo infibulation, since intercourse was believed to be harmful to the voice.[5]
- First-century writer Celsus (25–50 C.E.) describes the procedure in his medical encyclopedia, which commences something like a modern piercing: "The foreskin covering the glans is stretched forward and the point for perforation marked on each side with ink."[6] An echo of this practice carried on in modern Europe to prevent the "harmful effects of masturbation" in young men.[7]
- From Peru to Mexico, ancient Mesoamerica and South America had rich traditions of personal adornment, including elaborate plugs for enlarged earlobe piercings, and septum jewelry. Ritual piercings, particularly of the tongue and penis, were practiced in Olmec, Mayan, and Aztec cultures.
- The oldest known written reference to piercing the glans of the penis is in the *Kama Sutra*, an ancient Sanskrit text on the art of love dating back to around the first century C.E. It describes in detail a variety of penis inserts and pins as a means of enhancing sexual enjoyment for a man and his partner.[8]

Tribal Cultures

Among the body parts commonly pierced today, a few have substantial tribal antecedents from around the globe:

- **Labret:** The word *labret* (pronounced with a hard *t*) refers to an ornament worn through a perforation in the lip. It has been in our dictionaries since the nineteenth century, after explorers interacted with the Tlingit people of Alaska. Labret piercings have been practiced in diverse areas, including Papua New Guinea, Ethiopia, Amazonia, and the northwest coast of the United States.
- **Nostril:** This traditional piercing placement in India has also been worn by indigenous tribes in both North and South America.
- **Nasal septum:** A widespread piercing in Mesoamerica, South America, Papua New Guinea, Borneo, and elsewhere. Septum jewelry can be particularly frightening and impressive, making this a popular ornament in many warrior cultures.
- **Ear cartilage:** Popular among African tribal peoples such as the Fulani and Maasai, upper-ear piercings were also common among the Iban Dayaks of Borneo, who wore their ornaments for a fearsome appearance and to denote their status.[9] The

claws and teeth of leopards and bears were placed through the upper ears of successful hunters.[10]

- **Tongue:** Shamans of at least one aboriginal tribe in central Australia, the Aranda, wore tongue piercings. A hole the size of a small finger was ostensibly left by a spirit's lance as proof of the encounter and the attainment of shamanic status. A shaman must not practice for a year after receiving the piercing. If it closed, he would know his power was gone and he would not practice at all.[11]

- **Penis:** Many varieties of penis piercing and modification have been practiced worldwide, including the implantation of beads, gold bells, or other foreign objects under the skin of the penis in men of Southeast Asia. Japanese men have a tradition of inserting pearls under the skin. Australian aboriginal men sometimes insert small stones into incisions in the penis.[12]

Western Civilization

Unlike traditional tribal cultures, modern Western nations have not been a fertile ground for body piercing. Religion has had an intense puritanical effect on our relationships with our bodies, and biblical passages have been interpreted to mean that marking the skin is prohibited because the body belongs to God.

Westerners' attitudes toward body art changed during the early fifteenth through seventeenth centuries as travelers and explorers returned with tales from faraway lands where the savages painted, poked, and decorated their bodies. Sailors came home sporting earrings and tattoos. Among sailors' favorite ornaments were gold earrings, which were reputed to pay for a proper burial if the seaman washed ashore.[13] These masculine decorations eventually spread to soldiers, miners, and stevedores. There is also evidence that a number of upper-class men and women, particularly in the Victorian era, were inspired to flirt with piercings. A "breast-piercing craze" hit London in the 1890s, and the practice reportedly became popular among "seemingly sane, civilized Englishwomen."[14]

Sailors, Freaks, and Fetishists

Seafaring men had been decorating themselves for centuries, but prior to World War II, body art was still mostly limited to sailors and sideshow entertainers. During this time, however, there were a few body art pioneers who carried it further, mostly in secret. Ethel Granger, whose famous thirteen-inch corseted waist echoed the practice of decades past, was one notable fan of body piercing. Ethel's husband, Will Granger, assisted her by piercing her nostrils, septum, nipples, and ear cartilage. She was the first woman recorded in modern history to be so extensively pierced.[15] Body piercing was also used in the 1930s by the Great Omi, a famous sideshow performer, born Horace Ridler. He wanted something more extreme than the tattoos that covered his entire body and face, so he had his septum pierced by a veterinarian and inserted a variety of ivory tusks. He also had his earlobes pierced and stretched until the holes could accommodate jewelry the size of a silver dollar.[16]

Punks and Primitives

In the late 1980s we began to see the emergence of two divergent philosophies about piercing and other forms of body art. One harkens back to traditional cultures by emphasizing the spiritual and ritual meanings of body modification. The other philosophy, more visceral and modern, emphasizes the use of piercing and other body modifications for pleasure, pain, and rebellion. These approaches are not always conscious, nor are they mutually exclusive, and they both still have relevance today.

One of the most influential figures in the rise of modern body piercing is Fakir Musafar, the father of modern primitivism. Born as Roland Loomis in 1930, he grew up close to an Indian reservation in South Dakota, which inspired his imagination at an early age. Fakir is one of a few modern body art pioneers whose fascination with body adornment and modification and compulsion to experiment on his own body contributed to the existence of piercing as we know it today. He coined the term *modern primitives* to represent what he felt to be the connection between the practice of body modification and the spiritual use of piercing and other rituals, often taken directly from tribal practices. He views modern primitivism as an antidote to the superficiality of modern life. A handful of individuals—including Fakir—were deeply affected by the images of indigenous body art that appeared in *National Geographic* magazine. A number of these early devotees were inspired to emulate some of the modifications they viewed in those pages.

In 1989, Re/Search Publications released a book containing a series of interviews with body modification enthusiasts who were considered radical at the time. This book, *Modern Primitives: An Investigation of Contemporary Adornment & Rituals*, was highly influential. In it are interviews with Fakir Musafar and Jim Ward, and there's even a photograph showing the outline of my angel wings after my first major tattooing session. The interviewees frankly discuss their body modifications as expressions of their alternative sexuality. *Modern Primitives* was the first mass-market publication to address these subjects in a thoughtful and nonjudgmental manner, and it had a significant impact on the early growth of piercing.

Today, there are many modern primitives who enjoy exploring the mystical side of body modification. They often prefer traditional jewelry materials to high-tech metals, and they pay tribute to their ancestors or tribal cultures through their adornments.

Body piercing as an expression of rebellion and identity assumed a harsh manifestation when the punk movement of the late 1970s and 1980s embraced it. This faction was launched by working-class youth in Britain, and it quickly spread through the force and anger of punk rock music. Punk rockers shoved safety pins through their flesh to cause shock and disgust; their piercings and tattoos conveyed group solidarity and class angst. Like the sideshow performers of the past, they used self-injury as performance art. Punks raised public awareness of piercings and helped pave the way for later popularity.

Pleasure and Pain: The Gauntlet

The first groups to embrace body piercing as a modern lifestyle choice included gay men, BDSM practitioners, and others who used piercing as a profound means for expressing their alternative sexuality. Nipples and genitals were experimented upon with enthusiasm, and they remain a staple of the piercing industry today.

The field of body piercing as we currently know it would be quite different, or perhaps nonexistent, without the involvement and commitment of a group of gay SM enthusiasts in California. These pioneers formed a network of men with an interest in piercing, spearheaded by the organizational and networking skills of Doug Malloy (see "The Legacy of Doug Malloy," page 16). Meeting informally, they helped to usher piercing into the United States.

A leader of this group, Jim Ward, is regarded as the founding father of modern body piercing. With Malloy's encouragement and financial backing, he started a small piercing business at his home in West Hollywood in 1975. Inspired by too many late-night calls for piercing assistance and a desire to legitimize his work, Ward eventually moved to a storefront. In November 1978, Gauntlet Enterprises opened on Santa Monica Boulevard in West Hollywood—the first professional body piercing specialty studio in America.

Gauntlet's early clientele was from the local alternative communities and the T&P (tattooing and piercing) social club organized by Doug Malloy. Gradually public figures, including musicians, models, and actors, started to patronize the studio, followed by growing numbers of the general public. Initially Jim Ward made the jewelry himself on the premises, and piercings had an element of trial and error. An "installation" was free with a jewelry purchase. The jewelry designs (along with Ward's names for them), piercing techniques, and placements pioneered by Gauntlet established the foundation for today's body piercing industry.

It was Jim Ward, along with Doug Malloy and Fakir Musafar, who also produced the world's first professional publication dedicated to the subject, *Piercing Fans International Quarterly* (PFIQ). The inaugural issue of the magazine was published in 1977, and it had a run of fifty issues before it finally shared the unfortunate fate of Gauntlet itself in 1998. After having grown to encompass multiple retail branches, a jewelry manufacturing department, corporate offices, and a mail-order division, they went out of business. After twenty years in operation, a series of bad business decisions necessitated an infusion of outside capital. Subsequently, a hostile takeover led to Chapter Seven bankruptcy and permanent closure.

I received the first honorary "Master Piercer" certificate bestowed by Jim Ward, and I was the first to present an enthusiastic female face to the world as a piercing advocate. When the book *Modern Primitives* gained recognition, the press began to seek out professional piercers. As vice president of the original Gauntlet branch in Los Angeles in the late 1980s and early 1990s, I was in the right place at the right time to participate in a flurry of media exposure that helped to broaden the appeal of piercing in the United States.

Body piercing is a distinctly sexual form of self-expression for many piercees, and at times, this aspect of piercing has overshadowed its wider meanings and popularity. During the 1987 police raids in Britain referred to as Operation Spanner, sixteen men were arrested and charged with assault for private, consensual homosexual activities, which included body piercing. One of these "Spanner Men" was Alan Oversby, also known as Mr. Sebastian, who is considered by many to be the father of European piercing. An influential British tattooist and piercer, he was largely self-taught; and, like Jim Ward, he received some instruction from Doug Malloy. Oversby was arrested for performing a genital piercing on a client and sentenced for "assault occasioning actual bodily harm." The courts refused to hear the defense that the activity was consensual,

The Legacy of Doug Malloy

If you have ever heard that the Prince Albert piercing was named after the one worn by Queen Victoria's consort or that Roman centurions attached capes to their pierced nipples, you have been visited by the spirit of Doug Malloy. This name was the pseudonym used by Richard Simonton, a wealthy businessman who concealed his passion for piercing and his life as a homosexual SM practitioner from his family and professional associates. His deep enthusiasm for body piercing as a sexual behavior has had a lasting effect on the development of the piercing industry.

Malloy created two informal underground publications about piercing. One was a fictionalized autobiography that was available briefly as a booklet in the 1970s. The other, which has had an astoundingly enduring influence, was a leaflet entitled "Body Piercing in Brief." It contained descriptions of a dozen piercings—including their fabricated histories—with drawings by Jim Ward. This sheet aroused substantial interest in piercing and was widely disseminated by Gauntlet for many years. In spite of the problems Malloy's inventive stories have caused for researchers, Jim Ward emphasizes their importance, stating, "I sometimes wonder if people into piercing today have any deep appreciation of the tremendous impact Doug Malloy has had on their lives. . . . What was it that made him the center from which the whole modern piercing movement sprang? . . . No one before him had ever presented such a broad palette of piercing possibilities complete with history and lore. It didn't matter that he probably made up a lot of it. . . . It was a message a lot of people were waiting to hear whether they realized it or not."

saying, "Pleasure derived from the infliction of pain is an evil thing,"[17] illustrating the bias against alternative sexuality and piercing.

The Media Brings the Message

By the late twentieth century, the time was ripe for piercing to escalate in popularity and availability. As piercing became more popular within alternative groups in the 1980s, the press took notice, and this snowballed into even greater media attention. By the mid-1990s, widespread publicity in the form of print publications, television talk shows, news programs, and sitcoms fed the interest in the subject, and pierced celebrities put the cherry on the top. Piercing became part of our modern world; people were getting new holes poked all over the place.

Rock stars have had some of the greatest impact in bringing an awareness of piercing to the public. A defining event in the popularity of piercings was the 1993 launch of a popular music video by the band Aerosmith. The video for "Cryin'," which won an MTV Music Video of the Year award, featured actress Alicia Silverstone getting a navel piercing. According to my former apprentice Paul King, who portrayed the piercer in the video, the procedure was staged using a body double because the actress was still a minor. Ironically, she described navel piercing as "gross" during the video shoot.

After piercing's dramatic musical introduction, hordes of young women across the country sought to follow the new trend. The immense demand for piercing, however, occurred before a ready supply of skilled piercing professionals was available to do the job. With nowhere better to turn, would-be piercees swarmed the tattoo studios. Although tattooing and piercing are now perceived as similar types of activities, the tattoo community initially put up resistance to this new form of body modification. Many tattoo artists considered piercing to be repulsive and perverted. After an army of gals approached tattooists inquiring, "Do you do belly piercings?" they started replying, "Well . . . yes!" even though they did not possess the appropriate training, skill, or passion. Those young women in the early 1990s essentially inspired the creation of body piercing as a full-fledged industry. Driven by desire, the art was ushered into the Western world through brazen experimentation.

Throughout the 1990s and into the new millennium, navel piercing has maintained its widespread popularity, and other body piercings have followed suit, becoming acceptable with ever-broadening segments of the population.[18] Many emulate the influential fashion models, actors, musicians, and sports figures by wearing visible piercings, and even middle-aged professionals and parents have joined the ranks of the pierced, if not as openly. When the general public was first introduced to body piercings, they were shocked—even appalled. Nowadays, those same people seldom give piercings a second glance, and some of them have piercings of their own.

Media Impact

In 1990 the *National Enquirer* ran a story about body piercing with the humorous headline, "Bizarre New Fashion Fad Turns Folks into Human Pincushions." A photo showing my septum and tongue piercings was among those printed with the commentary.

Surely most readers of that article must have believed that piercing would be a short-lived craze, as reported. But the depth of attraction to body adornment proved far stronger than anybody might have imagined. This wacky article actually instigated the popularity of tongue piercings!

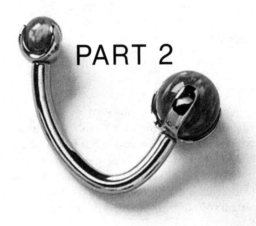

PART 2

Groundwork and Preliminary Considerations

Risks, Myths, and Warnings

Is Piercing Right for You?

You and Your Piercer

3

Risks, Myths, and Warnings

In our culture, body piercing is a lifestyle choice. Many young tribe members around the world, however, must comply with the body modification traditions of their societies. Under primitive conditions, without access to modern medical knowledge, proper sterilization, or antibiotics, these young people literally risk their lives to conform. (Imagine caring for your piercing, as some of these people do, with daily applications of animal dung!) Obviously, the dangers of piercing are different depending on the circumstances, but certain risks of body piercing are universal.

Is Piercing Risky?

A great deal of hype and hysteria about body piercing is perpetuated by the media and by conservative religious, medical, and educational communities. They describe piercing as a highly dangerous behavior related to everything from juvenile delinquency to cancer and death.

Usually, the only piercings that receive attention in the press are the problematic ones, which skew the statistics and magnify the perils. Thousands upon thousands of piercings heal without incident every year, but nobody hears about them because they are not newsworthy.

Educate yourself before getting pierced so you will be ready to deal with any problems that do occur. An introduction to the most common piercing risks is presented here. In-depth information on identifying and troubleshooting these and other complications is presented in chapter 16.

Piercing: Not a Do-It-Yourself (DIY) Hobby

At the beginning of the modern piercing movement, few competent practitioners were available. Lacking pros to help, people who felt the urge lanced their own bodies with heated sewing needles or common earrings. Even today, amateur or unethical hack piercers can be found who will pierce anything on anyone, *badly*. Young teenagers who cannot obtain parental permission for a piercing and those who cannot easily afford professional services in a studio often take this route.

Many online shops sell piercing kits, which advertise that they come with "complete instructions" and are "easy to use." Wrong! These are no safer than a home root-canal kit and must be avoided. A DIY piercing is often poorly placed and has a greatly increased risk of infection and other problems. Piercing studios are common now, so there is no longer any excuse for shoddy piercings.

Ear-Piercing Guns

In an optimal procedure, a highly trained professional gently creates a piercing with sterile equipment and inserts quality body jewelry. The guns used to pierce earlobes, ear cartilage, and sometimes other body parts do not meet these standards, so it is best to avoid them. Jewelry retailers use stud-gun piercing as a sales incentive: "Free Piercing with Purchase of Jewelry." The devices are also available directly to consumers over the Internet and in beauty supply stores. They may appear to be a cheap, convenient option, but there are a number of factors that make ear-piercing guns unsafe and inappropriate for body piercings—and even inadvisable for piercing ears.

These gadgets were originally invented for tagging cattle and other animals, and later adapted for use on humans. The gun forces a pointy earring through the skin, which causes *more* tissue trauma and discomfort than the razor-sharp needle used by body piercers. The one-size post length does not "fit all" and cannot accommodate a plump earlobe or any swelling; it is certainly not long enough to be worn in a body piercing. The stud earring typically employs a butterfly-style clasp that can inhibit the healing process and increase the risk of infection by compressing the tissue, limiting circulation, and trapping secretions and bacteria.

Blood from a piercee can *aerosolize* (become airborne in microscopic particles) and contaminate the inside of the reusable gun. These surfaces may come into contact with the next client's tissue, and it is possible to transmit disease in this way. Sometimes guns are "sanitized" between uses with alcohol or other disinfectants, but this does not kill all surface microbes. One outbreak of serious infections that caused several piercees to be hospitalized was attributed to a contaminated spray that was used to "clean" the gun between customers.[1] Most of these ear-piercing guns contain plastic parts that melt, so they cannot be processed in an *autoclave* (a machine that sterilizes equipment using heat and pressure) between clients. The gun manufacturers have attempted to address this issue by producing "one use" cartridges that contain the jewelry, but since these cartridges are inserted into a reusable device, they still pose a greater risk of infection than piercing with a sterile, disposable needle.

Other problems sometimes occur with these guns: the stud fails to fully penetrate the tissue on the first try, or the earring doesn't discharge from the gun, leaving the device stuck to the piercing. These situations require handling the tissue, and many gun operators do not wear (or even have access to) medical gloves. Many are teenagers who are not highly trained in procedure, placement, or sanitation techniques.[2]

Infection

Infection is one of the most frightening and potentially serious dangers associated with body piercing. Two distinct phases are of concern: If you get pierced in unsanitary conditions, or with unsterile implements or jewelry, an infection can be transmitted *during* the piercing. Or, if you fail to care for the wound properly throughout its healing period, you can get an infection *after* the piercing is done. Studies show that the risk of infection increases when either the piercer's technique or the aftercare is poor.[3]

The incidence of infection is difficult to calculate because there is no reliable information about how many piercings are actually being performed. Some smaller studies done on college campuses usually reveal more about the quality of nearby piercers than they do about the rate of infection for body piercing in general.

Our world is full of *microorganisms* (germs, including bacteria, fungi, and viruses). Many of these are harmless—or even beneficial—to us, but some are *pathogenic* (capable of causing infection or disease). We are all routinely exposed to countless germs, but many complex factors impact how they affect us, including the potency and amount of an organism entering the body, and how it gets in, as well as the strength of the immune system.

The viruses hepatitis B and C and HIV are examples of *bloodborne pathogens* (microorganisms that can cause disease when present in the blood). They are of particular concern because if the needles or jewelry are not sterile, there is potential for these serious bloodborne diseases to be transmitted during piercing.

HIV, the virus that causes AIDS, is quite fragile and dies quickly when exposed to air; there have been *no* documented cases of HIV transmission through piercing.[4] The hepatitis virus, however, is easier to transmit because it is quite hardy. Studies show that hepatitis B can live on a dry surface for at least seven days![5] Even though the virus is robust, improperly performed body art accounts for a very small proportion of hepatitis transmissions.[6]

Bacterial infections can range from minor skin eruptions to deadly infections of the brain or lining of the heart. Never ignore a suspected infection: left untreated, certain kinds that start out as trivial can become lethal. *Local bacterial infection* (at the site of the piercing) is the most common sort, and deeper, larger, or systemic infections in healthy piercees are fairly rare.

The medical field has developed specific infection-control practices, called *Standard Precautions* (formerly *Universal Precautions*), for dealing with blood or other potentially infectious body fluids and any equipment that could be contaminated with them. Safe piercers are educated about these procedures and adhere to them meticulously.

Health Conditions and Piercings

Certain medical conditions make piercings riskier, and in some cases inadvisable. Health problems that weaken your infection-fighting defenses, including diabetes, lupus, HIV/AIDS, and other immune system disorders, can make you slow to heal. You might be more vulnerable to infection, and if you do contract one, it could be more severe and harder to cure.

Some heart disorders make you susceptible to *infective endocarditis* (a potentially deadly infection of the lining of the heart or heart valves, previously referred to as *bacterial endocarditis*). If you have a history of this illness or serious cardiac problems like a valve replacement, an ethical piercer will require proof that you have consulted with your doctor before proceeding. If you ordinarily must take antibiotic *prophylaxis* (preventive treatment) before dental procedures, your physician may recommend this before piercing. Cardiac ailments are one of the few preexisting conditions that can increase the risk of a fatal outcome: if you are advised against piercing due to your health, heed your doctor's word!

Rashes such as eczema or psoriasis, scars such as keloids, and other skin abnormalities are less serious health issues. If you are considering a piercing in an area affected by one of these conditions, seek an evaluation by an experienced piercer and a piercing-friendly doctor.

Some states have regulations that require piercers to ask clients specific health-history questions on the release form before piercing, whereas other states have laws that prohibit piercers from asking certain health questions. Be honest about your medical history and respect a piercer who has the principles to decline to pierce you if the risk is unacceptable.

Allergies and Skin Problems

All sorts of bumps, lumps, and skin irritations can crop up around a piercing, coming and going as healing progresses and occasionally remaining permanently. Some of these are caused by mechanical stress against the piercing; others are caused by a cleaning product or jewelry material. Skin disorders can be difficult to diagnose, even for dermatologists, so experimentation is needed at times to identify and correct a problem. Conditions can also have a combination of causes, which further complicates diagnosis and treatment.

A nickel allergy can be triggered by jewelry made of inferior metal. This type of allergy can be serious and irreversible, which is one reason it is critical to wear only high-quality, inert jewelry (see "Jewelry Materials for Initial Piercings," page 74).

Migration and Rejection

Two rather distinctive piercing complications are *migration* (the piercing moves from its initial placement, then settles and heals in a new location) and *rejection* (the jewelry is expelled completely from the body). The piercing is likely to migrate when unsuitable or insufficient tissue is pierced, or if your jewelry is too small in diameter, thin in gauge, or of poor quality. Inexperienced and untrained piercers often make these errors.

Migration and rejection can also result from using a harsh aftercare product, following poor health habits, or experiencing excessive physical trauma or emotional stress during the healing period. And, unfortunately, sometimes even when everything is done properly, a piercing will migrate or reject for no known reason. This is simply a risk of placing a foreign object through your skin: it may not stay in the desired position.

Scarring and Permanent Physical Changes

A piercing has the potential to be a temporary adornment (especially when compared to a tattoo), because the jewelry can easily be removed. There is a risk, however, of irreversible changes to the body, including discoloration, a mark such as a scar, bump, or dimple, or a permanent hole.

Many piercings shrink or close quickly, but some piercings will remain open indefinitely without jewelry in them. The placement of the hole, the length of time you have worn the piercing, the thickness of the jewelry that was in it, and your individual tissue all impact whether or not your piercing stays viable after removing the jewelry.

Piercings that are stretched to large dimensions commonly leave significant voids that may be considered disfiguring; to correct them, plastic surgery is required. Stretching a piercing too quickly or attempting to expand unsuitably thin tissue leads to problems. One potential consequence of overzealous stretching is a *blowout* (part of the interior channel is pushed out, leaving an unsightly lip of flesh on one side of the piercing). This distortion will usually be a lasting reminder of your hasty actions unless it is surgically removed. Piercings that are stretched improperly can also suffer from thinning tissue that does not regrow. A worst-case scenario is tissue *necrosis* (death) and the loss of the piercing and some of the skin in the area. Jewelry that exerts excessive pressure against underlying bone can cause bone necrosis.

There are piercings that have a tendency to effect changes such as the hardening or thickening of the tissue surrounding the openings, and this can be irreversible. For example, nipple piercings are known for causing permanent enlargement, especially in *underdeveloped* (small) anatomy. Specifics are covered in chapters 10–13.

Scarring and tissue discoloration at the piercing site are relatively normal occurrences, especially if you have a history of darkened scars. This can happen even when a piercing is performed properly and heals uneventfully. Migration often leaves a small track of scarring or discoloration from where the piercing was initially placed. Rejection usually results in a split scar. Piercings of the ear cartilage are prone to disfigurement if a serious infection develops. The cartilage can collapse, causing a "cauliflower ear" appearance.[7]

Excessive scarring sometimes occurs in reaction to piercing, and it can be very difficult to resolve. If you have a history of problems with scarring or *keloids* (large growths of fibrous tissue), piercing is generally inadvisable. For more on this topic, see "Excessive Scarring," (page 209) and the subsequent sections in chapter 16.

Unfortunate Events

Accidents happen, and there is a risk of catching jewelry and tearing a piercing. An act as simple as taking off your shirt can be dangerous for a piercing on the torso, face, or ear. Strenuous workouts, airbags, pets, children—even sexual activities—can cause ripping or splitting. Obviously, healing piercings are more delicate and vulnerable to injury, but older piercings are still susceptible.

You must be aware of your jewelry and your movements, take steps to protect your piercing, and avoid activities that could lead to such accidents. If you engage in sports or other behaviors that pose a risk to your piercings, wear protective gear. See "Protective Patch," page 187, for details.

Jewelry that is too thin can carve through the flesh like a wire slicing a wedge of cheddar: hence, I coined the term *cheese-cutter effect* to describe this unpleasant (and largely preventable) occurrence. Wearing charms or heavy weights on thin-gauge wires makes trouble likely.

Somewhat less predictable incidents can take place when jewelry in oral or nasal piercings is swallowed or, more seriously, inhaled. The best way to prevent this is by wearing quality jewelry of the proper fit and checking the closure (bead or ball) daily to ensure that it is tightly affixed.

Dangerous Piercing Placements

Certain piercings should be avoided altogether because they are inherently risky or rarely heal. However, scores of photos of these placements and others can be found online. Simply because someone is willing to do a piercing on you or has done it on others doesn't mean it is safe or advisable. Preferring to err on the side of caution, I will not perform the following piercings due to their risky nature.

Less Obvious Risks

It's easy to understand that a piercing could become infected or snag on something and get torn, but some risks are subtler. A person with prominent facial piercings may be

Risky Piercings

Anatomy	Risk
Facial and Oral	
Eyelid	Scratched and scarred cornea, dry eye, blindness
Lip surface or chin surface	Migration, rejection, scarring
Horizontal (transverse) tongue	Excessive bleeding, nerve damage, tooth injury, gum injury
Tongue surface	Rejection, scarring
Cheek (I no longer do cheek piercings beyond the first molar)	Punctured parotid duct or gland, leaking saliva; see "The Worst Piercing Story," page 119
Lowbret and vertical lowbret (between cheek and gum line inside)	Gum and bone erosion, scarring
Mandible (below the tongue through soft palate to underside of chin)	Gum and bone erosion, leaking saliva, scarring
Torso	
"Outie" navel	Herniation, peritonitis
Nipple (male or female) if too small or too inverted to pinch up	Migration, rejection, scarring
Sub-clavicular (underneath the collarbone)	Uncontrollable bleeding, nerve damage, potentially life-threatening risk of pneumothorax (collapsed lung)
Female Genital	
Isabella (deep clitoral shaft piercing from bottom of the clitoris to the top of the hood)	Excessive bleeding, nerve damage
Princess Albertina (through the female urethral opening)	Bladder infection, migration, rejection
Male Genital	
Deep penile shaft piercing or trans-scrotal piercing	Excessive bleeding, nerve damage
Additional Areas of Concern	
Uvula (soft, fleshy extension that hangs at the back of the throat)	Loss of jewelry or needle (caught in throat or aspirated into lungs)
Piercing close to the surface through a small pinch of tissue	Migration, rejection, scarring
Piercing behind bone, tendon, or other anatomical structure	Excessive bleeding, nerve damage, loss of function
Anal piercing	Infection
Hand web, all *interdigital spaces* (between fingers or toes), anywhere on feet or hands	Infection (high risk), migration, rejection, scarring

Piercing and Acupuncture

One of my apprentices was a licensed practitioner of traditional Chinese medicine and acupuncture. He felt that a piercing of an acupuncture point might briefly treat or affect a condition associated with that particular point. But after continuous stimulation, the point would cease to be affected. He postulated that the point then relocates near the piercing site but is not obliterated. He is not the only acupuncturist to subscribe to this theory.[8]

subject to condemnation from society. This may take the form of relatively minor dirty looks or comments to more serious problems such as loss of employment, expulsion from school, or parental disapproval. At the most extreme, you could be disowned by your family. These are severe consequences that deserve due consideration if they are relevant for you. Piercings can also cause relationship problems with your spouse or significant other. More than one divorce has been blamed on a lack of piercing compatibility.

Another potential problem for people with visible body piercings is experiencing unwanted contact, like a pregnant woman who has complete strangers rub her distended belly. If you experience this problem, be polite but firm and explain that it is *always* appropriate to ask permission before touching someone you don't know.

Myths and Misconceptions

One big misunderstanding is that pierced individuals are all alike in some way. There isn't any one type of person that represents all piercees; nowadays piercing is for everyone. See "Who Gets Pierced and Why?" on page 6. Another frequent (and sometimes disastrous) misconception is that a piercer who posts a license or certificate must have some particular training or skill. Find out much more about piercers in chapter 5, "You and Your Piercer."

Luckily, most of the stories about uncontrolled bleeding or post-piercing paralysis are fabrications. Of course, *some* bleeding is a normal consequence of any piercing, though many do not bleed at all. There is no "special nerve" a piercer can hit to cause paralysis from any traditional body piercing. Nor is there any major artery located in the pathway of the popular piercing sites.

Throughout the body there is a network of nerves and blood vessels, and the larger of these tend to be located close together. They are also commonly situated in protected locations behind bone, tendon, and muscle, which is a good reason to never pierce behind such structures. And, fortunately, blood vessels and nerves tend to slide or roll when grabbed or poked at (which makes drawing blood a challenge at times). Piercers routinely puncture the smallest and most peripheral of the vessels and nerves with no ill effect whatsoever. This is a normal part of body piercing. See "What to Expect," page 182.

One misconception that remains widespread even in much of the medical community is that piercings always represent a pathway to the interior of the body. This is untrue! A healed piercing is a sealed channel of tissue from end to end (in medical terms, a *fistula*), and only when a piercing is healing, injured, or experiencing a flare-up, is it an open wound, or pathway into the body. See "The Wound Healing Process," page 181, for details.

You will find information throughout this book to clear up many mistaken beliefs about piercings:

- Many people think that sterling silver is a good metal for new piercings and gold is a bad one, but that's backward. Learn more in chapter 9, "Jewelry 101: Sizes, Shapes, and Materials," especially the section "Gold," page 76.

- You should not twist or move your jewelry all the time to prevent it from getting stuck, nor should you use strong antibacterial soap, alcohol, peroxide, or ointment during healing. See chapter 14, "Healing 101: Standard Aftercare," for instructions.

- Oral and genital piercings do not get infected more easily than other areas. Similarly, they are not always more painful or harder to heal. In fact some of the piercings in both of these areas are just the opposite. Read chapters 11 and 13.

- Body piercings do not always set off the buzzers in airport checkpoints. See "Metal Detectors and Security," page 250.

- Body jewelry can sometimes be left in for X-rays, MRIs, and medical examinations and procedures. See "Medical and Dental Emergencies and Appointments," page 247.

- Nipple piercings do not normally preclude nursing a baby. See "Nipple Piercing and Breastfeeding," page 253.

Minimizing Risks

You greatly minimize the hazards of piercing by becoming an educated consumer. Serious complications are extremely unlikely if:

- You are in good health
- You get pierced by a qualified practitioner who follows all hygiene precautions
- You wear quality jewelry of an appropriate material, size, and style
- You consistently follow sensible cleaning and care procedures

Oral Piercings and Yeast Infections

One common urban myth has led many piercers and piercees to be unnecessarily concerned about the safety of drinking beer or eating bread or certain other foods during the healing of a tongue or other oral piercing. The yeast in foods and beverages is of a completely different type than the yeast that causes yeast infections, and it has no impact on the health of a piercing.

The mouth normally contains many microorganisms. The growth of one of these, *Candida albicans* (a fungus), is kept under control by the presence of normal oral bacteria. But when the usual bacteria are not present, a *yeast infection* (an overgrowth of Candida) often occurs.[9]

Thrush (an oral yeast infection) cannot be caused by ingesting food or drink that contain yeast. In the case of healing oral piercings, thrush is almost always the result of overusing mouth rinse that contains alcohol. Strong products kill off the healthy, protective flora, resulting in an imbalance that allows the yeast to overgrow.

The Point

Living is dangerous, and none of us gets out of this alive, so enjoying your journey is important. If you want a piercing, learn all the facts, evaluate your health and other personal considerations, and weigh the risks. If you do go for it, get the job done properly and chances are you and your piercing will be just fine.

Is Piercing Right for You?

If you want to experiment with your appearance, piercing can be a suitable option because it isn't as drastic or lasting as a tattoo. Body piercings might intrigue you, but you may not feel sure you should actually take the plunge. You could be fearful of needles, worried about experiencing pain or anxious about taking off your clothes in front of a stranger. The suitability of piercings for your lifestyle or health status is a reasonable concern. If you are attracted to piercings but hesitate out of fear or perceived obstacles, this chapter will help you form realistic expectations, minimize unfounded worries, and encourage you to think carefully before making a final decision.

Responsibility and Commitment

Getting a piercing is kind of like adopting a pet: substantial maturity and patience are required to deal with it. Even the most resolute of piercees can feel challenged by the need to perform daily cleaning and to withstand the temptation to touch their piercing with dirty fingers for many months. Do you have the fortitude to wait half a year before changing your navel ring?

If you are lax about your health or hygiene, you are not a good candidate for piercing. You must support the healing process by taking care of yourself and keeping your environment—including your clothes and linens—clean. A nonstop party lifestyle will inhibit your body's ability to heal.

A certain level of financial solvency is also necessary because good body jewelry can be expensive. If the piece you are wearing is irritating your piercing or you lose a ball or some other emergency comes up, you may have to purchase new jewelry without advance notice. You must have the means to buy the best products and not borrow used jewelry from a friend (danger!) or pick up a cut-rate item at a novelty store. Quality body jewelry is not cheap, but it is indispensable.

Finally, emotional maturity and poise is needed to deal with adverse reactions. Will your feelings be hurt if people give you dirty looks or make disparaging comments? Can you handle having your relatives, friends, or coworkers express criticism or even disgust? If not, think twice about whether piercing is right for you, because not everyone will approve.

Ear Piercings ≠ Body Piercings

The earlobe seems destined for piercing. Throughout history, humans have adorned that humble bit of flesh with plugs, rings, and dangles. It is perfectly positioned for ornamenting the face without any troublesome veins or nerves getting in the way. The earlobe usually heals readily and tolerates most jewelry without complaint.

You may believe that the same trouble-free conditions apply to all piercings, but you are likely to run into problems if you have these unrealistic expectations. Simply having your ears pierced won't prepare you for the challenges of most body piercings. Only a few spots take as little as one month to heal, like the lobe does. Many sites take two to three months or more to heal, and the popular navel piercing has a healing time of six to nine months or longer (see the "Minimum Healing Times Chart" on page 276 for a complete listing).

Many body piercings are unsuited to frequent changes of jewelry. Some piercing placements and jewelry closures are difficult to deal with on your own, and you can end up damaging your piercing if you try. Earlobe piercings stay open well, once healed, but most other areas do not. Body piercings are different from ear piercings in many ways.

Healthy Bodies Heal Better

The healthier you are, the faster and easier you will heal. Remember: *your body* handles the healing process—not some magic lotion or potion you put on the piercing. Therefore, you should make an extra effort to pay attention to your health when getting pierced. Piercing is generally inadvisable in any of the following situations:

- You are sick or run down (especially if you are taking antibiotics or steroids)
- You have sensitive skin or are prone to scarring
- You are under an unusual amount of physical or emotional stress
- You are already healing other piercings or wounds
- You anticipate surgery or another medical or dental procedure

Lifestyle Considerations

Before getting pierced, think carefully about your lifestyle and circumstances. It is best to delay or forgo piercing if your current situation makes it apparent that you would have trouble healing.

- **Season/weather:** Heavy clothes over a piercing during cold weather can cause discomfort and complications. Pools, beaches, sand, and sunscreen all have the potential to irritate or infect. Swimming can expose your piercing to bacteria or chlorine and other harsh chemicals.
- **Physical activities:** Participation in contact sports make it challenging to heal a piercing due to friction, sweat, and trauma. Although it is possible to combine piercings with an active lifestyle, it is generally not a good idea to get pierced if you are a serious athlete, training for an event, or participate in rigorous sports that could pose a physical danger to your piercing.
- **Pending changes:** Traveling to places where water quality is poor or having plans that would necessitate removing your jewelry are big reasons to postpone your piercing.

- **Career path:** Whether your job is blue collar, white collar, or no collar, consider how piercings fit in with your work. Some food service industry jobs prohibit piercings. Construction workers and others whose employment involves lots of sweat and grime may have problems healing due to unhygienic workplace conditions. Or do you work in a professional capacity? Most employers still frown on visible piercings, particularly if you interact with the public. Many a piercee has had to choose between a piercing and a job. Conservative fields such as law or medicine tend to be especially unwelcoming to the visibly pierced. If you are a student contemplating a particular career or an employee interested in changing your current position, ask yourself if the piercing you desire is sufficiently discreet for you to land the job you want and keep it.

Concealment and Removal

Sometimes people get a new piercing and plan to take the jewelry out for activities or to conceal it at school, home, or work. Popping the jewelry in and out may sound simple, but it irritates delicate cells. Such abuse of the area often results in complications like scar tissue formation and migration. Touching your fresh piercing and jewelry during removal and reinsertion increases your chance of infection, too. One uninformed young man took his nipple ring out before daily football practice and then pushed it back in afterward. No wonder he had problems with discomfort and delayed healing!

Retainers and various jewelry alternatives are available to camouflage your piercing, though certain spots can be disguised more readily than others. Unfortunately, the most invisible retainers are unsafe to wear until after you are healed. Concealment issues are addressed in a separate section under each piercing, where applicable.

Obstacles

People who are interested in getting pierced may perceive other impediments. "I'm too old" and "I'm too fat" are two common concerns. Although age and weight can affect healing, most often these are emotional barriers that do not really preclude getting pierced. This kind of negative self-image can be disheartening and difficult to overcome, so a little reassurance may be in order.

Unless advanced age is causing you health problems and slow healing, age need not be a barrier at all. There are, in fact, people in their sixties and seventies getting body piercings—most often genital and nipple piercings! If you are older, you may feel concerned about looking foolish because body piercing is "a teenage trend." Rest assured, many mature adults have and enjoy body piercings.

Extreme obesity or emaciation can affect your health and therefore your ability to heal. Poor circulation, compromised immune function, and other medical problems related to weight are sound reasons to forgo piercing. You could still be a candidate, however, if you are healthy, committed to taking proper care of your piercing, and a competent practitioner deems your anatomy pierceable. One area of exceptional concern is the navel. If you are overweight, the avascularity of this area is even worse than usual, and the configuration of a heavy abdomen is often unsuited to piercing.

Certain placements require disrobing and revealing parts of your body, so piercers routinely see shapes of all types. Whether you are fat, thin, or in between, and even if you are modest by nature, a piercer worth his or her salt will put you at ease by acting in a manner that is professional and compassionate.

Kids vs. Parents

Parents and their children often have disagreements over the subject of piercing. Kids who want to get pierced may perceive their parents as too strict, while parents view piercings as evidence of rebellion or a sign that a child is "bad."

Piercees must be responsible and disciplined, but many young people lack these qualities, especially when faced with an extended healing time. Readiness cannot be determined by the achievement of a certain age, but young people should wait until their bodies are fully developed before getting a piercing below the neck. If their anatomy has not yet matured, a piercing could end up in an undesirable location by time the body has finished growing.

Parental attitudes vary, but even a mother who has piercings herself may not be ready to give her teen permission to get one. If you are an accommodating parent who agrees to go along with a nipple or genital piercing for your minor child (under the age of eighteen), take note: any piercer willing to perform this task has terrible judgment, poor ethics, and risks the possibility of being charged with sexual assault of a minor. Moreover, signing a consent form for your underage child to get an adult piercing could result in a charge of reckless endangerment of a minor against *you*.

Regulations for piercing vary on aspects such as minimum age requirements, the extent of parental involvement, and which piercings are legally sanctioned for minors. Studio policies also differ depending on the principles of the piercer. Some will pierce minors only with a parent present, even if the law is more lax.

Practical Advice for Parents

Maybe a desire to get pierced is a phase your child is going through—some young people *do* grow out of their interest in piercing—but try not to be judgmental. An interest in piercing does not automatically mean your child is obsessed with sex, into drugs, or gay. Piercings can fulfill the normal urge young people have to adopt a style that is different from yours and fit in with their friends. Think of the bright side: you might be able to negotiate, using a piercing as a reward for good grades or other desirable behavior.

In many cultures, getting a piercing or tattoo is an essential step into adulthood and acts to bind a family together. If you support your kid in the choice to get pierced, it might bring you closer together. And when you help him or her to find a quality piercer, you prevent the consequences of a do-it-yourself or hack job, which could result in expensive medical bills.

Practical Advice for Young People

If you sneak around behind your parents' backs to get pierced, you are proving that you cannot be trusted. It is against piercer ethics—and usually the law—for a minor to get pierced without the permission of a parent or legal guardian (not a friend's parent, yours).

If your mom and dad refuse to consent and you attempt to pierce yourself or have a friend do it, there is a very high risk of infection. You will get a bad piercing that will cause you endless trouble. Don't count on being able to hide it, either—fresh piercings are difficult to conceal. Your parents *will* find out. Showing them you are patient will help you earn their respect.

Relative Pain Levels and Sensations

Below is a general comparison of pain levels according to feedback from approximately 40,000 piercees—my customers. These describe *relative* intensity as perceived by the majority of my clients. Due to varying sensitivity levels and perceptions of pain, however, there are many exceptions and differences of opinion.

- *Easy:* earlobe, eyebrow, tongue, navel, fourchette
- *Easy to medium:* bridge, bindi, nasal septum, teardrop, most labrets, most surface piercings (on flat areas that lack a defined fold, flap, or protrusion of tissue), Prince Albert, guiche, scrotum, foreskin, lorum, frenum, pubic, vertical clitoral hood, horizontal clitoral hood, inner labia
- *Medium:* all ear cartilage, nostril, philtrum (upper lip center), tongue tip or sides, outer labia
- *Medium to intense:* triangle, nipple
- *Intense:* ampallang, apadravya, reverse Prince Albert, dydoe, clitoris

My clients most commonly describe the sensations from getting pierced as, "a pinch," "a sting," or "some pressure." Almost everyone I've pierced has remarked, "It wasn't nearly as bad as I expected!"

I have worked hard to become proficient at piercing swiftly and smoothly, factors that are largely responsible for the perceptions of my clients. Only when your piercer is experienced can you expect the sensations to be so mild.

Anxiety

The anticipation before piercing is often the worst part of the whole experience. Rest assured: your imagination is probably much worse than the reality. But your apprehension can make getting pierced far more harrowing than it needs to be. If you are unduly nervous or needle-phobic, prepare yourself by learning ways to deal with your fears. It will make your visit to the piercing studio more tolerable. Practice the "Breathing and Relaxation Techniques" on page 54 before your appointment.

Seek a piercer who will be supportive of your decision to conquer your fears and take you through the process with sensitivity. A good piercer will have a wealth of patience and understanding; he is not a therapist, however, so there is a limit to how much time and energy he can spend with you during a single piercing session.

Your piercer will be able to do a better job if you are not an emotional wreck requiring excessive support and reassurance. When he has to devote himself to consoling you, he is less able to focus on the technical aspects of his job. If you are so anxiety ridden that you panic and interrupt the procedure (ask the piercer to stop or grab at his hands), you make the situation worse and can cause a needle stick accident. If you cannot reign in your emotions so the piercing can be accomplished safely, your piercer should ask you to return at another time when you are composed and ready.

Expectation plays a role in the perception of pain and the experience of the piercing.[1] Prepare yourself by forming realistic expectations of the sensations associated with piercing.[2]

"Doesn't That Hurt?"

Pain is a very charged topic, and because it is subjective, even the most in-depth discussion leaves much to the imagination. Many people are concerned about being able to tolerate the pain they expect to feel during a piercing. This dread is a common reason people decide against getting one, even when they truly want it.

Some areas of the body are more sensitive, and certain piercings are generally accepted to be more intense than others. Nipples, for instance, are often described as tender, though usually more for men than for women. Then again, some piercees *enjoy* getting nipple piercings and do not find the procedure to be painful at all. Surprisingly, certain spots that are often imagined to be the worst, such as the tongue and genitals, can actually be among the least painful.

It is much easier to endure an instantaneous pain than one that continues for an extended period of time. The brief sensation experienced as a "pinch" can turn into "stabbed by an ice pick" at the hands of a less accomplished piercer, so choose wisely!

The sensation of getting pierced should begin to fade as soon as your jewelry is in place. For a few minutes afterward you might experience burning, stinging, or warmth—and a sense of accomplishment, of course. In the end you may perceive nothing more serious than discomfort.

Needle Phobia

Statistics show that at least 10 percent of the population is needle-phobic.[3] Even so, plenty of piercees are included in their numbers.

The "Badge of Courage"

Tattoos, scarification, and piercing all involve some degree of pain or discomfort, and visibly demonstrate that a person is capable of enduring it. Without pain, there would be little difference between this type of modification and dyeing your hair, for example. It is part of what sets modified people apart and makes us members of a shared community.

Although modern body piercing has roots in the BDSM community, few people get pierced because they want to feel pain. Even those who engage in consensual masochistic practices don't usually want to receive excessive pain from a piercer; they prefer it within the context of their relationships. Besides, piercing should be so quick as to be disappointing to the rare pain-seekers who try to satisfy their desires in a piercing studio.

Many people admit that they do enjoy the rush of adrenalin and endorphins caused by getting pierced. Some piercees relish the anticipation and excitement leading up to the event. Others derive a form of non-masochistic pleasure from the *sensation* of being pierced; even if it is intense, it might not be perceived as "pain." This is a subtle, but real, distinction. These are all natural highs that can be achieved through body piercing.

The Point

Now you can make a realistic assessment about whether piercing is right for you. Fortunately, the majority of obstacles are only perceived rather than genuine. If a hurdle is truly insurmountable, however, you must accept that reality. Consult your doctor if you have health concerns, or a piercer if you have questions.

5

You and Your Piercer

Many consumers drop by the nearest studio and get pierced by whoever is on duty at the time. Although this method is convenient, you cannot be assured of getting a safe piercing without learning certain facts about the piercer's abilities and hygiene practices. This chapter details exactly how to evaluate piercers and studios so you can make a sound decision.

Piercer Skills

Piercers are all the same, right? There can't be that much difference between one professional piercer and another, can there? If she has a licensed studio, and she charges money to do the job, she must know what she's doing. Right?

Wrong!

A license is no assurance that a piercer is competent. In some cases, getting a license simply requires paying a fee to a city or state agency. It does not guarantee that the piercer has received adequate training to perform the job properly. Even in regions with the most stringent laws, there is absolutely no focus on the skills of the piercer.

> **Wrong Answer**
>
> During one interview I inquired of an applicant, "Can you tell me why you want to become a piercer?" She responded, "It's the only job I can have with green hair." Needless to say, she did not get the job.

Your experience and your outcome (how well your piercing heals) are highly dependent on the proficiency of the person wielding the needle. Piercing is a hands-on profession that must be learned through practical experience. It can then be mastered only through practice, which commonly involves trial *and* error. No courses of study (not a single one!) are available from any accredited institution to confer a degree or prepare someone to work in the field. Sound instruction ideally involves a lengthy apprenticeship with a qualified mentor, but such opportunities for aspiring piercers are rare. Watch out for certificates that look impressive, because they do not always represent much formal education. See "Piercer Training," on page 267, to learn about piercer education.

Many so-called "professional piercers" have never had any particular training or are simply indifferent and sloppy. Some piercers lack passion or aptitude, and others are motivated by immature or inappropriate considerations.

Without specialized knowledge, a piercer is a menace; and without considerable savvy to evaluate prospective piercers, you will not be a safe consumer.

"I didn't know the quality of a good piercer till I actually went to one. I got my helix [ear cartilage piercing] at my old tattoo parlor, and I'm pretty sure none of them were piercers so much as tattoo artists with piercing needles. It hurt like a bitch, he stopped halfway into it, and then almost tore it out trying to close the ring, *and* dropped the ball on the floor but still put it in my ear. . . . When I considered getting my next piercing I was skeptical because of the last experience. I looked up as much as I could about piercers in the area. I came across [a piercer who] was great . . . made me comfortable; very informative; great experience, turned me on to a life of future piercings." R.

Skill-Level Scale

Imagine a scale from one to ten. At level one or level two, the piercer is a beginner. She may have pierced some friends, taken a brief course, or watched a "how-to-pierce" video. Getting pierced by someone this inexperienced isn't really a bargain, even if the price is cheap. She will take considerably longer to perform the procedure and cause you far more pain than she should. Novices don't know the best size or style of jewelry for you or how to optimally place a piercing to suit your anatomy. This affects not only the aesthetics of the piercing, but also your ability to heal. Neophytes also frequently have trouble inserting the jewelry once the piercing has been made. This causes undue tissue trauma, which further disrupts your healing, and it is also *extremely* painful. Finally, but importantly, piercers at this beginning level are less able to help you if troubleshooting becomes necessary later—and it probably will.

Further up the scale, a piercer has more skill. A piercer at level five has sufficient training and ability to accomplish your piercing adequately. This piercer may have completed an apprenticeship and gained some experience yet is still relatively unseasoned. There are finer points she has yet to learn and situations she may not be able to handle, depending on the difficulty of the piercing and challenges presented by your anatomy. This piercer can do decent job, but she is not the best you can get.

A piercer at level nine or ten is a true master. A piercing performed by a specialist with this superior ability is almost like a magic trick in which the hands move faster than the eye. The act is performed gently, and the piercing is perfectly placed to your build. This is art and science combined. A piercing by this expert is easy to tolerate, and you may even describe it as a pleasant experience. Should you require help during healing, she is versed in all there is to know, and you can rely on her to assist you.

In general, your pain level is inverse to the piercer's ability: the lower the skill level of your technician, the greater your discomfort or pain, and vice versa.

Some piercers have years of experience and yet they fail to pierce at a high level. She may not be applying herself to the task, or she may suffer from a lack of aptitude. Just because a piercer has been working at her job for a long time does not assure that she is proficient; some piercers are doing the same bungling job as always, ten years later.

Although this numbered skill-level scale is not a convention used within the piercing industry, it helps to illustrate how proficiency differs substantially from one piercer to the next.

Attitude and Ethics

A good attitude includes being professional, pleasant, and patient. Sometimes piercers fail to grasp that they are performing a service for you, not a favor! Your potential piercer must earn your trust by demonstrating her knowledge and competency. Don't settle for someone who does not fully answer your questions; if she is annoyed by your inquiries or exudes a "too cool" attitude, she is a poor choice.

Before taking your money, a piercer should be willing to provide a consultation to inspect your anatomy, discuss jewelry selection, the procedure, potential risks and complications, healing course, and aftercare guidelines. If a piercer cannot be bothered to attend to you politely before a piercing, it is even less likely she will be there for you if you need assistance later.

A poor attitude also prevents a piercer from gaining true mastery in the field. The piercer who takes her profession seriously is going to work harder to do a good job. The one who thinks she already knows everything, on the other hand, will not attempt to expand her knowledge or improve her performance.

If you are unimpressed by your local piercers, you may have to search a wider geographical area. Consider the following experience from a piercee in Arizona:

> "I was a little disappointed with my piercing experience. . . . I went in the shop with an excited, happy frame of mind. The guy who did it was obviously not the one who normally did the piercings; some girl was. He called her on the phone right from the front counter and told her she had a piercing; obviously the conversation didn't go well, because he just hung up and was *obviously* very irritated. He had me come around to the chair, marked my belly with a pen, and *wham!* just did it. I was expecting him to at least explain what he was going to do, talk to me for a minute, explain the different choices of jewelry . . . *something.* After he did it, I got up, he gave a *brief* aftercare speech, and sent me on my way. . . . I knew I needed more aftercare info. If I ever go to get anything else pierced, I'm going to find a different shop." A.

As well she should.

A piercer with sound ethics is committed to keeping her studio and equipment clean and honing her skills. Her actions are guided by honorable principles and a strong conscience, not the almighty dollar or an inflated ego. A professional with solid standards will refuse to bring out a needle any time it is inappropriate. Respect a piercer for declining to pierce you when she shouldn't; she's the kind you should return to when circumstances are right.

Studio Standards and Equipment Handling

Even the best piercer cannot do a good job without a studio that is properly set up and maintained for this specialized task. Professionals do not pierce out of a smoky nightclub, a friend's car, or their bathroom at home.

You have every right to inspect the environment and be assured of suitable *aseptic* (free of disease-causing microorganisms) conditions and hygienic practices before you have someone break your skin. If possible, make a preliminary visit to check out the studio before getting pierced. This gives you time to thoroughly evaluate the piercer and the premises. It also helps to alleviate nervousness that can cloud your judgment.

The way sterile equipment is handled in the studio is critical because if it is not done correctly, there is a risk of disease transmission.

Some mistakes are more obvious than others, so you must learn exactly what to look for. Use the following list to make an effective appraisal:

Setup and Sanitation Checklist

- ☐ Posting of state or local license(s). Check with your health department or other agencies to determine what kind of permit is required for piercing in your area, if any.
- ☐ A selection of body jewelry. A studio carrying only a handful of styles or sizes will be unable to meet the needs presented by the wide range of human anatomy.
- ☐ Cleanliness throughout! The premises and staff should sparkle. Smoking or drinking alcohol should never take place there.
- ☐ If studio policy permits customers to try on piercing jewelry—whether for ear or body—*run*.
- ☐ A public bathroom that is never used for cleaning contaminated piercing equipment.
- ☐ A hand-washing sink for the piercer. It should be stocked with liquid soap and paper towels or an air dryer, not reusable cloth towels.
- ☐ A separate room for performing piercing that has bright lighting and good ventilation. The piercing room should not be used for tattooing, haircutting, or anything except piercing.
- ☐ A *sterilization room* (separate enclosure for processing contaminated tools and equipment). The public should not have access to this area.
- ☐ Printed handouts containing detailed aftercare guidelines.

> **Dirty Deed**
>
> I once visited a studio where I observed a piercer accept cash payment for a job and then stuff the filthy bills into the drawer with her "sterile" piercing equipment. She did not appear to be aware of the fact that she had done something incredibly dangerous.

Vital Equipment: Sterilizers and Ultrasonics

An autoclave is required equipment in every piercing studio. Autoclaves are very expensive, but for sterilizing piercing equipment and body jewelry there is no acceptable alternative. Boiling in water, soaking in alcohol, or passing over an open flame definitely does not accomplish the job. Hospital-strength liquid disinfectants that reduce the number of microorganisms and chemical cold-sterilant solutions are not suitable substitutes for sterilizing equipment. Of course, simply *having* an autoclave is not enough: it must be operated and maintained in strict accordance with the manufacturer's instructions.

There must also be proof that the machinery is functioning properly, which is the purpose of *spore tests* or *biological indicators* (test strips containing heat-resistant spores). These are run through a sterilization cycle in the autoclave and then mailed away for evaluation by a laboratory to determine whether all the spores were destroyed. The results (pass or fail) are provided to the studio. A printout should be available for any prospective customer to see upon request. Any piercer without knowledge of spore tests or proof of results (at least monthly) is one you should avoid. The system in Europe is different, so you may not find spore tests there.

A flash-cycle cassette sterilizer is a special type of autoclave that is an acceptable alternative for sterilization in certain situations. The most popular unit in the United States is called a Statim. In Europe they commonly use a vacuum flash-cycle sterilizer. These are convenient because they have a briefer cycle than traditional autoclaves (less than ten minutes versus over half an hour).

The Statim is not designed for use on contaminated equipment, so it is best employed by piercers who use disposable tools or do freehand piercings (without metal forceps or receiving tubes; see "Forceps," page 58, and "Needle Receiving Tubes," page 59). If your piercer works with reusable piercing equipment, she must sterilize items that have been used on other clients in a regular autoclave before using the Statim to process her piercing setup. The piercer may then put tools and jewelry into the cassette and sterilize it in the Statim just prior to performing a piercing. She may work directly from the cassette, but she must not put used items back onto the Statim tray. This machine must also be spore tested. Good piercers are impressed, not annoyed, when clients are informed and concerned enough to ask about test results.

Even in studios where procedures are done only with disposable equipment, an autoclave must be used. A piercer cannot be certain that needles and body jewelry are sent in a sterile state or whether contamination occurs during shipping. Medical suppliers have stringent requirements for sterilization and packaging, but other industries are not held to the same standard. Needles or jewelry shipped in bulk packages must always be sterilized before use.

Another indispensable piece of equipment used in the studio is the ultrasonic unit (a machine that removes debris using agitation from sonic waves in liquid). Used piercing tools are run through a cycle prior to autoclaving. Some piercers claim to sterilize using an ultrasonic unit, but this appliance is not a substitute for an autoclave, so don't believe it!

New jewelry should be run through an ultrasonic unit to remove any polishing compound before sterilization, but a separate machine must be used—not the one that processes contaminated equipment. If the studio also does tattooing, there must be yet another ultrasonic unit for use with tattoo equipment.

The ultrasound machine has a high potential for environmental cross-contamination, especially if it is operated uncovered. It should never be located inside the piercing room or in a break room where food is prepared or eaten.

The above information should be considered a brief introduction to familiarize you with the equipment found in the piercing studio. It does not contain enough information to perform sterilization procedures, only to evaluate if the proper equipment is present and basic processes are being followed.

Equipment Checklist

☐ An autoclave sterilizer *and* current spore tests for it.

☐ Ultrasound cleaning unit(s) to suit the needs of the studio.

☐ A *sharps disposal* (a special container for safely discarding used piercing needles). If they don't have one, leave. They either reuse needles or fail to dispose of them properly. Both are inappropriate, unethical, and in some places illegal. Needles *must* be used on only one client and then carefully deposited in an approved container.

Equipment Handling and Hygiene Procedures

There are specific measures a piercer must follow to keep her studio hygienic enough to safely break your skin. Even if the autoclave is functioning properly, there are many potential pitfalls that could place you in danger.

New piercing needles and tools that are processed in an autoclave should be sealed into special individual packages before the sterilization cycle if they will be stored. To preserve their germ-free condition, these sterile packages must be handled *only* with clean gloves once they are removed from the sterilizer. They should be kept in a sanitary location (such as a closed cabinet in the piercing room) until used—within thirty days from the sterilization date marked on an internal indicator. Equipment that is not put to use within that time frame should be resterilized.

A simple request to see a sterile piece of piercing equipment can be very revealing about a piercer's aseptic procedures. Does the piercer put on medical gloves before touching it? If she does not wash her hands first, does she carefully pick up and don the gloves by touching their exterior only by the cuffs (to avoid transferring germs on her hands to the outside of the gloves)? Is there an indicator inside the package marked with a date? (One side of the package is usually made of clear plastic, and the other of paper.)

If a piercer holds a sterile tool or permits you to touch it with bare hands, it is considered contaminated. If she then returns the item to its storage place, she does not have adequate practices. The item must be resterilized after the package surface has been compromised.

Piercers need training and focus to consistently keep up with these protocols; even a small lapse can result in the spread of germs throughout the studio. Most piercers with a minimum of training are not aware of all the necessary precautions, and, unfortunately, neither are a number of experienced practitioners. To protect your health, you need to select a piercer who properly maintains the cleanliness of her studio.

Finding a Piercer

How do you locate a good piercer? Looking in the phone book or online for local studios is a logical first step. It is also a good idea to talk to people who have piercings and ask them if they have a piercer to suggest (or one you should avoid). Word-of-mouth referrals are standard in the body art field. Getting a reference from a friend who has had a good experience is an excellent starting point. Still, even a sterling recommendation is no substitute for personally assessing a piercer.

> "I went to this piercer, and he was really nice and everything, and he did an awesome job. But, he had some trouble getting the jewelry through so he had to pierce me twice. And, well, the piercing turned out crooked and then it rejected. He told me to use alcohol on it. But really, he's a great piercer!" J.

Internet Resources

The Internet is a valuable resource for locating a prospective piercer. When reviewing websites, consider whether the page looks professional and educational. Does it contain information on post-piercing care, studio policies, and a photo gallery of the studio's work? The piercings should look aesthetically appealing. Is there a focus only on wild and unusual placements, or do they show standard ones, too? If a website does not inspire your confidence, keep looking.

Websites like www.bmezine.com contain many postings about piercing experiences, both good and bad. These can help you learn what to look for, what to avoid, and whether a prospective piercer has a good reputation.

Portfolio

Ask to look at a photo album of piercings performed in the studio, including pictures of the placement you are considering. This is a graphic representation of a piercer's work and shows how you can expect your piercing to look. Try to determine if pictures of healed piercings are shown, particularly if you are considering an uncommon spot that is challenging to heal.

Check photos for apparent legitimacy; some studios have had their portfolios stolen. High-tech computer programs can allow devious people to alter photos of unhealthy piercings, or even add body jewelry onto an image of an unpierced person.

Ask to Watch

Some piercers and piercees are open to having a spectator present during piercing—even a stranger—so it doesn't hurt to ask. If you wish to observe, you may be asked to sign a waiver to protect the studio from liability. This may seem strange, but it is an accepted practice. Occasionally, the piercee feels just fine, but the onlooker passes out!

Notice whether the piercer appears confident and composed. Does she perform the piercing rapidly with steady hands, or is she slow and fumbling? Also consider whether she has a comforting "bedside manner." This demonstration reveals the experience you can expect for yourself, so be sure you like what you see. Learn about handwashing and piercing room protocols and procedures in chapter 8 to make a more comprehensive evaluation.

Medical Professionals as Piercers

Piercing is similar to certain medical practices, but simply because an individual is licensed to provide health care does not mean she is skilled at body piercing. There may be an overlap of skill sets, and knowledge of anatomy, *venipuncture* (drawing blood or inserting an intravenous line), and infection control is relevant to both endeavors. But you would never consider visiting a chiropractor to treat your toothache, or a gynecologist for an ingrown toenail. Similarly, it doesn't make sense to go to a nurse, chiropractor, dentist, EMT, or any other medical professional for piercing unless *specific* instruction in body piercing was part of her education.

Any medical professional who feels confident to pierce based on medical training alone demonstrates how little she actually knows about piercing. Even a talented brain surgeon is unsuited to the task without knowledge of jewelry size and style, placement, and piercing techniques.

Doctors do not ordinarily make the effort to learn about standard piercing practices or equipment. Some doctors use injectable anesthetics to numb the area, but this increases the potential for complications and is not necessary when a piercer is skillful. Frequently doctors pierce the skin, remove the needle, and then attempt to force the jewelry through the fresh channel because they do not know about the special piercing needles that facilitate jewelry transfers. Whether you get pierced badly by a novice *or* a doctor, excess tissue trauma makes the aftermath more painful and healing more difficult, and the placement of the hole is seldom optimal. Finally, physicians are often unaware of the industry standards for piercing aftercare and may advise use of products that are unsuitable for healing this unique type of wound.

Still, there are some good piercers who are also medical personnel. These individuals, however, have sought out information and instruction on piercing as practiced by professionals in the industry.

Trust Your Instincts

Your instincts are a valuable tool, and you should listen to them when it comes to selecting a piercer. Still, you have to distinguish between normal apprehension about getting pierced and a feeling of mistrust for a piercer. This a good reason to pay the studio a visit before scheduling your piercing.

If you encounter a piercer who acts unethically or makes you uncomfortable in any way, you have the right to say, "Stop." You can leave. Trust your intuition and *never* stay in a situation that feels wrong. This isn't a haircut. Your health is at stake. Any of the following should cause warning bells to clamor and are reasons to call off your piercing:

- If you don't feel safe or comfortable
- If a piercer touches sterile or used piercing equipment without wearing gloves
- If a piercer does not have up-to-date spore tests or does not know what they are
- If a piercer or other staff member makes sexual innuendos or behaves unprofessionally
- If a piercer reeks of liquor or permits (or drinks!) it in the studio or you spot track marks or other signs of drug abuse

The Association of Professional Piercers

The Association of Professional Piercers (APP) is an international nonprofit health, safety, and education organization. The piercers who are "Professional Business Members" meet certain personal and environmental criteria. They uphold a safety agreement that encompasses minimum standards for using quality jewelry, maintaining cleanliness, and behaving professionally. The APP has an educational website, www.safepiercing.org, that includes information about piercing and member listings.

The APP is a respected and reliable resource that has set the standards for the industry. Anything described in this book as "industry standard" refers to the APP. The APP, however, does not monitor the "artistic merit" of member piercers. This means that you can be confident that its members maintain an acceptable level of hygiene, but no claims are made about the actual skills of the piercer. Still, APP members have at least one year of professional experience, and they are clearly among those piercers who are most conscientious about doing a good job.

It is reasonable to ask any piercer who is not a member of the APP, "Why not?" Does he fail to come up to the organization's standards, is he unfamiliar with his industry's professional association, or he is apathetic? All of those are poor qualities in a piercer.

The association has members who agree to comply with certain standards, but it is not a certifying agency. Any piercer stating he is "APP certified" is claiming a status that is unauthorized by the organization.

While it isn't often discussed openly, there are sadistic individuals in many professions, including medicine, dentistry—and body piercing. These people enjoy inflicting pain upon others nonconsensually. Unfortunately, a sadist in the piercing field is poised to receive a lot of joy from her work. Unless you are a willing masochist, stay far away from any piercer with a reputation for being very painful, or if word around town is, "she likes to make it hurt."

Pricey Hack Job

A mother took her teenaged daughter to one of the most respected dermatologists in her state to get a navel piercing. The teen brought her own jewelry, which the doctor swabbed briefly with alcohol instead of autoclaving to ensure sterility. After piercing her, the doctor dropped the jewelry-closure ball on the ground, picked it up, wiped it again with alcohol, and put it onto the ring in her fresh piercing. He advised her to use hydrogen peroxide and antibiotic ointment for aftercare and keep a bandage on it for five days. *None* of this is accepted practice in the piercing industry. He charged $120 for this service, which didn't even include the jewelry. This girl knew that the doctor did not adhere to standards of professional piercing, but her mother refused to listen because, she felt, "doctors know best."

Should You Travel?

Truly outstanding piercers are relatively rare. If you are lucky, you will find a top-notch pro nearby, but the closest qualified piercer may be three hundred miles away. How do you determine if you should go through the extra effort and expense to travel for a piercing?

If your plans are modest—for instance, you want a single tongue piercing—the most reputable local piercer might suffice. It is also convenient to use a nearby studio for routine jewelry changes and any piercing emergencies that occur. On the other hand, if you are a serious piercee with ambitious plans for unusual piercings, a highly experienced piercer is a necessity. And if you are planning to get a genital piercing, you must find an indisputable authority, even if you have to save up for a while and travel far from home. See "Genital Piercings: Selecting the Right Piercer," page 134, for more information.

The Point

A good piercer can be a resource and an inspiration, but a bad one can cause you agony and infection. Don't settle for a less-than-competent practitioner, an impatient piercer with a condescending attitude, or a so-called "professional" who doesn't adhere to appropriate hygiene protocols. You must be confident that your piercer is safe and qualified in every aspect.

PART 3

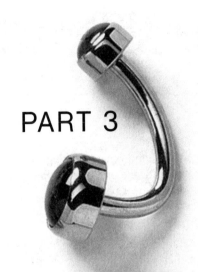

Piercing Preparation

Picking and Preparing

At the Studio

Piercing Procedures

Jewelry 101: Sizes, Shapes, and Materials

6

Picking and Preparing

There is nothing quite like getting a new piercing. Selecting the specific placement for your jewelry and preparing for the procedure—both mentally and physically—can be an important and fun part of the experience.

That Irresistible Urge

Deliberation and preparation before a piercing help to assure the best possible results, but there is no doubt that many a piercing is acquired on the spur of the moment. Experienced piercees often describe feeling an irresistible urge for a new hole—*now*. For some piercees, fulfilling this deep craving can involve months of research and decision making. Others simply head over to their favorite piercing studio with a sudden yearning. Both methods can result in a decent piercing, but especially for novice piercees, some forethought should produce a more predictable and positive outcome.

Decisions, Decisions

When considering a particular piercing placement, think about whether it appeals to you on other people. Deeper motivations aside, most piercees choose a piercing because they like the way it looks. You may first experience the desire to be pierced and then think about what parts of the body are pierceable and how wearing jewelry in the various spots will suit your appearance, lifestyle, and other factors. Sometimes you will be inspired, consciously or not, by seeing a certain piercing "in the flesh" or in the media.

> "For me, it's something that I really feel I want. No one factor plays into it, because I never feel I want a piercing until I have subconsciously taken all those factors (and more) into consideration." E.

Anatomy (physical structure) and *aesthetics* (physical appearance—especially when considered pleasing) are the two most critical issues for deciding on placement. The primary practical consideration is whether you have suitable tissue to support a specific piercing. You can attempt a preliminary evaluation for yourself, but your piercer will ultimately determine the appropriateness of your build for the piercing you desire. The second matter is far more subjective: will it complement your appearance? If your piercer gives you the go-ahead based on your anatomy, and even gives you a thumbs-up as his personal opinion, you will ultimately be the one to decide on the aesthetics for yourself.

Anatomy

People and their pierceable body parts come in a tremendous range of shapes and sizes. Examine the ears of a few friends to see how different they are from one side to the other and from person to person. The variations may be subtle, but the distinctions are vital when it comes to the safety and success of piercings. A few areas are universally pierceable, but even common spots like the eyebrow, tongue, and navel are not safe or possible for everyone. Try not to get your heart set on a piercing until you consult with a piercer, and be open to alternatives he may suggest if you are not configured for the one you have in mind.

Aesthetics

Jewelry will bring attention to the area in which it is worn. If your ears resemble those of Dumbo the Flying Elephant, you might not want all eyes drawn to them with conspicuous jewelry. (Or maybe you do!) Perhaps an eyebrow piercing to bring the focus away from your large ears would be preferable? Conversely, if you have never liked the shape or size of your nose, you might consider customizing your nostril with jewelry to make it more pleasing to you. Then again, if you have a lovely nose, why not embellish it with a glimmering jewel? Whether used to downplay, modify, or highlight a particular feature, your piercing can be personally empowering and gratifying. Gaze in the mirror and envision how a piercing will look on you. Would a ring or stud be best? Does a subtle ornament suit you or would bold jewelry look better? Ask some trusted friends for their opinions. A professional piercer is also a good resource if you have doubts or concerns.

Symmetry is another matter to contemplate. You may prefer only *midline* (in the center) placements like traditional navel or tongue piercings. If you got only one nipple pierced, for instance, you could feel lopsided. You might have a fondness for an asymmetrical style, or an inclination toward balanced asymmetry in which you have multiple smaller piercings on one side, and a single stretched hole on the other, for example. These are simply personal preferences; other than the anatomical and practical considerations, there isn't one correct way to place your piercings.

If you already have other body art, think about how the new piercing and jewelry will look and what overall effect you wish to achieve. You might like a fierce style, with multiple large-gauge piercings, or perhaps you want a more understated appearance. The placement should be your primary focus and the jewelry secondary, because the ornament can be changed, but the location of the hole cannot—at least not without getting another piercing. Don't forget that leaving some unpierced *negative space* (an area in between) usually looks best.

The aesthetics of piercing is a deeply personal matter, and it can be a highly charged one. Some people find *all* piercings disturbing or disgusting. Of course, the most important thing is that *you* are pleased with the appearance.

How Much Is Too Much?

Opinions on this range from one extreme to the other, and what is too much for one person will be not nearly enough for another. Only you can say what feels right for you. But at what point do piercings become excessive? Certainly, if they negatively affect function in any way—including your ability to be employed—that can fairly be considered "too much."

Harsh Judgment

One *Newsweek* columnist was so repulsed by piercings that she commented in an article, "When I can read the latte menu through the hole in my server's earlobe, something is seriously out of whack. The first time I saw this I nearly blew my lunch into the tip jar."[1]

Piercings tend to be most aesthetically pleasing, and more widely accepted, when they are placed with a focus on accent and enhancement. If your piercings begin to take over, it may be time to slow down and take a good look at your external appearance. And if you're getting lost in a sea of metal, perhaps some scrutiny of your motivations is warranted.

In addition to aesthetics and function, health considerations are also important. If you feel compelled to get one piercing after another regardless of your ability to heal or a medical condition (mental or physical), then this is also piercing overkill. There is, however, no way to pin down a precise number that pushes one over the edge to "excessively pierced."

The Consultation

A consultation with a piercer is helpful if you have questions about your suitability for a piercing or just can't make up your mind about which spot to choose. It's also a good way to get acquainted with a piercer, evaluate his professionalism, and see if you develop a comfortable rapport. An appointment might be required, or you may be able to walk in without a prior arrangement.

A qualified professional will be able to evaluate your anatomy, make suggestions about what will work with your build—or not—and explain why. Your jewelry options can also be covered so you can get a whole picture of how the piercing will look. Most shops do not charge a fee for this service, but if a consultation is done during a separate visit from your piercing and takes up much of the piercer's time, you may want to tip him.

Anticipa-a-tion!

The anticipation of an upcoming piercing can be exhilarating—even addictive. Lots of piercees describe their pre-piercing expectation in positive terms:

> "It's not a bad nervous feeling that I get; it's kinda like that feeling you get while you're waiting in line for a roller coaster." M.

After a number of piercings, the intensity of nervous anticipation may decrease, a fact some piercees lament:

> "I don't get jittery anymore, which is something I don't like. It's more fun for it to feel like you've actually *done* something rather than approaching it with a resounding 'eh.'" A.

Preparing for Your Piercing

You've done your homework and made your appointment. You are excited but apprehensive, too. You can't help but worry at least a little: How much will it really hurt? Is it going to look good on me?

There are a few extra things you can do to prepare. By readying yourself physically and mentally and by gathering the supplies you'll need, you play an active role in making sure your piercing experience will be great.

Supplies

Some of these items may be provided free or sold by your piercer. Find out what cleaning products your piercer suggests and whether they are available at the studio to determine what else you might need to purchase. If you obtain the things you will use beforehand, you won't be searching the shelves of a drugstore when you should be basking in the afterglow of your new piercing instead. You may want to buy:

- A piece of fruit or juice to have after piercing to stabilize your blood sugar
- Panty liners or sanitary pads to contain bleeding after female and male genital piercings (see chapter 13 for more information)
- Mild soap, non-iodized sea salt, and an appropriate soaking container for body piercings
- Paper towels for drying your piercing after bathing
- Shaved ice, popsicles, or ice cream, if you're getting a tongue or lip piercing
- Alcohol-free antiseptic mouth rinse for cleaning an oral piercing

The Piercing-Ready Body

Pay attention to your health and do what you can to enhance it prior to piercing. It's prudent to avoid drinking alcohol the night before your appointment, as it could cause you to bleed excessively, and a hangover will surely intensify any discomfort you experience. For obvious reasons, do not take any medications that have a blood-thinning effect, such as aspirin, Advil (ibuprofen), or Aleve (naproxen). Avoid large doses of caffeine for several days prior to piercing. Vitamin E may also thin the blood. Know the properties of herbs, supplements, or alternative remedies you're taking to avoid increasing your risk of bleeding. If possible, stop using anything questionable two weeks before your piercing. Herbs that have blood-thinning effects include chamomile, licorice root, ginkgo biloba, ginger, garlic, ginseng, goldenseal, and many others. Vitamin K supplements help to support optimal clotting. They are available at health food stores. Take them according to the package instructions for two weeks prior to the piercing, unless it is inadvisable due to a health condition.

Have a dental exam and teeth cleaning in the weeks before getting an oral piercing. Your mouth will be sparkling fresh, and this can also help avoid a dental emergency during healing. The first few months (when the lining of the channel is forming) are critical.

You'll feel best if you are rested and clearheaded on the day of your piercing appointment. Pay attention to your personal hygiene as a courtesy to your piercer and to safeguard your own health. It is polite to refrain from eating garlic and onions before an oral piercing and to brush your teeth shortly before entering the studio. Spend some extra time cleaning your ear, nose, or whatever area will be the focus of your visit. Unless you customarily do so, you don't usually have to shave the area to be pierced; however, trimming the hair nearby can facilitate the piercing process.

Give some thought to the clothing you will to wear to the studio if you have to disrobe. Dress for comfort and practicality. If you're getting a navel piercing, wear low-cut pants or other attire that makes it easy to reveal the area. Avoid clothes that would obscure or rub your new jewelry; a bodysuit would not be convenient. If you will be getting an ear or facial piercing, put up long hair so it doesn't get in the way.

Have a Snack

Eating a light meal one to two hours before your piercing is one of the simplest yet most effective things you can do to be physically prepared for your piercing. This helps to assure stable blood sugar levels during your visit and provides your body with some fuel reserves to prevent lightheadedness. Even if you feel as though you are too nervous to eat, have a small snack or smoothie, but avoid eating heavily right before piercing or you could experience nausea or vomiting.

The Piercing-Ready Mind

The following may help to minimize your anxiety level during a visit to the studio:

- Do something relaxing the hour before your appointment.
- Be confident of your decision to get pierced and your choice of piercer.
- Remind yourself that the piercing takes only a few moments of your life; it will pass quickly.
- Practice breathing and relaxation techniques (page 54) to use during your piercing.

The Point

You have done your research and selected a piercer and a spot to pierce. By preparing yourself mentally and physically, you've moved a step closer to the exciting event. Next you will learn all about what takes place in the studio before the piercing, during the process, and through its aftermath.

7

At the Studio

When the time finally arrives, piercing day is an exciting one. No matter how well prepared you are, feeling at least a little bit nervous is normal. But a good piercer will do everything possible to put you at ease and make your experience in the studio a positive one. This chapter covers the piercing process from your point of view as the piercee.

Moral Support

Feel free to have a friend or family member join you at the studio for support and possibly to drive you home if you have any concerns about being able to operate heavy machinery afterward. You should ask about the studio's policies, however, if you want to bring your whole bowling team, have someone hold your hand, or join you in the room during your piercing. Some piercers have rules against admitting visitors.

Children tend to be distracting for both you and your piercer. They are best left at home or in the retail area with a friend or relative for supervision. The piercing room is not a suitable environment for young children due to the presence of sterile equipment. Used tools and a biohazard waste bin are also common items in the piercing room. These are potentially dangerous areas for a child—especially when the adults are focused on other matters.

How to Be a Good Piercee

Piercers are justified in expecting appropriate behavior from their customers. When visiting a piercing studio you should show respect to the piercer by:

- Demonstrating a commitment to caring for your piercing
- Being educated about the process, sober, and mentally prepared—not unduly anxious or hysterical
- Understanding that piercing is a very individual matter and that the jewelry or placement that worked for your friend may not be right for you
- Arriving on time if you have an appointment
- Being cognizant about what you touch to avoid contaminating the premises

How Much Does It Cost?

Prices for piercings vary depending on the difficulty of the placement, experience of the piercer, jewelry material and style, store policies, and customary fees in your geographic area. The cost of the piercing, jewelry, and aftercare products all factor into the total expense.

Call local shops to get an idea of the average price for the piercing you are considering. The cost should never be the sole determining factor for selecting a studio. You will be paying someone to put a needle through your body—go for verifiable expertise, not the cheapest rate! Similarly, a high price doesn't guarantee superiority; overcharging is sometimes done to cover up poor quality.

The fee may be a package deal that includes piercing and basic jewelry and sometimes an aftercare product, too. Studios that offer a wide assortment of jewelry often use a separate price structure for the piercing fee and jewelry because different styles and materials vary in cost.

If you wish to purchase jewelry from another source or bring in your own (or someone else's) previously worn jewelry, you will need to have the piercer's approval prior to your appointment. Many studios have rules against using so-called "outside" jewelry for initial piercings; this is a reasonable policy that helps them maintain quality control.

The most popular areas, such as ear, nostril, tongue, and navel piercings, sometimes cost less than nipples or genitals. Most single body piercings will be in the $30 to $60 range. You can expect to pay around $75 to $100 for a genital piercing. A discount may be offered if you get multiple piercings done in the same session, because the piercer's expenses are minimized when she performs more than a single piercing per tray set up. Avoid a piercer who charges an exorbitant fee for male genital piercings and a pittance for female piercings, or vice versa. This is an indication that something is amiss! The fees should be approximately the same for both genders. Also think twice about any piercer who charges excessively high prices (for example, $100 extra) for genital piercings. This is often done because the piercer doesn't like to do them or is unskilled, which are good reasons to go elsewhere.

Apprentices do not provide the same level of service as experienced professionals. So, if you get pierced by a novice but are charged the same fee as for a pro, you will be paying with your cash (and your body) to train a student piercer. This shouldn't be your burden unless you make an informed decision to participate in a piercer's education—and if you do, a break on the price is appropriate.

Tips and Other Fees

Some shops charge a minimal fee to sterilize jewelry purchased elsewhere, to change your jewelry, or to give you a consultation. More often, these services are provided for free, especially when you buy something, get a piercing, or schedule an appointment for one. Whether you are asked to pay for such services or not, it is courteous to give the piercer a tip if she spends much time attending to you.

If you are pleased with your piercing experience, tipping your piercer is appropriate unless the establishment has a policy against it. Signs to that effect or tip jars may be in evidence to guide you. If you aren't certain about the prevailing custom in your area, you can ask whether tips are accepted. Piercers perform a personal service similar to those provided in salons and spas, and they are usually happy to receive a token of your appreciation. Although tipping is not as common in Europe, if you reside in North America, you can apply the same guideline you use for tipping in restaurants, though anything short of pocket change is courteous. If you are low on cash or tipping is not standard where you live, you can always return later with some cookies or other small gift if you feel inspired to express your sentiments. A good piercer will always do her best whether a tip may be forthcoming or not. One of the best ways to show you are pleased is by spreading the word about your great piercer to your friends and associates.

Piercing as Ritual

Getting a piercing can be an intensely altering experience that echoes the traditions of primitive societies. You should be aware that a piercing does change you. When you come out of a studio with a new piercing, you are a different person, with a different body, than when you entered. The way your modification affects you and any meaning you impart to it is entirely up to you.

Today, body piercing commonly functions as a visible way of cutting the apron strings that connect child and parent. As a youth enters adulthood he can take ownership of his own body by receiving a piercing without the involvement of his parents. This rite of passage is practiced—consciously or not—by many of today's young piercees.

You can use your piercing as a sacred celebration of a joyous occasion like a birth or marriage or as a solemn commemoration of a death. Your ceremony may draw upon the customs of your ancestors or tribal peoples, but it need not have historical precedence to be filled with special meaning. Merely connecting your personal intentions to the transformative nature of the event can bring a profound sense of value and importance to your piercing.

Many piercers are amenable to incorporating personal rites into the piercing encounter, provided their clients discuss it with them first. A good piercer will act as a facilitator without imposing her own agenda on the process, leaving room for you to create your own significance. Your experience does not have to include elaborate words or actions. An act as simple as reciting something during your piercing—aloud or in silence—can have a powerful and lasting impact.

Studio Preliminaries

Be cognizant of what you touch while in the studio to avoid contaminating yourself or the premises. The most rigorously hygienic shops have a strict zero-tolerance policy on handling all piercings and worn body jewelry. Any piercing, regardless of age, can flare up and ooze potentially infectious bodily secretions. This discharge can be transferred to your hands, and then to surfaces in the studio. Someone with a fresh piercing (or a cut finger) can encounter the contaminated spot. This represents a possibility for transmission of disease-causing microorganisms. Do not be offended if you are asked to stop handling your piercing or jewelry and wipe down or wash your hands. Don't be insulted if a piercer puts on gloves to handle jewelry that has been in your body, even if you haven't worn it lately. The worst-case scenario is that nobody working in the studio seems to care what anybody touches, because this is an indication of potentially perilous ignorance or indifference.

When you arrive, inform the person at the counter that you are planning to get pierced or that you have an appointment to do so. Let her know which piercing is of interest. If you haven't had one already, you may be given a brief consultation to check your suitability and to determine jewelry size. In a well-stocked studio you may be shown a selection of possibilities. Jewelry should be chosen for your anatomy and placement and should never be based solely on whatever is left in stock. In the best studios you will get detailed descriptions of the material and design features of the suitable jewelry options plus a demonstration of how each piece opens and closes. Be suspicious if you are permitted to choose jewelry without guidance, because size and style are crucial aspects for successful healing.

Do Little Harm

When selecting your jewelry, remember this key principle: do a minimum of damage and preserve the maximum number of nerve fibers by starting your piercing with the thinnest serviceable gauge. The smaller and more sensitive your anatomy, the more important this advice is. I perform piercings no larger than 10 gauge, though many piercers make holes that are much bigger, or use the pierce-and-stretch method (see page 228). However, the same results are available with less risk if you can be patient and stretch over time.

Unpackaged display jewelry is not sterile. If you select an item that is taken directly from the showcase, it must be run through a sterilizer before being inserted into your new piercing. If the studio does not have a short-cycle autoclave such as a Statim, this will delay your piercing for thirty minutes or longer. For items that are placed onto jewelry rather than through your body (such as a captive bead), a soak in a strong disinfectant solution may be sufficient.

Pick up care products such as mouth rinse or soap and sea salt if they don't come with your piercing package and you haven't stocked up already. The piercer or shop personnel may discuss the aftercare guidelines with you and request payment (or this might be done after the piercing).

Sign on the Dotted Line

Before piercing, you can expect to fill out a waiver or release form and present valid identification for proof of age. Ethical piercers are unwavering in their demand for the proper documentation. Even if you look well over the age of majority, it is common for piercers to look at your ID and to photocopy it onto your release form. Check with the studio for specific requirements if you are underage. Your parent or guardian should also be asked to present identification to prove the relationship between you. If you and your accompanying adult do not have the same last name, records may be requested such as guardianship papers, a divorce decree, or proof of a legal name change.

The paperwork you encounter will depend on the studio's policies and local laws. You may be asked what you've most recently eaten and when, and if you've ingested any medications, recreational drugs, or alcohol. Disclose pertinent medical history that could affect your piercing experience or healing course. If you have sensitivities or allergies, especially to iodine or latex, call attention to this verbally in addition to noting it on your release form so your piercer can make substitutions for iodine skin prep or latex medical gloves. These forms are essential for protecting both you and your piercer. Any studio that does not require this type of paperwork is a fly-by-night operation.

You may have to wait for the piercer to ready herself and set up the cleaning and marking supplies, sterile instruments, and jewelry that will be used for your piercing. Some piercers invite you in to observe their preparations, while others prefer to use this time to focus and prime themselves for your procedure.

Follow Me, Please

Next, you will be taken to the piercing room. It may resemble a medical office with a doctor's examination table and stirrups, or a dentist's chair. Don't be put off if this area seems a little cold or sterile—it's appropriate for a hygienic room to seem that way. A piercing room could have an earthier ambiance, but it must have surfaces that can be disinfected and are easy to keep clean.

Your piercer should show you a specific place to put your personal belongings. Be careful not to plop your sunglasses or bag onto a sterile tray or contaminated surface such as the biohazard trashcan. To avoid causing a distraction during your piercing, turn off your cell phone and any portable electronic devices, unless you discuss this with your piercer.

You will need to remove or adjust your clothing to expose the area for cleaning and marking. Your piercer will indicate where and how you should position yourself. You may need to change positions several times. Depending on the piercing placement, you might, for example, be marked while you are standing and pierced while you are reclining. A good piercer will guide you along; you won't have to wonder what is about to happen. Tell her if you have a preference for more information, or for less.

Piercers, like health-care personnel, should have a professional demeanor when dealing with unclad bodies. Your piercer should not make you feel self-conscious or uncomfortable by staring or acting improperly while you are undressing. Many studios have a policy against leaving clients alone in the piercing room, so you may not be permitted total seclusion while you undress. However, you should have relative privacy and be well away from other customers and staff.

You Want It Where?

Now is the time to reiterate the placement you have in mind and the effect you wish to achieve with your piercing. Mention any future plans you have for stretching or adding more piercings in the area, as this affects the best location for the current hole.

Your piercer will mark the prospective spot after cleaning the tissue. This step is critical because once the piercing has been made it cannot be repositioned. Take your time to consider the mark or marks carefully; envision how your jewelry will look. Bring in a friend for another viewpoint if you need help. Don't be afraid to request a change if you are not satisfied, or at least ask your piercer why she selected that spot. A good piercer will be able to explain the reason a particular location was chosen—and why the one you requested is less ideal.

For precision, I make my dots the same size as the jewelry gauge I will be inserting. Some piercers draw lines or crosses instead of dots; if you can't tell exactly where your piercing will be placed, ask your piercer for clarification. (I can't help but wonder: if a piercer's mark is much larger than the hole she is about to make, is she aiming for somewhere *specific?*)

Once you are both pleased with the proposed location for the jewelry, your piercer will begin the procedure. After making the mark(s), she should put on fresh gloves before touching the instruments used for piercing. Depending on the area and her piercing style, she may use her fingers or a tool to support the tissue for piercing.

Breathing and Relaxation Techniques

The conscious use of breath is a simple, time-honored technique for managing stress, pain, and anxiety.[1] Most piercers will at least instruct you to take a deep breath right before inserting the needle and have you exhale while the piercing is made. If she fails to coach you, you can still do this for yourself as the procedure commences: Breathe in through your nose slowly and deeply, filling your lungs. Exhale through your mouth even more slowly; completely empty your lungs. Try to let all your muscles loosen and relax as you maintain your focus on each calming breath. Keep your breathing controlled and deep until your jewelry is in place—don't hyperventilate.

Visualization or distraction can also help. Close your eyes and picture yourself walking on the beach. Enjoy the warm afternoon sun heating your skin and the gentle breezes caressing your hair. Hear the waves breaking on the shore nearby and imagine smelling and tasting the salty sea air. Use any pleasant scenario you like and try to engage as many senses as possible; stay focused on this throughout the procedure.

Another technique is to hold a friend's hand or grasp an object. This will help you to avoid concentrating on the piercing and transfer the tension elsewhere.

A Quick Stick

Next is the actual piercing. Some people prefer not to look at the needle; others feel it is important to observe it in order to know what is happening and maintain a sense of control. Try your best to stay absolutely still.

Ow! The piercing should be one brief—though possibly sharp—sensation.

Okay, maybe it did pinch a little, but most piercees find the pain was so fleeting that it was over before they even realized it was starting. Next, the piercer will insert your jewelry, pushing the needle out as she does so. A little maneuvering may be needed to get the jewelry in and securely fastened. This part of the procedure is sometimes more uncomfortable than the needle stick, especially if your piercer is not skillful. Try to breathe deeply and stay relaxed. As the adrenaline and endorphins pump through your system and then dissipate, it is not uncommon to feel light-headed. Don't worry; it will pass quickly. Alternatively, enjoy the brief rush while it lasts. Your piercer will clean up the area, offer you a look in the mirror, and bandage the area if you are bleeding. Congratulations! You did it.

The Aftermath

When the piercing is all done, your piercer may offer you a glass of water or other beverage and some candy. It isn't a bad idea to accept; or, if you brought juice or a piece of fruit, have it now to stabilize your blood sugar. During the aftermath, you may experience some sensations such as aching or stinging, though seldom much pain—or at least not for long. These feelings can remain or return intermittently throughout the rest of the day. Analgesics are not suggested prior to your piercing due to their tendency to increase bleeding; however, you may wish to take some ibuprofen afterward to diminish any discomfort and swelling.

If your piercer did not discuss aftercare prior to the piercing, it should be covered at this point. Ask questions until you feel clear about how to take care of your piercing, what products to use, and how often. Take as much time as you need in the studio to relax and recover. If you don't feel steady, be honest with yourself and your piercer.

Arising before you are ready can result in a serious injury if you fall. Your piercer should be happy to let you remain for as long as you need before you depart.

Understandably, you could be distracted during your visit to the studio and may not recall all the details of the aftercare later, even if the piercer discussed them at length. Take a copy of the printed care guidelines with you and when the excitement of the piercing has subsided, review the aftercare sheet.

Make a Note

While you are in the studio, ask your piercer the exact dimensions of your jewelry and write them down. A lack of accurate information can present challenges down the road if you need to change your jewelry or buy replacement parts. For instance, if you lose a ball, you'll need to know the gauge of your jewelry. It might also be beneficial to write down where you made your purchase, because not all parts are compatible, especially with threaded jewelry. If you need to adjust the fit of your initial jewelry or you decide to change the style, it is helpful to know the size and other specifics.

Record everything you can: the gauge (thickness), the length of the post (if it is bar-style jewelry) or the inside diameter (for ring-style jewelry), the ball size, the material, and the studio or piercer. Keeping notes about your healing course or trials with different care regimens can also be useful. Use the "My Piercings and Jewelry Chart" (page 274) to keep track of the particulars. Keep this book handy and you will have a complete log whenever you need it.

Joining the Tribe

Piercing can bring a tremendous sense of satisfaction and joy provided that all aspects are handled properly. It can be an awesome experience in the true sense of the word. You may have an urge to show off your new piercing and celebrate your status as a changed person. Unfortunately, friends and family might not fully understand the depth of your experience, nor appreciate your taste in body art. If that's the case, you may want to turn to an online community such as BME (www.bmezine.com) or Tribalectic (www.tribalectic.com) to discuss your piercing with like-minded people. Membership to the BME website can be gained by submitting a written description of your piercing. Writing such an account enables you to relive and internalize your piercing experience and share it with others who can appreciate it.

The Point

Now that you know about the details involved in a visit to the studio, you are almost fully prepared to get your piercing. However, we have touched only briefly on piercing procedures, so read on to learn about the tools and techniques piercers use.

Piercing Procedures

Once you've decided on the piercer and the placement, filled out the paperwork, and entered the piercing room, what will the piercer do? Although it's not necessary that you know every detail, familiarity with the common equipment and procedures can help you form realistic expectations and evaluate whether your piercer is working in a manner consistent with accepted practices. This chapter introduces you to the instruments and technical aspects of piercing; it is *not* an instructional manual on how to pierce. Always patronize a competent professional; *do not attempt piercing at home.*

Setup

Your piercer must thoroughly wash his hands with soap and water, dry them with disposable towels, and put on clean medical gloves before touching you or any piercing equipment. If he doesn't wash his hands, or use a waterless cleanser of the sort used in medical facilities, he shouldn't perform a piercing. A hands-free sink is best, but if he touches the faucet handles to turn on the water, then he should use paper towels or his elbows—not his clean hands—to turn it off. Next he should don a new pair of gloves.

If you have a latex sensitivity or allergy, remind your piercer before he puts on gloves. Informed, responsible professionals stock gloves made of nitrile or other latex substitutes. Sterile gloves are not essential for a safe procedure, though in a few places they are mandated by law. In the healthcare field, clean medical exam gloves are considered adequate for drawing blood and inserting intravenous (IV) lines,[1] and standard piercing industry practice deems them suitable for performing body piercing.

Your piercer may apply a disposable self-stick barrier film that is changed for each client as part of the piercing room preparations. He may place it on a light or other fixture he will need to touch or adjust during your procedure. Once he is gloved, he should handle only his piercing equipment (including cleaning and marking gear), the area of your body he will be piercing, and barrier-covered protected zones in the piercing room. His gloves must be changed if they touch anything else. To perform a piercing safely, several pairs are needed during the course of a setup, piercing, and cleanup.

Before he begins the process, your piercer should assemble all the supplies he needs on a clean tray. The tray should be disposable, autoclavable, or have a disposable plastic-backed paper liner, like those used in a dentist's office. An alternative is the Statim setup described in "Vital Equipment: Sterilizers and Ultrasonics," page 37.

Piercing Tools and Techniques

The tools and techniques used by your piercer will depend on his style and the type of piercing you're getting. One tool that all piercers must use is some type of piercing needle. In the United States, extremely sharp, beveled-tip hollow needles are expressly made for the purpose of body piercing. Quality needles are razor-sharp; they pierce most tissue with a minimum of force. The needle is usually held and pushed through by hand, though some piercers use a needle holder or pusher. Good needles are crucial for a comfortable procedure. Piercers sometimes say, "Your skin is really tough," to excuse a slow or botched piercing, but that is seldom the problem when top-of-the-line needles are used.

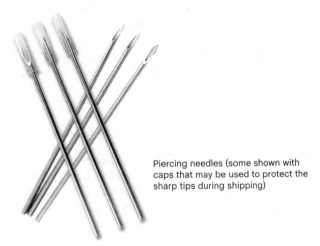

Piercing needles (some shown with caps that may be used to protect the sharp tips during shipping)

Piercing needles come in a range of sizes to suit the preferences of different piercers; I favor a needle about two inches long for most piercings. Needle thickness is expressed as its *gauge* (a numerical standard of measurement for the thickness of wire). Needle gauges correspond to those used to describe the thickness of body jewelry. For both needles and jewelry, the higher the number, the thinner the item (see "Gauge Measurements," page 67). It is standard practice to use the same gauge needle and jewelry for most piercings. Needles also come sized in odd measurements, called *half gauges*, which some piercers use for certain techniques that are discussed later.

Curved needles are also available. They are designed for piercings in areas where a straight needle does not conform well to the anatomy being pierced or the area surrounding it. If a curved needle will be used, it must be manufactured with a smooth arc and not bent with pliers in the studio.

Like all instruments in the traditional piercing setup, sterile needles should be stored in individual packages. Just before the contents are used, the wrapping should be opened carefully to minimize the potential for contamination.

To avoid the gratuitous use of the word "needle" in the studio, I use the abbreviation "P.N." for piercing needle, or simply refer to it as a "piercing instrument." If you are sensitive, I spare you the distress of having a needle called to your attention or even hearing about it by name. Should you want to see it or talk about it, I will certainly oblige, but any piercer who forces you to look at a needle against your wishes is treating you in an abusive manner. It is not required that you see the piercing instrument, and if you are needle-phobic, this would be unnecessarily traumatic.

Both the American-style needle and the cannula type (described immediately below) can be safe for body piercing when the technician is trained to use them correctly.

Cannulas

Outside the United States, the *cannula* or *catheter needle* (a needle covered with a flexible plastic sleeve) is frequently used. In some countries, it is illegal for piercers to use American-style piercing needles because they are considered medical devices. The sharp tip of the cannula makes the piercing, and when the needle is withdrawn, it leaves the hollow casing in the piercing channel. This method requires an extra step if jewelry is to be inserted in the same direction the piercing was made: sterile scissors must be used to cut off the attached hub (part of the equipment that is needed when the cannula is used for its intended medical purpose). The jewelry is fed into the plastic casing inside the piercing channel, the sheath is then withdrawn and the jewelry is in place. This may result in a little more bleeding because the hole made by the cannula is slightly larger than the jewelry.

Corks

Some piercers place a small sterile cork on the exit side of the tissue for support during the piercing, and to receive the needle. A potato, carrot, or piece of Styrofoam is not acceptable to serve this function. (Yes, some so-called "professional" piercers have used these objects. If your piercer reaches for a vegetable, run!)

Forceps

Forceps (a medical grasping tool) can be used to hold and support the tissue to assist a piercer in making a quick, safe, and accurate piercing. A variety of shapes, sizes, and styles are available, though forceps are not suited to all areas of the body, and not all piercers use them. *Pennington forceps* (a triangular-jaw clamp) are commonly used for body piercings, and a larger oval-headed model is often used for tongue piercings.

Forceps secure and compact the skin but should never cause pain or excessive trauma to your tissue. The tool should not leave scratches, deep grooves, or cause a contusion (though bruising in the pierced region is a normal consequence of the piercing itself). The pinching sensation from forceps is sometimes considered "the worst part" of a piercing, but, in the hands of a skilled technician, the tool seldom causes more than a moderate pinching feeling. Further, clamps limit the circulation, which may have a slightly numbing effect or at least a distracting one. When they are removed, you may feel more sensation than when they are put in place, and this is apt to occur if they are left on longer than usual. Tighter or denser tissue might feel more sensitive when clamped.

The piercer carefully positions the jaws of the forceps on your tissue so the marks for placement are lined up evenly on each side. When he pierces with the needle square to the jaw of the forceps, he will hit his mark on the exit side; your piercing will be placed in its intended position. A good piercer will get the forceps on and off quickly, leaving them as loose as possible while they are still secure. Manipulation of the tool once it is attached to you is unnecessarily painful and can be damaging, so he should move it very little once it is clamped in place. I find that forceps with a relatively small head provide the best support for many piercings.

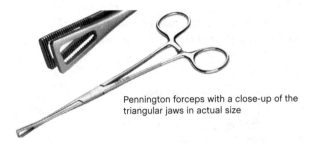

Pennington forceps with a close-up of the triangular jaws in actual size

Forceps are often left in place until after the jewelry has been inserted into tongue and some labret (lip) piercings. The forceps must have a large enough head for the barbell or labret stud ends to fit through, so the clamp can be removed. Otherwise, the tool will be attached to your body by the jewelry.

An alternative style is *slotted forceps*, which have a segment of the jaws removed so that they can easily be taken off after jewelry is in place without being opened or fitting over the barbell ends. I don't use this type, because if the piercee jumps or pulls back during a piercing, which happens occasionally, the forceps could slide right off.

Traditional metal forceps are reusable following appropriate decontamination and sterilization processes. Recent innovations include various types of disposable plastic clamps designed specifically for piercings.

Needle Receiving Tubes (NRTs)

Needle receiving tubes serve a similar purpose as forceps but are used in areas where clamps don't fit or aren't practical. The NRT is a hollow tube with a *lumen* (space inside) large enough to accommodate the needle; it supports the tissue on the exit side during the piercing procedure. Some have flared ends, and others are angled to better conform to the shape of the anatomy. Receiving tubes in metal, shatter-resistant glass, and disposable hard plastic come in various diameters and lengths.

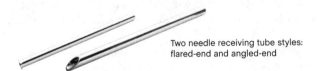

Two needle receiving tube styles: flared-end and angled-end

NRTs are commonly used for septum piercings and certain ear cartilage piercings such as the rook and daith. Many piercers use a large version inside the nose when performing nostril piercings. A considerate piercer will warm the tube by rolling it between gloved fingers before placing it against sensitive anatomy.

In addition to offering support, the tube also functions as a protective sheath by enclosing the sharp tip of the needle. A receiving tube can also be used to cap the needle during a jewelry transfer, even if the tube isn't used for support during the piercing.

Techniques

Depending on the area being pierced and the style and skill of your piercer, you will experience some of the following techniques during your piercing.

Freehand Piercings

Freehand piercing (done without tools other than a piercing needle) can be a valid approach, but it is more risky for the piercer due to the possibility of a needle stick accident. Instead of using forceps or a receiving tube, the piercer supports the area with his hand, so his fingertips are dangerously close to where the needle exits. The needle can jab the piercer's finger as it exits your tissue. Executing a procedure swiftly and placing the piercing accurately are more challenging using the freehand technique, but some piercers do an impressive job with this approach.

This method was not originally considered standard in modern body piercing. Tools were believed to be more or less indispensable for most placements. However, this practice has developed over time, and for some piercers, freehand is the traditional way.

Unfortunately, there are also piercers who perform freehand piercings due to a lack of instruction, a dearth of equipment, or reasons of ego. Some consider it a point of pride that they perform only freehand piercings. In reality, however, a piercer can work very quickly, gently, and safely whether using tools *or* performing a freehand procedure. It all comes down to training and experience.

The U.S. Occupational Safety and Health Administration (OSHA) has issued the following statement, which calls the technique into question:

> "The practice of 'freehand' piercing without the use of forceps or other available engineering and work practice controls to prevent contact with the used end of the piercing needle violates 29 CFR 1910.1030(d)(2)(i), an important provision of the bloodborne pathogens standard that requires that engineering and work practice controls shall be used to eliminate or minimize employee exposure." [2]

The method, however, is not prohibited if some type of "engineering or work practice control" is used, such as a device to cover the tip of the needle, or to protect the fingers.

The primary consideration of your piercer should be to use an approach that will provide a safe procedure, a pleasant (or at least tolerable) experience for you, and a precisely placed piercing. Carefully interview a prospective piercer about his training, piercing philosophy, and level of experience if he performs only freehand piercings. If he believes that forceps always cause tissue damage, he never learned to use clamps properly. Make sure he is not self-taught or minimally experienced before you let him pierce you.

Tissue Manipulation

Skin that is taut or inflexible can make the procedure more challenging for both you and your piercer. This simple but effective step loosens and prepares the area to make the piercing as comfortable as possible.

For forceps or freehand: The piercer performs highly localized manipulation by gently lifting and rolling the flesh between his fingers for ten to thirty seconds. It might go on for a minute or longer if your tissue is especially dense or tight.

For NRTs: He can prepare the area with a form of tissue manipulation for the septum and ear cartilage piercings that use an NRT, though for a slightly different reason. This technique helps to compact the tissue and also seat the NRT so that it does not slip during the piercing. He places a sterile swab or fingertip at the point where the needle will enter and puts the tube into position at the exit; he applies pressure from both sides while massaging in a barely perceptible circular motion.

Illumination

Your piercer might illuminate certain areas with a penlight or other bright light to check for visible structures such as veins and arteries in the proposed pathway of the piercing. He may do this during marking, right before the stick, or both. The tissue and forceps might be adjusted to move vessels out of the way, or the placement of the piercing might be altered.

Compression Technique

This technique is used for piercings of the cartilage, including the ear (above the soft lobe) and nostril. As soon as the piercing is done and the jewelry is in place, the piercer uses sterile gauze or cotton swabs to apply firm pressure on both sides of the piercing for fifteen seconds to a minute, as if attempting to staunch bleeding, even if no blood is present. This simple technique is intended to reattach the surface tissue to the cartilage underneath. It helps reduce the likelihood of localized ear cartilage and nostril bumps during healing. I do this for all of the cartilage piercings described in chapter 10. If your piercer is not familiar with this simple technique, describe the practice and ask him to perform it on you.

Anesthetics

In some parts of the world, particularly in the United Kingdom and Europe, a topical or injectable anesthetic may be administered prior to piercing, although it is certainly not necessary. In the United States, it is illegal for nonmedical personnel, including piercers, to offer anesthetics.

Basic Piercing Procedure

Below are the basic steps your piercer should follow. Unfamiliar terms are listed in the glossary and discussed in detail later in the book.

- **Clean the area to be pierced,** usually with Betadine or Techni-Care surgical scrub for body piercings or a germicidal mouth rinse for oral piercings. Cleaning inside and out is required for *orofacial* piercings such as the upper or lower lip. In the United States, alcohol is not normally used as a sole skin-cleaning product for piercing, though it may be used before the surgical scrub. Betadine and other iodine products occasionally produce skin irritation reactions, though the sensitivity is usually to ingredients other than the iodine, and true iodine allergies are reportedly a myth.[3] Also contrary to popular lore, an allergy to shellfish or seafood does not increase the likelihood of sensitivity to iodine.[4] If you have a history of trouble with topical iodine, remind your piercer prior to skin prep and he will use an alternate product.

- **Mark the placement** with an alcohol-based pen like a fine-point Sharpie, a surgical marker, or disposable items such as a sterile toothpick with a drop of *gentian violet* (a purple water-based fungicide also used in surgical markers). If a pen is used to mark you, your piercer should give it to you or dispose of it; he should not reuse it.

  - This part of the process should never be rushed. Don't hesitate to request adjustments until you and your piercer feel the marks are perfectly placed. With the exception of the nostril, vertical clitoral hood (VCH), and Prince Albert (PA), one dot for the entry and one for the exit are usually marked.

- **Secure the tissue**, either with forceps, a receiving tube, or fingers.

- **Pierce the tissue** with a sterile, disposable piercing needle. Ideally, this should last a moment and be done with a single, swift push. Stopping halfway through is inappropriate because every extra movement of the needle causes needless discomfort.

- **Insert the jewelry,** pushing the needle out with the jewelry. This should also be done in one smooth movement. The needle should not come all the way out of the tissue before the jewelry has completely passed through the channel.

- **Close the jewelry** with a captive bead, threaded ball, or other closure. Some jewelry, such as a nostril screw, does not require this step.

- **Clean up,** wiping the area clean if there is any bleeding, and using saline or sterile water if Betadine was used for skin prep (iodine can irritate skin if it is left on for an extended period of time). I favor foil-wrapped saline towelettes because they are effective for clean up, don't irritate, and instantly help to diminish the stinging sensations that often follow piercing. Alcohol should *not* be used; it is irritating and painful on a fresh wound.

  - Your piercer should carefully dispose of the needle directly into the sharps disposal container as soon as possible following your piercing.

  - Any reusable instruments such as forceps should be placed into an appropriate storage container (often in a germicidal liquid) for subsequent sterilization.

  - Disposable items and paper products used in the procedure should be placed in a clearly marked biohazard waste can.

  - Your piercer cannot clean the premises with the gloves he wore during your procedure; they are considered contaminated. He must put on a new pair after he discards the tray set up that was used during your piercing. The table or chair, tray, and other surfaces that were contacted but not autoclaved or disposed of should be cleaned with hospital-grade, hard-surface disinfectant.

Proceed with Caution!

The following things should *never* happen during a piercing (and if they do, bolt!):

- Your piercer asks you or your friend to hold the forceps with unwashed, ungloved hands.
- The forceps are locked tightly onto your body.
- The forceps are left hanging from your body, even momentarily.
- The piercer drops something on the floor (such as a tool he is still using, or your jewelry), then picks it up but does not change gloves and replace or resterilize the item.

Other Tools

There are a number of specialized tools, including pliers and hemostats, designed to facilitate the insertion and removal of body jewelry. These metal instruments must be sterilized between clients. They also have the potential to scratch and damage jewelry or pinch tissue, so they must be used carefully. Because of this, it's a good idea for a piercer to use his fingers instead of one of these tools, when possible. But for tasks that can't be done by hand, these tools work very well. For more information, see "Jewelry Tools," page 221.

Insertion Tapers

Also called *insertion pins*, *insertion needles*, or simply *tapers*, these tools are used to facilitate jewelry insertion and to stretch piercings to a thicker gauge (see "Insertion Tapers for Jewelry Changes," page 220, and "Stretching," page 224). They look similar to needles, but there are differences. Tapers are not sharp, though they may be a little pointy in the thinner sizes. Also, they are solid, not hollow like piercing needles. The back end is formed into a concave, convex, threaded, or other shape to fit with specific styles of jewelry. Using the right type is key to ensure the successful transfer of jewelry into a piercing. They come in every standard jewelry gauge and are sized by the measurement at the thicker end. The thinner tip is usually two gauge sizes smaller than the larger end to assure a smooth gradation over its two inches or so of length. Tapers are commonly made of implant-grade stainless steel, though acrylic and other materials are also used.

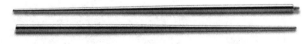

Pin-coupling and concave-end insertion tapers

Insertion tapers are occasionally used during the piercing process for putting in certain styles of jewelry. When the piercing is made in one direction but the jewelry must be inserted from the opposite side (for a gem to face the right way, for example), a taper can be used. A lubricated taper will push out the piercing needle, then help to transfer the jewelry into the piercing so that the ornament is situated correctly.

In the unfortunate event that your piercer fails to get your jewelry all the way through your tissue during a jewelry transfer, tapers can sometimes be used to locate the channel. It may be easier for your piercer to first pass a thinner taper through, then follow it with an insertion taper the gauge of your new piercing, and, finally, insert your jewelry.

The Point

You have an excellent idea of what to expect in the studio and throughout the piercing procedure. You are primed for a fantastic experience. Still, there is a great deal of valuable information about jewelry that has not yet been discussed. Round out your knowledge in the next chapter, and when the time comes to select body jewelry for a new or existing piercing, you will be versed in all the details.

9

Jewelry 101: Sizes, Shapes, and Materials

Though much of the focus in piercing is on where and how to place the hole, a vital factor for uneventful healing is having the right foreign object in your wound—the jewelry. The more you know about body jewelry, the better your chances of getting a quality piece that will be safe for healing.

All That Glitters

From functional to flashy, the choices for body jewelry seem almost infinite. Only certain styles and types, however, are suitable for healing. Without knowing what to look for, you can easily be seduced into getting jewelry that is inappropriate (or even harmful) to a fresh piercing. Every element of the jewelry—its size, design, material, *and* quality—affect your chances of having a healthy piercing.

Earrings, Nipple Rings—What's the Difference?

Simply put, earrings are not meant for wear in body piercings. The thin wires can cause cutting, migration, or rejection. For safety, body piercings require jewelry that is thicker than most earrings. In addition, both stud earrings and hoops that have a straight post meant to pass through the lobe are too short for body piercings—and even for some ear piercings. Many hoop earrings have parts that would poke and irritate if worn in other areas of the body. Even fine jewelry earrings manufactured from quality materials are not made in the appropriate styles or sizes. Good designs for fresh piercings are simple, made of uniform thickness, and have secure closures so they do not detach unintentionally during regular activities such as bathing and sleeping.

If you lack information about body jewelry, naturally you are going to buy whatever appeals to your sense of fashion or fits your budget best rather than what is optimal to wear in a new piercing. And some piercers prefer to sell you what you like rather than what you need, especially if you want an item with a higher price than a basic model that is superior for healing.

Choosing jewelry for piercings differs dramatically from shopping for a ring to wear on your finger. The look of the initial piece must always be secondary to safety aspects that affect compatibility with your body. There are countless options to wear after your piercing has healed, so you can change to a trendier, flashier, or smaller ornament later.

So why can't you pick just any piece of jewelry you like?

- The material may not be safe for a fresh piercing, either because it cannot withstand sterilization or it may cause skin sensitivity, allergy, or infection due to incompatibility with the body.
- The design and manufacture may be poor, leading to irritation of the fresh wound.
- Shoddy jewelry may have dysfunctional closures, like beads or balls that fall off easily, resulting in lost jewelry and accidental piercing closure.
- The size and shape may not be right for your anatomy, and ill-fitting jewelry can cause inflammation, embedding, and other problems.

The Body Jewelry Boom

Many of the body jewelry styles we wear today have roots in the ornaments worn by primitive peoples in their piercings. The designs were modified and modernized by Jim Ward, who introduced most of the basic pieces that remain in use today.

In the past few decades, body jewelry has become a big business, and now it is mass-produced around the globe. Improvements such as the introduction of high-tech metals and advanced production methods mean that the finest goods now approach aerospace precision in their quality.

Unfortunately, the explosive popularity of piercing has also brought on an epidemic of inexpensive, poorly made body jewelry—much of it from overseas. A lot of the eye-catching novelty jewelry is made of inferior materials using substandard manufacturing processes. Uninformed retailers and uncaring piercers are selling these shoddy goods, and uneducated consumers are purchasing them and wearing them in their piercings, sometimes with regrettable consequences.

The Basic Shapes

There are two basic shapes of body jewelry: The *ring* (a hoop) and the *barbell* (a post with a ball or other closure on each end). Variations on these two forms comprise the most popular and functional styles that are suitable for the majority of fresh piercings.

There are two basic types of rings, though they are very similar in appearance:

- Captive bead ring
- Fixed bead ring

And there are two basic styles of bars:

- Straight barbell
- Curved barbell

A closed captive bead ring
and an open fixed bead ring

An unscrewed (open)
circular barbell

A straight barbell and
a curved barbell

Another common style is essentially a combination of a ring and a barbell; it is circular in shape, but the closures work like those on a barbell. For practical purposes, we'll call this ring-style jewelry:

- Circular barbell

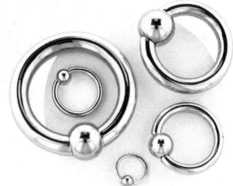

Even though a studio's selection of body jewelry might be vast, the majority of items will simply be adaptations and modifications of these simple styles.

Sizes and Measurements

Body jewelry sizes can be confusing because of the gauge system used to measure the thickness and the tremendous array of sizes and shapes. A clear, detailed ruler or *caliper* (measuring instrument) can come in very handy.

A selection of captive rings in a range of different gauges and diameters

Each piece of body jewelry is measured using two dimensions:

- **Gauge** (thickness)
- **Length** (for the post of barbells, curved barbells, nostril screws, and similar designs) or *inside diameter* (for ring-style jewelry)

Gauge Measurements

The thickness of body jewelry made in the United States is measured using a system called *American Wire Gauge* (AWG) or *Brown & Sharpe*. (See "Gauge Conversion Chart," page 275.) According to this system, the lower the number, the thicker the material, so 20 gauge is thin and wiry, whereas 4 gauge is very thick (and not a standard size for a new piercing). The thicker the jewelry, the bigger the jumps between sizes. In practice, when we refer to a 14-gauge captive ring, we are talking about the thickness of the metal that passes through your skin.

Supply and Demand

During the late 1980s, one of my biggest challenges as manager of the Gauntlet was stocking an adequate supply of jewelry for our piercing needs because only one company in the country was making body jewelry at the time—ours. That's certainly changed!

To compare, most conventional earrings are around 18 gauge, though sometimes they are as thin as 20 gauge. The common initial minimum size for below-the-neck piercings is a little thicker: 14 gauge. Somewhat confusingly, the gauge sizing system for medical needles is not the same one used for piercing needles and jewelry. A 16-gauge medical needle and a 14-gauge piercing needle are similar in size. More sensibly, perhaps, in Europe sizes are generally measured in millimeters.

Diameter or Length

In the United States, body jewelry is measured by fractions of an inch. Rings are measured across the inside diameter, at the widest part. Barbells are measured by the

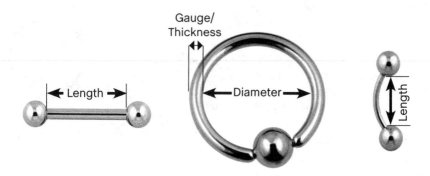

length of the bar, from one end of the post to the other. Balls or other ends are never included in the measurement.

The length of a curved bar is figured by measuring straight across from one end of the post to the other. The dimension of the curve is not taken into consideration; so a bar shaped with a deeper curve than another will have a little more room on it, but this is not reflected in its length.

The beads in captive rings and the balls for barbells are also measured by diameter at the widest point, in fractions of an inch or millimeters. Generally the smaller the ring diameter, the smaller the ball, though some styles play with proportion to achieve different effects.

Ring diameters start at $1/4$ inch in the thinnest gauges, though rings that tiny are not common. Due to practical issues and manufacturing limitations, a certain range of sizes is typically available in each gauge. For example, thin gauges are wobbly and unstable in large diameters, and thick wire cannot be bent into tiny diameters. A well-stocked studio, however, has many sizes on hand to offer you the best possible fit for your anatomy and piercing placement.

Conscientious piercers carry barbells in increments of sixteenths of an inch for optimal fit, from $3/16$ inch up to well over an inch if ampallangs or apadravyas are performed in the studio.

Ring-Style Jewelry

Captive Bead Ring

A popular style of basic body jewelry is the *captive bead ring* (CBR), also called a *captive, captive ring,* or *ball closure ring* (BCR). This metal hoop uses tension to hold a *captive ball* or *captive piece* (a removable bead or ornament) in a gap between its ends. This piece is drilled with dents or holes into which the ends of the ring are seated. The captive piece

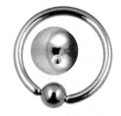

A captive bead ring with a close-up of a captive bead

can be made of the same material as the ring or from a contrasting one. There are thousands of different beads and other captive pieces available in a range of colors, shapes, and designs. The smaller ones can be safely interchanged during initial healing.

A well-made CBR has a smooth circular shape and ends that are convex to ease insertion and hold the bead firmly. The tips should look even and finished—not like someone filed them in a garage with a handheld rasp.

The captive ring opens by forcing the hoop to widen slightly, which releases the tension on the bead, allowing it to come free. It closes by snapping the bead in between the tips, engaging the spring tension of the ring. For this jewelry to be closed securely, the gap between the ends of the ring must be slightly narrower than the captive piece it holds. When the metal is *annealed* (a process used to improve a metal's properties), the beads in an average-sized ring can be removed or changed without the use of tools (see "Annealing," page 79).

Use the following technique to make changing the bead easier:

- **To remove the bead**, grasp the ring between the thumb and index finger of one hand (at three or nine o'clock, with the bead at twelve o'clock) and hold the bead between the thumb and index finger of the other hand. Draw the bead and ring in opposite directions.

- **To insert a bead**, hold the jewelry the same way as for bead removal. Make sure that your fingers do not obscure the drills or dents on the bead. Start by seating the dent of the bead onto the side of the ring that you're not holding. It is usually best to do this by feel rather than trying to look at it. Use leverage on the ring, via the seated side of the bead, to ease the second dent of the bead into place. It should "snap" into position, though the bead may still spin freely.

To remove the ring from the body without pinching the tissue, the gap may need to be wider than the one left by removing the bead. In this case, the ring itself will need to be bent open somewhat. To avoid warping the ring, it is usually best to twist the hoop in a coil shape, rather than simply pull the ends of the ring apart. With the exception of swapping out your bead, seek professional assistance for any ring changes that are necessary during healing.

Before attempting to change your own bead, practice with jewelry that you are not wearing. In the event that you can't manage the job, you will need to get help from your piercer, or purchase some ring expanding pliers (RXPs) (see "Jewelry Tools," page 221). Beads made of fragile materials like natural stone or glass can be chipped during insertion, so the use of RXPs is suggested.

The CBR is a simple design that has several advantages: it is extremely versatile, secure *when properly fastened*, and easy to manufacture. One disadvantage is that it is possible for the ball to fall out and become lost. The ring can follow, and your piercing can shrink—or even close. This type of ring can also be awkward for the uninitiated to handle and may take strength and dexterity to operate, depending on the gauge, diameter, and quality. The CBR is made in other shapes and forms (such as square, teardrop, triangle, D-ring, and so on), but these are best for healed piercings.

Fixed Bead Ring

The *fixed bead ring* (or simply *bead ring*) and the captive ring are almost identical in appearance; but, as indicated by its name, the bead is permanently attached to one end (see photo on page 66).

The jewelry twists open and closed for insertion and removal. On a quality piece, the bead is drilled so that the open end of the ring fits into it securely. When both ring and bead are the same material, you may not be able to tell the two styles apart without attempting to spin the bead. If it moves, it is a captive bead ring.

Fixed bead rings lack versatility, but one advantage of wearing them is that you can't possibly lose the bead. This is one reason they are popular in gold, which is pricey. This style is mostly made in thinner gauges that are easier to manipulate for insertion and removal. Depending on its material, quality, and size, a fixed bead ring may require tools such as brass-jaw pliers for opening and closing. Another disadvantage is that bead rings are unsuited to frequent changes. The metal can become disfigured from overuse, and excessive opening and closing will cause brittleness and, ultimately, breakage. For a nominal fee, gold can be re-annealed by a jeweler to restore it, but this must be done before the piece breaks. When your ring feels more difficult to bend, you will know the time has come for a treatment.

After repeatedly bending a fixed bead ring, it can become harder to get it to stay securely shut. The open end of the ring may unfasten, pop out, and sit in front of (or behind) the bead. Also, you may see a small gap between the end of the ring and the bead even when it is closed. To redistribute the tension properly, open the ring slightly and carefully squeeze the ring together as if to make it smaller. Then, bend the ring as if to close it, but go further so that the open end passes over to the opposite side of the bead. (If the end of the ring sits in front of the bead, bend it to the back, or vice versa). You should then be able to close it tightly.

Threaded Jewelry

The following sections introduce *threaded* jewelry that uses screw threads for their closures. These styles have male *screw threads* on one side. These fit into a female hole that is *tapped* (drilled out) with the matching thread pattern on the other. The processes for creating these closures on high-quality barbells makes manufacturing them—and other threaded jewelry—costly and complex, especially when compared

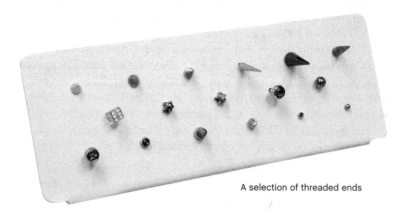

A selection of threaded ends

to captive rings. Threaded items tend to be either cheap junk or relatively expensive, well-made pieces.

An advantage to threaded jewelry is that the ends can be replaced with jewels, spikes, and other ornamental pieces. Some manufacturers make jewelry with only one end that can be removed, but the sort with two interchangeable ends is far more versatile. Threaded ends can be switched safely, even while a piercing is healing.

A disadvantage of threaded jewelry is the possibility of an end unscrewing and the jewelry falling out. Wear quality products and regularly check the tightness of all threaded pieces to prevent this problem.

Circular Barbell

This style functions the same way as a barbell—the end (or ends) screw off and on, but it is manufactured in the shape of a ring. People may call it a "bull ring," or "horseshoe" (see photo on page 66).

The circular barbell is simple to insert and remove because no bending or tools are needed. An additional benefit is that the inside diameter can be adjusted by spreading or narrowing the gap between the balls. This is especially useful for areas in which a precise fit is required during healing. Your piercer can easily widen a circular barbell to form a *C* or *U* shape to conform better to your anatomy. A good circular barbell is costly when compared to fixed or captive bead rings, due to the expense of machining the threading.

> ### Handy Tip
> To assure your threaded jewelry does not come unscrewed, use Loctite or other *thread-locker* products, which are available at hardware stores. After your piercing is healed, put a small dab on the threads, tighten the end in place, and carefully wipe away any excess. Use regular strength unless you never want to take out your jewelry.

The *captive circular barbell* is a useful style in which a captive bead is inserted to fill the gap between the two ends, forming a complete ring. This variation has three beads: two on the circular barbell, plus the captive in the center. The middle bead is secured by tension, the same way the bead is held in place on a captive ring. A bead of the right size that is inserted correctly will not fall out easily. This reduces the possibility that your circular barbell will catch on a partner's jewelry or other object. It serves the added function of preventing the threaded ends of the circular barbell from unscrewing. However, it limits your ability to adjust the ring diameter, which becomes reliant upon the size of the captive bead.

Depending on your anatomy and the size of the jewelry, this style could get a little heavy for a fresh piercing. If it becomes uncomfortable, simply remove the middle bead during healing.

Ring-Style Jewelry: What's the Difference?

Circular barbells cannot be manufactured in the thinnest gauges because of the threading. Other than the design features described, no practical distinctions exist between these different rings. They may be worn interchangeably on all piercings that use ring-style jewelry. I suggest the circular barbell as preferred initial jewelry for several piercings. For details, see the descriptions of individual placements in part 4.

Bar-Style Jewelry

This basic jewelry style includes many straight and curved versions of a post with two ends.

Barbell

The second most common body jewelry style is the barbell, along with its variations. The basic barbell is shaped like the classic dumbbell found in a gym: a straight bar post with two spherical ends (see photo on page 66). Barbells are a good choice for piercings in areas where ring-style jewelry would be unwieldy, uncomfortable, or unsafe. Straight barbells are suited to tongue, nipple, and a number of male genital piercings.

In order to fit properly, a barbell worn in a new piercing must be long enough to accommodate tissue changes such as swelling or *development* (see "Post-Piercing Nipple Development," page 131). A bar that is too short can cause discomfort, swelling, embedding, and healing problems. A post that is too long can catch and cause trauma, which also leads to troubled healing. Often a longer post is used at first and then downsized to fit more snugly once healing is complete.

The ball size of a barbell is also critical to its fit. The balls must be big enough to avoid becoming embedded but not so large as to be irritating or to cause the jewelry to be pushed away from the tissue.

Curved Barbell

The terms *banana bell, L-bar, bent bar, curved barbell,* and simply *curve* all refer to a barbell that is shaped to form approximately one-fourth of a circle (see photo on page 66). It should be a manufactured piece with a smooth, consistent curve. This popular variation of the straight barbell is suited to areas like the navel and eyebrow, where a ring can be obtrusive, but a straight barbell doesn't conform well.

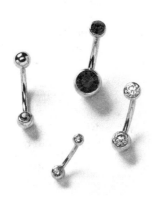

A selection of jeweled navel curves, a popular style for navel and VCH piercings

Jeweled Navel Curve (JNC)

This bejeweled variation is designed for vertical piercings. A set crystal or gem is affixed to the bottom of the post; this allows the stone to face forward when the jewelry is in place. Only the top can be interchanged with a matching or contrasting stone, ball, or other threaded end. The smaller gems are safe for wear in some fresh piercings, but the version with large gems is too hefty for healing.

Good quality is extremely important. If the stone falls out (a common problem with lower-end products), dirt and germs will lodge in the cavity left by the missing gem, increasing risk of infection. The entire piece of jewelry will need to be replaced.

Threadless Jewelry

The majority of bar-style jewelry is threaded, but an alternative type is the threadless "snap-together" barbell patented by NeoMetal. This design has a special pin coupling on the removable end. The slightly bent pin straightens out when inserted into the hole in the barbell post. This produces a spring-tension force that holds the two pieces together. Threadless jewelry is available in gauges smaller than most threaded jewelry, and it is well suited to facial piercings. The tiny sizes may be referred to as *mini-barbells*. The threaded variety is superior for oral piercings, which undergo stressors such as eating and chewing gum. Otherwise, both closure styles are usually acceptable if they are quality products.

Threadless snap-together jewelry is an alternative to threaded styles

If a barbell doesn't unscrew, try pulling instead. The threadless design is available in many of the variations described above.

J-Curve

Also called a *J-bar*, this style looks very much like a jeweled navel curve when it is worn, and it is suited to the same areas. Generally both ends are threaded, so it is more versatile. The J shape projects the lower end of the jewelry forward, allowing the ornament on the bottom to be more visible, which is especially useful for piercees with a deep navel.

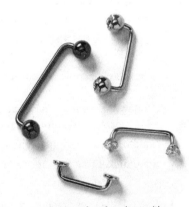

A selection of J-curves with gem and ball ends

Surface Bars

This modified barbell is designed for piercings on flat areas of the body. It is shaped like an open staple, with a straight bar post between two short legs or *uprights*. Often the legs are at right angles to the bar, but for some areas, one or both may have a different angle. The bar post should rest at a uniform depth under the surface with the uprights at 90-degree angles to the tissue. This should reduce pressure, distortion, and irritation during healing. Bars used for Christina piercings have only one upright leg. Discs, gems, or other threaded pieces screw onto the ends of the bar. An accurate fit is crucial; the jewelry must be

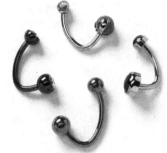

A selection of surface bars with flat discs, balls, and gem ends

the perfect length to encompass the tissue between the entry and exit of the piercing, and the barbell ends must not sink into the skin, nor should the legs protrude more than a millimeter beyond the surface.

Other Shapes

Although captive rings, barbells, and their variations are appropriate for the majority of piercings, some areas of the body require jewelry that is designed or adapted for the anatomy. One example is the *nostril screw*, a modified post style with a corkscrew tail that rests against the inside of the nostril (see photo, page 94).

Another style is the *labret stud* or flat-back barbell, which is popular for wear in oro-facial piercings (see photo on page 79). This is a short barbell with a flat disc on one end to reduce contact with the teeth and gums. See chapters 10 through 13 for more details about anatomy-specific jewelry.

Jewelry Materials for Initial Piercings

Only a few materials are considered safe for wear in a fresh piercing. A primary consideration is that the jewelry must be able to withstand the heat and pressure of autoclave sterilization; therefore, metal is the most common material for initial jewelry, although plastic and glass are also occasionally used. Another crucial factor is *biocompatibility*: the material must be well tolerated by the body and local tissues to avoid causing trouble healing, allergy, irritation, and infection. Finally, the human body is a harsh host, so only materials that are highly corrosion resistant fare well in the flesh.

Many metals are actually *alloys*, mixtures of different elements that have been combined to achieve certain properties that their components do not have on their own. Very few, however, are suitable for piercings, because they would react negatively to the body chemistry if worn adjacent to open tissue. The materials suggested for wear in initial piercings by the Association of Professional Piercers are listed below (see www.safepiercing.org for updates). The metals with *implant designations* have numbered codes that represent a precise standard for the alloy and its quality as determined by the American (now International) Society for Testing and Materials Standard (ASTM) and/or the International Standards Organization (ISO).

- Steel that is ASTM F-138 compliant or ISO 5832-1 compliant
- Implant-certified titanium (Ti6Al4V ELI) that is ASTM F-136 compliant or ISO 5832-3 compliant
- Commercially pure titanium that is ASTM F-67 compliant

The following are materials that have been proven through practical application to be suitably biocompatible for initial piercing:

- Solid 14-karat or higher yellow or nickel-free white gold
- Solid nickel-free platinum alloy
- Niobium (Nb)
- Inert, low-porosity plastics such as Tygon Medical Surgical Tubing S-50HL or S-54HL, PTFE (Teflon), or Bioplast
- Fused quartz glass, lead-free borosilicate, or lead-free soda-lime glass
- Nickel-negative EEC Nickel Directive compliant steel (European standard)

Metals

The steel and titanium grades listed above are highly biocompatible and very unlikely to cause irritation to a piercing and the surrounding skin. However, making jewelry with them presents challenges because the usual techniques and tools for working gold and silver cannot be used to manufacture steel or titanium body jewelry. These harder metals have higher melting points, and they must be machined with high-tech equipment rather than crafted by a jeweler's hand. They also require a great deal of polishing to be made smooth enough to wear in the body.

The implant-designation metals are used in medical applications such as bone pins and screws and joint replacements. They have been designed and tested for safe long-term wear in the body. Cheaper jewelry is frequently described as "implant grade," but this is often a false claim. You can't tell by looking, so how can you be sure?

Mill certificates, mill test certificates, or simply *mill certs* are documents that provide evidence of a specific grade of metal (with an ASTM or ISO code designation). By law, manufacturers of steel and titanium body jewelry must provide these to their customers (for example, your piercer) upon request. Ask your piercer/jeweler about her metals and if she has copies of mill certs to demonstrate the grades). You don't need to understand exactly what the numbers mean, but mill certs should warrant that the steel or titanium is one of those in the metals list. It is not possible to know whether the piece of jewelry you're buying is from the batch indicated on the paper, but the presence of a certificate showing a recent date and the appropriate material means you have at least a chance of getting the right metal.

Since you cannot be certain of the origin of any individual piece of jewelry, the best thing to do is shop with a reputable company and follow the guidelines presented in "What to Look for in Quality Body Jewelry," page 78.

Implant-Designation Steel

Steel is the most prevalent metal used for body jewelry in the United States. It is less expensive than gold, and it is often less costly than titanium. Steel body jewelry is very durable, but in large sizes it can be quite heavy.

Many grades of steel contain irritating components and have a high risk of causing problems. The particular alloy listed above (ASTM F-138 or ISO 5832-1 compliant) is chemically inert and created not to react with the surrounding tissues or immune system. It is well tolerated by almost all piercees.

Titanium

Titanium body jewelry is growing in popularity and availability. Like steel, titanium is usually alloyed with other materials when used for jewelry. Unlike steel, however, almost all titanium body jewelry *is* made from implant-grade metal, because of its frequent use in medical and dental applications. Titanium jewelry must have a high-polish mirror finish because the naturally porous surface can disrupt the delicate cells of healing piercings.

Titanium is lightweight—about half the weight of steel—extremely strong, corrosion-resistant, and durable. It can be beautifully colored using an *anodizing* process that changes the way the surface refracts light. In its natural, polished state this metal appears similar to steel but is a bit darker in color. When anodized it can range from a brownish shade to yellow, green, blue, purple, and even multicolored. Titanium is very pretty, but depending on the body chemistry of the person wearing it and whether it is worn in a friction-prone area, the color will eventually fade. This is not harmful, but it may be disappointing. However, you might be able to find a studio with an anodizing machine that can recolor your jewelry.

Implant-certified titanium is considered the most inert of the body jewelry metals. For those concerned about nickel sensitivity, this is a good choice because there is no nickel present in the titanium alloy used for body jewelry.

Niobium

Niobium is an elemental metal in the same family as titanium. It can be anodized in lovely colors in the same way. It does not have an implant-grade designation, so some piercers feel it should be worn only in healed piercings, although it has been widely used with good results for many years. High-quality niobium appears to be safe and inert for most piercees and is accepted by the APP for initial jewelry.

Niobium can be blackened through a heating and cooling process. The charcoal-colored finish is permanent; it will not fade like other colors of anodized titanium or niobium. Only high-polish niobium should be used for initial piercings; matte-finish pieces are rough and porous.

Gold

Gold has a long history of use within the body. Its use in modern dentistry also attests to its safety. Still, specific implant designations do not exist for gold. It comes in many different alloys, so use caution when making a purchase, especially since gold is significantly more expensive than most other body jewelry materials. *Cheap gold is never good gold.* However, a high price tag alone does not guarantee quality or acceptability for wear in body piercings.

The term *karat* refers to the purity of gold. Pure gold, or twenty-four karat gold (24K), is highly biocompatible, but it is too soft for body jewelry. It must be alloyed with other metals. Out of twenty-four parts of metal, eighteen karat (18K) indicates that eighteen parts are gold and six parts are other elements (75 percent gold and 25 percent other elements).[1] Some piercers sell fourteen karat (14K) gold, which is about 58 percent gold. Regardless of how many karats the gold is, the jewelry is safe to wear in the body only when inert elements are used in the alloy.

If there is too much silver, copper, or other reactive material in the mixture, even eighteen-karat gold can be problematic. Much of the white gold used for body jewelry is alloyed without nickel; for whiteness it contains palladium, an inert element in the platinum family. Colored golds such as pink and green should be avoided, since they usually include irritating elements.

Acidic body fluids can react with certain alloys and cause a dark discoloration of the metal. Frequent use of a gold-polishing cloth will usually resolve this problem. Gold is durable, but excessive exposure to chlorine (in pools and hot tubs) can cause gold jewelry to become brittle.

Gold has an undeserved reputation as being unsafe for initial piercings, but when it is alloyed for wear in the body, it works very well. Because of its high cost, many piercers do not stock a large selection of gold jewelry, so you may need to place an advance order if you wish to start a piercing with it. Regular fine jewelers are often unfamiliar with the need for inert alloys, smooth surfaces, and safe closures. Consult a piercer about the exact requirements before you place an order or purchase gold jewelry.

Platinum

Platinum is a completely inert precious metal that is 60 percent heavier than gold. It is rare: ten tons of ore must be mined to obtain just a single ounce of platinum. It has a rich, bright-white color and is very strong, but it is prohibitively expensive for most piercees. Platinum is difficult for jewelers to work with, in part due to the metal's extremely high melting point. When alloyed with an inert element such as palladium, it is a good choice for body jewelry, but platinum is seldom stocked in body art studios and will probably need to be custom-ordered for you. Many piercers are unfamiliar with platinum, so you must find one with a lot of jewelry savvy to carry or order it for you.

Nontoxic Plastics

Certain inert, high-tech plastics make good alternatives to metal body jewelry. Tygon Medical/Surgical Tubing (silicone) and PTFE (Polytetrafluoroethylene—a form of Teflon) are flexible, autoclavable plastics that are widely accepted within the industry for use in fresh piercings. Tygon should be changed out every few months, as it stiffens and discolors over time. Some states have legislation prohibiting the use of such plastics for initial jewelry, even though years of successful use show that they are safe for piercings. While Tygon meets some standards for medical use and biocompatibility, it does not meet FDA requirements for use as an implant material.

Tygon is commonly used for surface piercings (see "Surface Piercings," page 237) in areas that lack a pliable fold of tissue. The tubing's remarkable flexibility makes it more comfortable to wear than metal. These materials can also be worn as jewelry substitutes during medical procedures that require you to remove metal from your body (see "Retainers," page 248).

A newer product in this family has recently joined the ranks of alternatives to metal jewelry. *Bioplast*, a flexible plastic that was developed specifically for body piercings, was included in the APP's 2008 update for acceptable initial jewelry materials. It is biocompatible, nonporous, and capable of being sterilized in an autoclave at up to 250°F (121°C). It is inexpensive and can be cut to fit. Unlike standard PTFE, which is white, Bioplast is available in colors and comes shaped into curved bars, circular barbells, and nostril screws. It is also more flexible than PTFE. A labret stud design with a flat back is also made, and this softer material seems kinder than metal to delicate oral tissues. Metal barbell balls, gems, and other ends press fit, self-thread, or use a special converter or threading tool to attach onto the plastic posts.

Jewelry to Avoid in Fresh Piercings

Some common body jewelry materials are suitable for healed piercings but are not suggested for new piercings. Others materials are safe only for jewelry that is not worn through pierced tissue.

Acrylic

Acrylic is not suggested for initial piercings because it is not ordinarily autoclavable and may have some safety risks for long-term wear. Acrylic is fragile in the smaller gauges used for fresh piercings and can break with normal use.

Glass

Certain types of glass are very inert and autoclavable; this jewelry can be suitable for wear in new body piercings. The area of concern is the fragility of the material in small sizes. The sturdier tube or plug styles in 10 gauge or thicker are safe for some piercings.

Natural or Organic Materials

Natural materials such as bone, horn, and wood are popular for wear in piercings, but they are unable to withstand the heat of an autoclave. They tend to be porous and cannot hold a finish smooth enough for exposure to open tissue, and in thin gauges they are too fragile for safety. It's true that countless primitive peoples around the world have used such materials for their initial piercings for centuries, but safer options are available in today's high-tech societies. Our urban environments and immune systems differ dramatically from those who speared their bodies with eagle claws and porcupine quills. They also had much higher early mortality rates than we do nowadays. While it may be appealing to use natural materials and reenact ancient piercing rituals, today's Modern Primitive is advised to wear these items only in healed piercings. See "Natural Materials," page 232, for information on this type of jewelry for healed piercings.

Sterling Silver

Sterling silver is not suggested for use in fresh piercings or even healed piercings other than the earlobe (if tolerated). It has a tendency to tarnish, and this is an irritant to the body. The dark discoloration is a form of dirt, corrosion, and rust that can permanently stain your skin (see "Tarnish Tattoo," page 211).

Gold-Plated, Gold-Filled, Gold-Overlay, Vermeil, or Rolled Gold

All of these techniques involve coating a base metal with a layer of gold to create an affordable piece of jewelry with the look of gold. The problem is that the gold surface (which is *very* thin—measured in millionths of an inch)[2] can wear or chip off, leaving the body exposed to the metal underneath. Never wear any gold body jewelry that is touted as less than 14-karat solid gold. This isn't as critical when you are wearing a necklace or bracelet, but in a body piercing, there is the potential for serious consequences.

Fashion and Novelty Jewelry

This inexpensive junk can be trendy or cute, but these pieces are machine-manufactured in massive quantities, and they are not hand-finished or inspected. Novelty jewelry is sold in discount stores, kiosks, and shops that do not perform piercings. Piercers selling it should be avoided because they either don't know enough to steer clear of it or have fallen prey to the lure of the dollar. You generally get what you pay for where body jewelry is concerned. Don't go for the cheap stuff: it isn't worth the risk to your piercing and your health.

What to Look for in Quality Body Jewelry

Quality jewelry differs significantly from the cut-rate goods, but the products are often similar in appearance. The following explains what to look for to identify good jewelry.

Finish and Polish

To be safe for healing, metal body jewelry must have a *mirror finish*—a high-shine, super-smooth surface. Wearing body jewelry that has nicks, burrs, tooling marks, or scratches can cause severe complications. When jewelry has an uneven surface, the new cells that are formed during healing grow into the irregularities. Then, when the jewelry shifts or moves, these areas tear. As this cycle is repeated, scar tissue forms and healing is delayed. A faulty finish can also introduce bacteria into the wound and cause infection.

Annealing

Annealing is a heating and cooling process that improves the properties of a material. In the case of body jewelry metals, it helps make jewelry pliable enough to bend fairly easily. This procedure can also be performed to refurbish gold rings that have become work hardened. The material is heated to specific temperatures and cooled at particular intervals. Glass can also be annealed to improve its durability.

Cheap captive and fixed bead rings are not annealed. If you cannot bend a ring (up to 14 gauge or so, in average diameters) with your fingers, then it is probably not annealed. Jewelry that is not annealed will be harder—or impossible—to insert and remove without tools.

Internal and External Threading

Most straight, curved, and circular barbells have ends that connect via the use of tiny screw threads. On *internally threaded* pieces, the part of the jewelry that passes through your skin is smooth, and the threads are on the removable end, such as the ball or spike. The end screws *into* a hole in the jewelry that has been drilled or *tapped* with the matching thread pattern, to receive it. This allows for the safe, comfortable passage of metal through your body when you take your jewelry in and out. According to the APP standards, body jewelry for initial piercings must have internal tapping (no threads on the posts) starting at 18 gauge.

An externally threaded barbell and an internally threaded labret stud

Alternatively, *externally threaded* jewelry has the screw pattern cut into the *post*, and the ball or other end is tapped with a matching hole to receive it. This comparatively rough surface may be passed directly through the tissue to insert and remove the jewelry. There are ways to put the threads inside a needle during piercing and special tapers that are sometimes used during jewelry changes. Without this safeguard, inserting this style can be like running a small metal file through your body if the channel is tight.

Internally threaded jewelry is more difficult to manufacture. Machining the screws tiny enough to fit *inside* a 16- or 14-gauge post (and tapping the post to receive them) is much more challenging than simply cutting screw threads into the jewelry post, as with the external threading style. Internally threaded jewelry therefore costs more, but it is usually worth the extra expense. Manufacturers who produce high-end internally threaded products are more likely than the bargain-basement guys to use implant-grade materials. Some companies do make quality pieces with external threads, which are fine for healed piercings that do not have tight channels; but, for initial piercings, internal style jewelry avoids any possibility of scraping your piercing with screw threads.

Buying Body Jewelry

What does all this really mean when it comes to buying body jewelry? You'll buy most jewelry for initial piercings in a studio, often after a consultation with a piercer. Jewelry can also be purchased from reputable manufacturers via the Internet. Unless you are an experienced piercee, you should always confer with your piercer prior to ordering, because body jewelry can be expensive and is usually not returnable due to sanitation issues.

Discuss your options prior to getting pierced and let your piercer be your guide when deciding on jewelry. Ask the important questions: What is the material and grade? What is the gauge and diameter, or length? Is the jewelry annealed (if it's a ring), or does it have internal or external threading (if it's a bar)?

Your Body Knows the Difference

Body jewelry quality varies widely, from heirloom pieces of finely crafted gold with genuine diamonds and gemstones to inferior metals that can turn your skin green and infect you. Some of the cheap stuff is fashionable and attractive, but once you know the difference, is that *really* what you want for your body? I remember the sign Jim Ward posted in the jewelry case at Gauntlet many years ago. It bore a sensible statement in calligraphy on parchment: "The bitterness of poor quality remains long after the sweetness of low price is forgotten."

The Point

Congratulations! You have amassed a great deal of knowledge about body jewelry styles, sizes, and materials. You are prepared both mentally and physically, and you know what to expect in the studio. The time has come to delve into a detailed discussion about each of the common piercings.

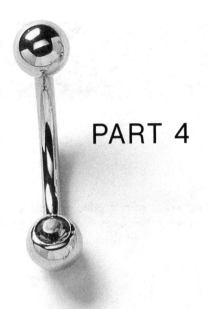

PART 4

The Holes

10

Holes in Your Head:
Ear, Nose, and Facial Piercings

The anatomy above the neck has a wealth of pierceable placements. Some, like the eyebrow piercing, are modern innovations. Many, however, have long histories in tribal cultures, such as piercings of the lips, nose, and, of course, the ears.

Earlobe Piercing

- Healing time: 4 to 8 weeks
- Initial jewelry style: Ring-style (bead ring, captive bead ring, and circular barbell) or bar-style (straight barbell, labret stud, mini barbell, or nostril screw)
- Initial jewelry gauge: 20 to 10 gauge
- Initial jewelry size: From $5/16$-inch to $5/8$-inch diameter (rarely larger), depending on jewelry gauge and weight

Piercing of the *lobule* (the fleshy portion of the earlobe) has become a mainstream part of our culture, at least for women. It has a rich tradition and lore that spans every inhabited continent. This universal ornamentation crosses the gender barrier and can signify femininity or masculinity. Earrings have been seen on everyone from Mr. Clean to prostitutes, pirates, and society ladies.

Ancient Piercing

The University of Pennsylvania Museum displays a statue from Iran, circa 3500–2900 B.C.E., of a female head with multiple ear piercings.

Earlobe Piercing: Choice of Jewelry

You have a vast choice of jewelry to wear in your earlobes, but one type is not recommended: regular earrings. For the comfort and the safety of your healing piercing, quality body jewelry is far superior when compared to cheap costume jewelry and even pricey traditional-style earrings. Earrings with a straight posts tend to painfully jab you behind the ear, especially when you are sleeping or using a telephone. The metal used in ordinary earrings is often substandard, potentially leading to allergies, and the post length is sometimes too short.

More sizes and styles of body jewelry are safe to wear in ear lobe piercings than any other placement. The main concern is to avoid heavy rings, since they can cause delayed healing, scarring, or thinning tissue.

Earlobe Piercing: *Placement*

The typical ear piercing is located in the center of the lobe. The angle of the piercing can range from parallel to your face to perpendicular to your ear, depending on your anatomy and preferences. I like to place the piercing slightly higher than the midpoint of the lobe because the flesh is very soft and the hole tends to settle a little over time, especially if you wear large or heavy jewelry. Still, the placement for earlobe piercings can be dictated almost entirely by aesthetics because there are few anatomical safety issues, unlike in most other areas. Earlobes are prone to problems only when the piercing is placed in an extreme location, such as at the bottom of your lobe, where there is too little tissue, or at the juncture of your earlobe and your face, where some blood vessels may be present.

Let your piercer know during marking if you have a particular vision for the look of your piercing or if you plan to stretch the hole after healing. He might want to move the placement a little higher, depending on your goal size.

Placing a pair of earlobe piercings so that they appear symmetrical can be trickier than you might think; the left ear is often remarkably different from the right. Multiple earlobe piercings along the rim of the ear are common and relatively socially acceptable. Further up the ear, where the tissue becomes dense, you have cartilage, which is very different. The assertion, "The higher up the ear you go, the more it hurts and the longer it takes to heal," is true for many piercees. For more information about cartilage piercings, see the following section of this chapter.

Earlobe Piercing: *Procedure*

Once the placement is marked and agreed upon, I use forceps to secure the tissue for the piercing. Some piercers prefer a freehand or receiving tube method. Any of these techniques can be used successfully to pierce the earlobe. I normally make the piercing from front to back. There is seldom significant bleeding or discomfort, though a 10-gauge earlobe piercing is more likely to bleed than a thinner gauge.

To avoid the potential for disease transmission and other problems, do not get your ears (or anything else) pierced with a gun. See "Ear-Piercing Guns," page 21, for more information on their dangers.

Earlobe Piercing: *Hygiene*

Although earlobes generally heal quickly and easily, contact with dirty telephones can cause an infection. Stay away from public phones, and keep your own phone(s) clean while you are healing any piercing of the ear. If you get only one ear pierced, use the other for the phone, and rest the unpierced side on your pillow if you do not sleep on your back. Practice the "T-Shirt Trick" on page 185 to keep your pillow clean.

The ear is not concealed or protected by clothing, so there is a chance you could touch the jewelry without even realizing it. You must avoid this for uneventful healing.

Earlobe Piercing: *Healing and Troubleshooting*

The same care that is suggested for body piercings should also be given to ears. Even though a variety of solutions and products are marketed for use on ear piercings, they are not among the top options. The reasons are explained in "What Not to Use on

Your Piercings," page 191. Four weeks is as fast as the healing period gets, so resist the temptation to change your jewelry prematurely.

The earlobe is the area of the body with the highest incidence of the cheese-cutter effect. This can be triggered by a specific pulling incident, or it can occur over time from wearing jewelry that is too heavy on a thin gauge. Wear jewelry that is thick enough to prevent this undesirable vertical expansion of the hole. Unfortunately, plastic surgery is the only way to repair tissue that has been damaged in this way. If the hole hasn't migrated too close to the edge of the lobe, ask your piercer about using an *eyelet* (hollow tube–style jewelry) to line the tissue (see photo, page 241). This could allow you to wear dangling jewelry without further harm.

You must be careful when having these areas repierced. The new location should be slightly off to the side so it doesn't merge with the old hole or repaired tissue due to weakness in the tissue fibers. The area should be well healed from any such procedure for several months prior to repiercing.

Earlobe Piercing: Changing Jewelry

Locating the hole in the back of your ear can be challenging when swapping jewelry. Some piercees find it easier to insert jewelry from back to front, depending on the style. *Never force jewelry through.* If you have trouble changing your own jewelry, see your piercer for assistance.

All of the suggestions offered for the nostril can also be used to conceal earlobe piercings. See "Nostril Piercing: Concealment," page 96.

Earlobe Piercing: Stretching

The earlobe is the most easily and commonly stretched piercing on the body, and the one that is expanded to the largest dimensions.

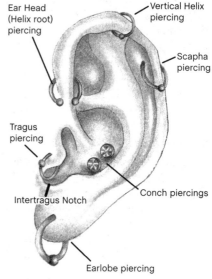

You may be able to safely stretch up one gauge as soon as two months after piercing if you have a speedy, uneventful healing period. For more information and instructions, see "Stretching," page 224.

Earlobe Piercing: Retiring

At some point, you may consider *retiring* your piercing (removing the jewelry to abandon the piercing). Once fully healed, the hole may shrink, but the vast majority of earlobe piercings will stay viable indefinitely without jewelry in place. Only the nasal septum, Prince Albert (male genital piercing), and inner labia have an equal likelihood of remaining open.

Ear Cartilage Piercing (Helix or Scapha)

- Healing time: 3 to 9 months or longer
- Initial jewelry style: Ring-style, straight barbell, mini barbell, or nostril screw

- Initial jewelry gauge: 18 to 14 gauge, occasionally as large as 12 or 10 gauge
- Initial jewelry size: ⁵/₁₆- to ¹/₂-inch diameter ring-style jewelry; bar-style jewelry is anatomy-dependent (commonly with a post length of ⁵/₁₆ or ³/₈ inch)

Like the earlobe, ear cartilage piercing has been practiced widely throughout history and around the planet. While still not as prevalent as lobe piercings, cartilage piercings continue to gain popularity and acceptance in Western culture. Because the cartilage lacks *vascularity* (blood supply) of its own—the circulation is in the surrounding tissues only—these piercings are quite tricky to heal.

The contours of individual ear anatomy vary considerably, and so do the options for placing a cartilage piercing. Jewelry can be situated nearly anywhere along the rim of the ear where the denser tissue begins, and higher—right up to the top of the ear. Aesthetics play a big role in selecting the placement.

The piercing can pass through your *helix* (the curled outer rim of the ear) if it is pronounced enough. Or you can pierce at the base of the helix where it joins the *scapha* (the flatter portion of the cartilage from which the helix curves). Depending on your anatomy, this sometimes allows a ring to rest parallel to your ear. If you pierce a little farther in on the flat of the scapha you can wear a stud there, or a ring large enough to encircle your helix, though this will be uncomfortable for healing if the jewelry has a large diameter. Yet another possibility is a vertical helix placement at the top of the curve if you have sufficiently defined cartilage. The piercing can be angled outward slightly, so if you wear a ring, it will lay gracefully. These locations are all in the realm of traditional or ear cartilage piercing placements. See pages 87–92 for more exotic placements.

Your piercer may use illumination to check your ear for visible blood vessels, which are easy to detect and avoid. Don't try to sidestep the cartilage by piercing a pinch of skin close to the edge. These tend to migrate or reject because they are situated in too little tissue and the pressure from hard cartilage behind them pushes the jewelry out. If your piercing is so superficial that a tiny ¹/₄-inch diameter ring fits, the placement is too shallow.

> **Happy Surprises**
> *Reinsertions* (inserting jewelry in a hole that was left empty) are almost always successful for earlobe piercings if the channel was healed before it was abandoned. If I were the gambling sort, I would have won many times over the years by betting piercees that I could put in jewelry painlessly and without repiercing, even when the client was completely certain a hole had closed forever. I never did wager—but I'd have been a winner every time. I have seen plenty of surprised smiling faces, however, which is even more rewarding. Get help from a piercer or purchase an insertion taper, as you can cause injury by trying to force jewelry through a hole that has shrunk. See "Will It Close?" page 231, and "Repiercing after Loss," page 215, for more information.

Ear Cartilage Piercing: Procedure

Forceps or a receiving tube may be used to support the tissue for piercing. A freehand procedure with or without a cork backing is also common. Many piercees find that ear cartilage piercings sting or pinch. I've had some cartilage piercings that I would describe as very sensitive and others that I barely felt.

Ear Cartilage Piercing: Watch out for Bumps Ahead

Cartilage piercings require gentle treatment and patience. There is a tendency for this area to develop small bumps around one or both of the openings during healing. Generally these are localized areas of inflamed excess scar tissue. Bumps can form because the surface tissue is pushed away from the cartilage by the needle during piercing. If the exterior layer does not get pressed back into place, the body has a tendency to fill in this space by producing excess cells. If your piercer practices the compression technique (see page 61) to reattach the tissue after piercing, this will reduce your chances of forming a bump.

Don't Shoot!
Piercing the ear cartilage with a stud gun is illegal in some regions.

Ear Cartilage Piercing: Gauge-up Procedure

When performing ear cartilage piercings, many piercers (including me) use a needle one gauge (or one-half gauge) larger than the jewelry. This technique is intended to promote the comfort and healing of the piercing by allowing your body to form a small cushion of scar tissue, so the theory goes. This may be more comfortable and make healing easier because the jewelry does not press directly against the dense cartilage. Your piercing may bleed a little more if it is performed with a larger needle. Some piercers have success with the same-gauge technique.

Ear Cartilage Piercing: Healing and Troubleshooting

You *must* minimize trauma and pressure to successfully heal cartilage. Try sleeping on a soft pillow that you can shape so there is no direct contact with your ear. Snagging your jewelry on a brush or your hair will cause irritation. Avoid getting hair styling products on the wound and jewelry, as these products can also cause trouble.

Healing ear cartilage takes time and patience, even when you are taking proper care of the piercing and wearing high-quality jewelry. The piercing seems healed and then regresses; this cycle usually repeats for an extended period of time—sometimes a year or longer. Since they can be challenging to heal under the best of circumstances, it is vital to make sure no aspect of your ear cartilage piercing is substandard.

Ear Cartilage Piercing: Changing Jewelry

To facilitate the insertion of new jewelry, support the tissue on the exit side as you try to transfer a new piece into place. Even fully healed cartilage piercings may respond poorly to frequent jewelry swaps or attempts at introducing novelty jewelry.

Ear Cartilage Piercing: Stretching

Ear cartilage is *not* pliable, and stretching a hole in it can be tricky and feel tender. It is imperative to wait until the initial healing is complete and the hole is settled before making an attempt to stretch. A large opening in the cartilage is extremely difficult to achieve by traditional expansion methods; few piercees have the requisite patience or pain tolerance. See "The Dermal Punch," page 240, for information about an alternative tool that is used to create larger holes.

Ear Cartilage Piercing: Retiring

Ear cartilage piercings in average sizes usually leave an inconspicuous mark when jewelry is removed, unless troubled healing caused excess scarring. Once established, some ear cartilage piercings will remain viable for an extended period without jewelry present, though the hole usually shrinks, making it difficult and painful to reinsert jewelry. Sometimes the channel closes completely when jewelry is removed, even if it was pierced for a long time.

Ear Cartilage Piercing: Variations

The information above applies to all variations of the ear cartilage piercings described below. Details and differences are outlined for the most popular "exotic" cartilage placements.

Ear Cartilage Variations: How Much Does It Hurt?

Many piercees are especially anxious that an exotic ear piercing such as a tragus, rook, or daith will be painful due to the relatively thick, hard cartilage of those areas. However, some piercees report that these are *less* tender than a traditionally placed helix piercing. In the hands of a capable piercer, you may feel less of a sting (though perhaps more pressure) from some of the cartilage piercing variations.

Ear Cartilage Variations: Techniques

A forceps, receiving tube, or freehand procedure is suitable for specialty ear cartilage piercings, depending on the specific placement and the preferences of your piercer. The gauge-up technique is common for all the variations.

The Tragus Piercing

- **Description:** Frames the small protrusion of cartilage that juts out from the face over the opening of the ear canal
- **Healing time:** 3 to 9 months or often longer
- **Initial jewelry style:** Straight barbell, mini barbell, or ring-style
- **Initial jewelry gauge:** Usually 18 or 16 gauge; possibly 14 gauge or larger for those with substantial anatomy
- **Initial jewelry size:** Most commonly 3/8-inch diameter, though 5/16-inch or 7/16-inch is sometimes used

Tragus Piercing: Placement

A ring should rest comfortably in the *intertragus notch* (the groove above the earlobe at the bottom of the opening to the ear canal). Depending on the angle of your tragus, the piercing is usually placed relatively perpendicular to the tissue. It must be set well in from the edge, in a natural crease of the skin, if possible.

I often see tragus piercings with rings that are either too large or too small. The ring must not be so large as to get caught on the *antitragus* (the rise of cartilage above the earlobe, next to the intertragus notch). An improper fit is not aesthetically pleasing, and a ring that doesn't hang down properly can cause irritation. Wearing ring-style jewelry can be problematic if your tragus is as wide as it is tall. A small barbell is best for a wedge-shaped tragus.

Tragus Piercing: Procedure

Piercers use a variety of methods for tragus piercings, from backing the tissue with a bent cotton swab to the more common forceps method. For this piercing, I use both forceps and a receiving tube: I make the piercing from front to back, passing no more than the bevel of the needle through the tissue, then I cap the piercing needle with the receiving tube for a safe jewelry transfer in the same direction.

The Conch Piercing

- **Description:** Done in the deep bowl-shaped central shell of the ear
- **Healing time:** 3 to 9 months or longer, commonly 6 months or more
- **Initial jewelry style:** Preferably a barbell, since a ring is subject to excess trauma; it must be wide enough to clear without binding the edge of the ear
- **Initial jewelry gauge:** Most commonly 14 and 12 gauge, with 16 and 10 gauge less frequently used
- **Initial jewelry size:** A ring with a ¹/₂- to ⁵/₈-inch diameter is usually large enough for a piercing placed an average distance from the edge of the ear. Barbell length can be as short as ⁵/₁₆ inch for slim cartilage, but some cartilage in this area is hefty enough to require a ⁷/₁₆-inch post.

This piercing has been practiced by a number of groups, including the Mangebetu tribe in Africa and a sect of Hindu Yogis from India.

Conch Piercing: Placement

The *concha* (conch, or shell of the ear) is large enough that the placements can be divided into lower (sometimes called *sadhus*, especially when large gauge jewelry is worn), mid, and upper conch piercings. Piercers may refer to *inner conch* (true conch piercings) and *outer conch*, which are really piercings of the scapha or antihelix. Fairly large blood vessels are frequently located in these areas, and illumination can be used to map them during marking so they can be avoided.

Conch Piercing: Procedure

The conch piercing is generally performed with a receiving tube or the freehand method. Alternatively, septum forceps (described on page 99) can be functional for this piercing, depending on your anatomy and the dimensions of the clamp.

The Rook Piercing

- **Description:** Placed in the small ridge of cartilage that originates near the face in the upper part of the ear
- **Healing time:** 3 to 9 months or longer, commonly 6 months or more

- **Initial jewelry style:** A ring or curved bar
- **Initial jewelry gauge:** 18 or 16 gauge, seldom larger
- **Initial jewelry size:** Rings or bars in 5/16- or 3/8-inch diameter

This placement is credited to California piercer and innovator Erik Dakota. It was publicized in Fakir Musafar's *Body Play* magazine in the early 1990s.

Rook Piercing: Placement

The rook is placed an area technically called the *inferior crus of the antihelix*. Some ears do not have a pronounced enough ridge. The piercing may be placed vertically, or at a more outward-leaning angle. The jewelry can frame the center of that ridge or be placed closer to your face. If you start with a bar, the angle of the piercing must suit your anatomy and the shape of the jewelry. If not, the bottom ball will press against your ear and cause discomfort and healing problems.

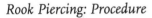
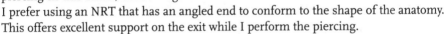

Helix piercing

Inferior Crus of the Antihelix

Rook piercing

Helix Crus/ Daith piercing

Antitragus piercing

Snug piercing

Rook Piercing: Procedure

A piercer must be skilled in order to put a piercing in this small, dense ridge of tissue.
I prefer using an NRT that has an angled end to conform to the shape of the anatomy. This offers excellent support on the exit while I perform the piercing.

Rook Piercing: Healing

If you spend a lot of time with a telephone or headphone pressed against your ear, you will find the rook is not a practical or comfortable piercing. If the piercing is too shallow, migration and rejection are common.

The Daith Piercing

- **Description:** Placed in the cartilage adjacent the face at the inner origin of the helix
- **Healing time:** 3 to 9 months or longer
- **Initial jewelry style:** Ring-style or curved bar
- **Initial jewelry gauge:** 18 or 16 gauge, rarely 14 gauge or larger
- **Initial jewelry size:** 5/16- or 3/8-inch diameter

This innovation is also credited to Erik Dakota. The name *daith* (rhymes with moth) reportedly comes from the ancient Hebrew word *da'at*, meaning "knowledge."

Daith Piercing: Placement

This piercing rests deep in the shell of the ear at the root of the *helix crus* (ridge of cartilage just above the ear canal that fades down into the conch). Most ears are configured with a pierceable crest at this location. It is a subtle but attractive piercing because of its concentric appearance; the jewelry frames the tissue and, in turn, the ear frames the jewelry. When placed properly (according to Dakota), the lower part of the ring seems to come directly out of the ear canal.

Daith Piercing: Procedure

The daith is tricky to perform due to its almost internal placement. I use an angled receiving tube. A short or bent tube may be needed to fit in the limited space. Some piercers use a curved needle to pierce this area. Hemostats are helpful to handle the jewelry for insertion and closure.

Daith Piercing: Healing

The daith can be an easy ear cartilage piercing to heal because it is protected by the surrounding anatomy. You still must keep dirty phones away, but most piercees find they can sleep on a healing daith without discomfort or irritation.

The Ear Head Piercing

- **Description:** Placed at the upper juncture of the ear and the head
- **Healing time:** 3 to 9 months or longer
- **Initial jewelry style:** Ring-style, barbell, or mini barbell
- **Initial jewelry gauge:** 18 to 14 gauge
- **Initial jewelry size:** 5/16- to 7/16-inch ring diameter, although a 1/4-inch post may fit; seldom is a post longer than 5/16 inch needed

Ear Head Piercing: Placement

This piercing is placed in the relatively thin cartilage at the *helix root* (the juncture where the helix meets the head). It is usually angled fairly parallel to the face. A ring can frame the area, or the end of a short barbell can be displayed there. The remainder of the barbell tucks into the curl at the front of the helix where it forms from the face.

A small percentage of people have a divot called a *preauricular pit* (a natural channel that can have some depth) in this region. This avenue can be expanded into a piercing only if you have no history of swelling or infection in this spot. For comfort and the success of your piercing, show your piercer where eyeglasses or sunglasses rest over your ears to assist in appropriate placement during marking.

Ear Head Piercing: Procedure

As with most of the other exotic ear cartilage piercings, I use the receiving tube technique. An angled tube conforms well to the anatomy in this region. If the tissue is pliable and pronounced enough, forceps may be used.

The Antitragus Piercing

- **Description:** Placed in the small, relatively vertical lip of cartilage above the ear lobe formed by the lower frontal rim of the conch
- **Healing time:** 3 to 9 months or longer
- **Initial jewelry style:** Ring-style, curved bar, mini barbell, or barbell; bar-style jewelry may be more comfortable
- **Initial jewelry gauge:** 18 to 14 gauge; 12 gauge used rarely for well-developed anatomy
- **Initial jewelry size:** Minimum diameter of $5/16$ inch (commonly $3/8$ inch, but $7/16$ inch is sometimes needed)

Antitragus Piercing: Placement

Anatomy is variable in this region, but many ears have a pierceable protrusion in this cartilaginous rise opposite the tragus, framing the intertragic notch. The piercing should just encompass the solid ridge of cartilage. If the piercing is placed too deep, it can unintentionally pass through to the back of the ear, which will cause problems healing. If the area is small and undefined, it is best left unpierced. The angle must be considered in relation to your placement and jewelry selection. The tissue is vertical, so ring-style jewelry will rest toward either the tragus or the edge of the ear.

Antitragus Piercing: Procedure

I perform this piercing using forceps to support the tissue, and if I pierce toward the ear, I use a needle receiving tube to encase the needle during the jewelry transfer.

The Snug Piercing

- **Description:** A horizontal piercing that frames a vertical protrusion of cartilage called the *anithelix*
- **Healing time:** 3 to 9 months or longer
- **Initial jewelry style:** Curved barbell, occasionally a ring for well-defined anatomy
- **Initial jewelry gauge:** Sometimes 18 gauge, but more commonly 16 or 14 gauge
- **Initial jewelry size:** If the tissue protrudes with good height but is narrow, a $3/8$-inch ring could be safe; the minimum diameter is the same for the curved bar.

Snug Piercing: Placement

This piercing goes through the same anatomical ridge where a rook is placed but farther from the face where the antihelix is vertical—usually across from the tragus. Many people do not have an outcropping to their cartilage in this location. Even if the tissue does protrude, it must be solid or the piercing will come through behind the ear. On well-developed anatomy, this can penetrate some the thickest cartilage that is pierced. As such, it can be more tender than most exotic piercings and take longer to heal.

The curved barbell will be the least obtrusive jewelry. This is not a phone- or pillow-friendly piercing.

Snug Piercing: Procedure

This piercing is suited to the forceps procedure. If you do not have a tall enough ridge of tissue to clamp, then you are not a good candidate for this placement. Even if forceps won't be used, this is a reasonable standard for judging the suitability of your anatomy.

Nose Piercings

Two main piercings are done in this region: the nostril (on the side) and the septum (in the center).

High Nostril piercing

Traditional Nostril piercing

Septum piercing

Before visiting the studio, give your nose a good blowing with a tissue or two. Breathe through your mouth during skin prep because the cleaning product can smell quite strong.

After the piercing, some tearing of your eyes, sneezing, or bleeding is perfectly normal, so if your piercer doesn't provide a clean tissue for you to hold, ask for one. Do not to touch your face with dirty fingers after the area has been prepped; if it tickles or itches, use the tissue.

You must postpone a nose piercing if you have a sinus infection or respiratory illness. However, if you have sinus allergies you still might be able to get a nose piercing, because normal nasal mucous does not appear harmful to healing.

During healing, you must be careful when you blow your nose. Maintain hygiene by touching the area only with clean hands and disposable tissues, not reusable hankies. You must also be gentle, because undue roughness and friction can cause complications. Once you are healed, blow your nose at will. Just wipe off your jewelry, too.

> **A Classic**
>
> Curious onlooker: "Say, how do you blow your nose with that jewelry in it?" Piercee: "Very carefully."

The nose functions as a filter, and this is obvious if you've ever blown your nose and seen black contents in your Kleenex afterward. Avoid exhaling smoke through your nose and French inhaling while healing a nose piercing. If you spend a lot of time in dusty or dirty environments, extra saline soaks (see "The Soak" and subsequent sections starting on page 188) are advisable. Soaks also help to minimize the formation of a cementlike crust on the jewelry from the normal secretions of both piercing and your nose. Submerge your nose into the cup of saltwater solution. The warm liquid helps soften the matter, and cotton swabs are perfect for removing stubborn particles. Fingernails should *never* be used.

The Nostril Piercing

- **Description:** Placed on the side of the nose, usually seated in a niche called the *supra-alar crease* (where the nostril naturally flares)
- **Healing time:** 3 to 4 months or longer
- **Initial jewelry style:** Ring-style, nostril screw, or mini barbell

- **Initial jewelry gauge:** Rings 20 gauge or thicker, up to 12 gauge for a large piercing; 20- or 18-gauge nostril screws with a head (gem, ball, or other ornament) 1.75 mm or larger; or 16 gauge, with a head 2 mm or larger
- **Initial jewelry size:** Ring diameters commonly ⁵/₁₆ to ⁷/₁₆ inch; post length on nostril screw or mini barbell is anatomically dependent and must have room for some swelling

Nostril piercing is second in popularity only to piercings of the ear. Many indigenous populations in the Americas, Africa, and India have worn nostril piercings throughout the ages. In Western culture, nostril piercing is primarily an aesthetic placement and does not ordinarily indicate marital, financial, or other status, as it often does in other regions.

Nostril Piercing: All about Jewelry
The ordinary straight-post earring style with a press-on backing is dangerous if worn in the nostril because its sharp end aims right at your septum, where it can cause damage if bumped. A backing can harbor bacteria and secretions from your nose and the piercing, which increases your risk of infection. Stud earrings often call unwelcome attention to the interior of your nose, but they fall out easily if worn without the bulky backing.

A number of popular jewelry styles are much better suited to the nostril, and each has its own advantages and disadvantages. The placement and angle of the piercing is closely connected to the way jewelry fits in the nostril.

Nostril Piercing: The Ring
The higher the piercing is placed on your nose, the larger the ring must be to fit. A ³/₈-inch ring is an average diameter for this area; to wear it, your piercing must be placed just shy of that distance from the edge of your nostril—unless the channel angles downward a little on the inside. However, if the angle is too steep, this will cause the ring to stick out too far from your nose. Ring-style jewelry works well for healing, but if you require an adornment that is more discreet, you will prefer a stud style initially. If you start with a stud but want the option to wear ring-style jewelry later, carefully plan the height and angle of the placement with your piercer.

Nostril Piercing: The Nostril Screw
The nostril screw is a stud modeled after a traditional East Indian design. The ornament displayed on the exterior rests atop a straight wire post that passes through the piercing; the tail terminates in a curl that rests flat against the interior of your nostril. This keeps the jewelry in place without requiring a backing. When properly sized and shaped to fit you, the jewelry is comfortable and is not visible inside your nose.

Nostril screws are less conspicuous than rings and they work well for healing, but *only* when properly adjusted to fit your nose. Pre-bent nostril screws do not take into consideration whether the jewelry will be worn on your left or right side, nor the individual thickness and shape of your nose. Ill-fitting nostril screws can cause serious problems, including embedding, tissue damage, and substantial discomfort. Your jewelry should be bent or adjusted for your anatomy.

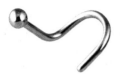

A simple nostril screw topped by a small ball (shown larger than actual size)

Nostril screws set with gems are a very popular style for nostril piercings, and many of the stone settings are flat in the back, where they attach to the post. For the stone to rest properly on your nose, this, too, must be factored in with the angle of your piercing and the shape of your nose. On a nostril of average shape the same angle will often suit both a ring and a stud set with a gem.

Nostril Piercing: The Mini Barbell

A flat disc backing on a mini barbell minimizes jewelry on the interior of the nose, and it eliminates the need to bend or adjust the jewelry. The press-fit style with a removable end is versatile, as different gems or shapes can be interchanged with the help of hemostats to hold the post. Some piercers may not be familiar with this jewelry, but it is an excellent option for piercees who do not find nostril screws to be comfortable.

Nostril Piercing: The L-Bend Style

Some piercees prefer a modified nostril screw, the *L-bend*, which lacks the curl on the inside portion of the wire. This makes the jewelry easier to insert (which is convenient when you change yours frequently), but it is also more likely to fall out. After you are healed, this style can work well if you are careful not to dislodge it. A normal earring post won't be long enough to form into an L-bend; specialized jewelry is still required.

Nostril Piercing: The Nose Bone Style

The *nose bone* is a short, straight post that consists of a gem or other ornament worn on the exterior and a small ball (approximately one-half to a full gauge size thicker than the post) on the inside. This requires you to stretch the piercing somewhat to insert and remove the jewelry, which has the potential to damage your tissue. They only work in a healed piercing if your skin is pliable. If not, they can be dangerous to the health of your piercing. The nose bone is not a safe design for a healing piercing.

Nostril Piercing: Placement

The traditional placement for a nostril piercing is at the crease line on the side of the nose. A big smile accentuates this feature to help pinpoint the spot. This area is often thinner than the rest of the nose, so it may heal faster and feel less tender when pierced. The jewelry will rest in a natural niche, where it nestles most gracefully. I find it aesthetically pleasing when the placement of the piercing forms a relatively equilateral triangular shape with the opening of your nostril, from end to end.

Depending on your preferences, other placements are also possible: higher or lower, closer to the tip of your nose or your face. The backing of a nostril screw or mini barbell will be visible when the piercing is too low, even if the jewelry is properly sized. Multiple nostril piercings are another possibility. Due to space constraints, you will achieve the most attractive, comfortable results when you decide on an overall plan before your first piercing is made.

Nostril Piercing: Procedure

The process often makes your eye water—usually just the one on the same side as the piercing. A small percentage of nostril piercings bleed freely for several minutes, though many bleed a single drop, and others not at all.

I support the nostril on the inside with either closed forceps or a large receiving tube—*not* a cork, which would distort the tissue (and definitely not a carrot, which I once saw in a "how-to-pierce" video!). Forceps should not be clamped onto your nostril, as they distort the area excessively and are uncomfortable on the dense tissue.

The piercing is usually made from the outside in, with the needle carefully guided so that it doesn't poke the inside of your nose. Optimally, your piercer will perform the compression technique (see page 61) to reattach your tissue to your cartilage and stop any bleeding.

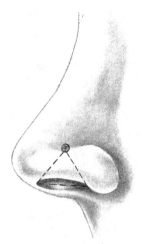

Traditional nostril piercing placement with the "pleasing triangle"

Nostril Piercing: Healing and Troubleshooting

The dense tissue takes months to heal, but the nose is less subject to trauma than many other pierced areas. Keep eyeglasses and sunglasses clean and don't let them rest on the jewelry.

Some redness or swelling is common during initial healing. If your nostril screw is sized correctly, it will accommodate a usual amount of puffiness. If the jewelry appears to be sinking into your tissue, a possible resolution is to apply a tiny piece of Micropore paper tape, available at drug stores. To keep the head of the nostril screw propped above the surface of your tissue, follow the instructions in the first bullet point of "What to Do for Hypertrophic Scarring," page 209–210. This can allow the skin to shrink back around the post and heal. Change the tape daily until the swelling subsides.

If this technique is unsuccessful in dealing with the problem, see a piercer right away to discuss your options. If your jewelry has made a large hole by sinking well into your skin, you may have to wear a ring for the remainder of healing. Even switching to a stud with a longer post, a larger head, or both may not help. Handle the problem promptly or the tissue can rapidly grow over your jewelry, and you will have an embedded piece that requires surgical removal.

Nostril Piercing: Changing Jewelry

Once your piercing has fully healed, with a little patience and practice, you may be able to change nostril jewelry yourself, though many piercees prefer to get assistance from their piercer. To remove a nostril screw, it must be twisted *and* pulled, following the curve of the corkscrew. Most nostril screws are tiny and can be tricky to handle, especially at first. Inserting a nostril screw is a little like riding a bicycle: when you move too slowly, it doesn't go smoothly. Once the tail portion is through the nostril, a swift twisting motion to get the post through the tissue is often best. The hard part can be passing the tail all the way through the channel before it curves—and finding the inside surface, since you can't see it. If the screw is made with too short or tight a tail, it can be nearly impossible to insert, even if the straight post is long enough.

Nostril Piercing: Stretching

Nostril tissue is challenging to stretch, but most piercees are happy with a small hole. If you have designs on a large one, take your time, and be aware that the lack of tissue elasticity in the area may mean an enlargement is permanent. The comments in "Ear Cartilage Piercing: Stretching," page 86, also apply to the nostril.

Nostril Piercing: Concealment

After healing, if you need to conceal your piercing, you can wear a tiny, flat disc that has been painted with skin-tone nail polish. See "DIY Retainers," page 248, for details on the technique. Another option is a nostril screw topped with a very small dome or ball of flesh-colored acrylic. These can be used for fresh piercings if they meet the safety requirements for minimum size, implant-grade post material, a custom fit, and the ability to withstand the heat and pressure of sterilization.

Clear glass and quartz nostril screws are made for concealment, but they are fundamentally unsuited to a healing piercing since the shape cannot be customized. Use caution even when trying them in healed piercings, as they can be fragile, and if they don't fit well, the inflexible material may irritate your piercing.

Retainers in high-tech, inert plastics are also available for post-healing concealment. The plastics are more forgiving than the harder materials, and they are not breakable. Depending on dimensions and design, they may not stay in place well.

Nostril Piercing: Retiring

Many piercees find a nostril piercing does not stay open long without jewelry in place. The hole can shrink in the time it takes you to remove, wash, and dry your jewelry and try to put it back in place. If you like the piercing, leave jewelry in at all times.

If you abandon a nostril piercing, you will have minimal scarring if you wore the usual small-gauge jewelry and your healing was uneventful. The residual mark ordinarily resembles an enlarged pore. Troubled healing could leave substantial scarring.

Nostril Piercing Alternative Placement: High Piercing Placement

This variation is placed *much* higher up the side of the nose in the softest, thinnest part of the upper cartilage—but not too near its juncture to the bone. They are usually done in matched pairs. The piercings should be placed at a 90-degree angle to the tissue; a long L-shape nostril screw is the jewelry of choice. A ring is not suited to this placement. Bring your glasses to the studio so they can be factored in during marking. Eyewear can irritate these piercings and make them hard to heal.

Some initial bruising, bleeding, and swelling is common, and you can expect a rocky healing course if you mistreat them at all. Seek a top-notch pro, because this is a challenging piercing to perform.

The Septum Piercing

- **Description:** Placed in the tissue that divides the nostrils
- **Healing time:** 4 to 8 weeks or longer
- **Initial jewelry style:** Ring-style, commonly a circular barbell, or a septum retainer

- **Initial jewelry gauge:** 16 gauge minimum, but 14 or 12 gauge is preferred, and 10 gauge only on large anatomy
- **Initial jewelry size:** Ring diameters of ³/₈ inch, ⁷/₁₆ inch, or ¹/₂ inch.

The nasal septum piercing can conjure depictions of colorful ethnic peoples wearing bones or feathers from the center of the nose. Alternatively, it can evoke harsh images of leather-clad punks and counterculture eccentrics with fierce bull rings. However, in our Western world, college professors, military personnel, and a host of so-called "ordinary" people also sport this piercing. Really, they do.

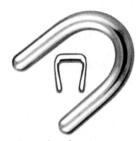

Two styles of septum retainers; the small one is actual size

How can this be, with a piercing that sits in plain sight, right in the middle of the face? The secret of the septum piercing is that it can easily and effectively be concealed inside your nose so that only your dentist knows for sure. (When someone is poised to look up your nose with a bright light, it will be somewhat visible.)

Septum Piercing: Placement and Jewelry

A traditionally placed septum piercing is not in the cartilage that divides the nostrils. Instead it rests in a *sweet spot* (a location optimal for piercing) in the soft, membranous tissue just below the cartilage but above the skin. On most individuals this will be well up into the nose, toward the tip. The traditional placement passes through minimal tissue; in fact, it is some of the thinnest skin that is pierced on a human body. The piercing should be positioned in this location for comfort (both during the procedure and for the wearing of jewelry), ease of healing, and optimal concealment.

The size of the septum's sweet spot does not necessarily correlate with the overall dimensions of one's nose; a large nose can have a small pierceable area. Rely on your piercer for input about the initial jewelry gauge; you can always stretch it later.

Unfortunately, not all piercers are aware of the optimal placement or the technique needed to pierce it. Even slight asymmetry can make it very difficult to achieve a straight piercing. At times, a ridge is present that prevents securing a receiving tube in place for the procedure. The proper location for the piercing is very specific, and on some individuals it is extremely small. The piercing goes into the hidden recesses of the nose, so it is tricky for your piercer to see what he is doing. Even accomplished professionals often find the desired results are elusive. Seek an expert if you want a well-placed, aesthetically pleasing septum piercing.

If you are able to openly wear facial jewelry, a captive or fixed bead ring is suitable. The size should be proportionate to your nose and not so large as to interfere with eating and drinking. A ¹/₂-inch diameter is a reasonable maximum for most people. A very large, heavy ring could be dangerous to your front teeth when you run or jump!

A septum retainer is effective for concealment because the U-shaped piece of metal flips up and hides inside your nostrils. Though acceptable, a retainer is not the best initial jewelry because it can get knocked out during cleaning, nose blowing, or sleeping. Also, it isn't as attractive when you do want to show off your piercing. Short barbells or plugs with O-rings are sometimes used as retainers, but these are difficult to clean and don't show even if you want them to, so they are not the best options.

The circular barbell is a functional and versatile style because it can hide like a septum retainer if you are not free to reveal your piercing, but it is also attractive when you want to put your jewelry on display. A small diameter (usually ⅜ inch) circular barbell is superior for concealment, comfort, and safety. The gap between the two balls allows your ring to be flipped up, so that the jewelry hides in your nose, but a ring that is too large will distort you nostrils from the inside. On most builds, a circular barbell will be as hidden as a septum retainer; however, if your nostrils flare higher than your septum, some metal will show. If you require maximum concealment, charcoal-colored jewelry is best because it is darker and less reflective than shiny steel.

Your piercer can widen the gap on your circular barbell so you can wear the jewelry up with the balls still in place. It should have a snug fit when inside your nose so it won't fall down at inopportune moments, though this makes it a little challenging to change its position.

Septum Piercing: Anatomical Issues

A *deviated septum* is a fairly common condition in which the tissue between the nostrils is displaced. There is often a raised ridge on one side and a concave crease on the other. This may be in the area where the piercing should be placed. It might not be impossible to get a straight piercing if this is the shape of your anatomy, but it is a lot more challenging. There is a tendency for the ring to sit further into the crease and the other side to ride up on the ridge so that the ring rests askew. Whether your septum is deviated or the piercing simply happens to turn out crooked, using clean or gloved fingers, you can twist the jewelry in the desired direction. If done frequently (ten to twenty times a day) during the first few weeks of healing, and *if* the piercing was placed in the sweet spot of soft tissue, it can often be coaxed into the desired position.

If you have had an injury, cosmetic surgery, or other alteration to your anatomy, tell your piercer so he can take this into consideration. Excess bleeding is sometimes a consequence of piercing postsurgical nasal anatomy. If you have a deviated septum, an asymmetrical nose, or otherwise challenging build, this piercing might still be worth a try. If your piercer is willing, you trust him, and you *really* want the piercing, go ahead; it won't leave any visible mark. The worst-case scenario is that you'll end up taking it out afterward. Perhaps you can negotiate with your piercer for a refund if you aren't pleased with the results. If an expert does not believe you are suited to the piercing and feels he cannot achieve acceptable results, consider a different placement.

In general, septum piercings have an undeserved reputation for being painful, but the ones that are placed in the sweet spot are not often described as intense. Many piercees hardly feel more than pressure. But, if your septum tissue is thicker than average, you have altered or challenging anatomy, or your piercing is placed incorrectly, it could feel much more tender.

Septum Piercing: Procedure

After cleaning, your piercer may mark dots inside your nose or guidelines on the undersurface to help him visualize the correct placement during the procedure. At the very least, he will need to put gloved fingers into your nose to feel the septum for the proper spot to pierce.

For the procedure, some piercers will seat you in a chair, but I prefer you *supine* (on your back) on a flat exam table. I position you so that your head hangs backs over the edge of the table. It is not particularly comfortable to hyperextend your neck this way, but it gives me an excellent view of the area from above and behind you—and I don't keep you that way for long. It is worthwhile to get the best placement.

I use an NRT for septum piercings. Tissue manipulation is invaluable, especially if there is any irregularity to the area. The nasal septum has a soft tissue membrane on each side, and this structure is quite mobile. If the tools aren't seated securely, they have a tendency to slip during the procedure, causing a crooked piercing.

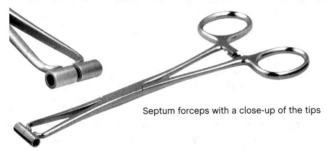

Septum forceps with a close-up of the tips

Special *septum forceps* have a short piece of receiving tube soldered onto each end, and this clamps onto the area. Precise positioning of this tool is crucial for a well-placed piercing. Regular forceps are not at all suited to the septum because they painfully crush the skin in the center of the nose, which is much wider than the tissue that must be secured and pierced. You should never be subjected to having ordinary Pennington forceps placed onto your nose for this piercing. Either septum forceps or the NRT can be used successfully when the technician is skilled at the procedure.

Septum Piercing: Healing and Troubleshooting

Your eyes may water and your nose may run for several minutes following the piercing. Some piercees report feeling the urge to sneeze, but they seldom do. Of course, bleeding is common, too, but it rarely lasts longer than your visit to the studio. The gauge-up procedure may be used for septum piercing, and when the needle is larger than the jewelry, the piercing is more apt to bleed.

If your piercing comes out crooked and adjusting it by manually twisting the jewelry during healing doesn't seem feasible, your piercer may offer to take out the jewelry and pierce you again. It is only advisable to be repierced right away if the first placement was very far off from where it should have been. Otherwise, a repiercing in the same session is apt to go right back in the same place as the first piercing, unless the entry and exit sides are swapped.

Septum Piercing: Septum Stench

Once your piercing is healed, you may encounter *septum stench* (the pungent, rotten odor that comes from the sebum that accumulates in healed piercing channels). It is a normal secretion from piercings throughout the body (see "Normal Piercing Secretions," page 182). However, because your septum piercing is inside your nose, the distinctive aroma is obvious when the smelly substance is present. Don't worry: only you can smell it!

The daily use of soap and water will help to diminish the smell. Wash and rinse as you rotate the jewelry under running water. Some piercees find natural materials such as wood or bone are superior for minimizing odor. A soak with a drop or two of lavender essential oil added to the water will provide a fresh, relaxing scent. Read more about the uses for lavender in chapter 15, "Alternative Aftercare."

Septum Piercing: Changing Jewelry

After the initial four- to eight-week period, septum piercings are usually well healed and the jewelry can be changed. The main challenge of swapping your septum jewelry is that you cannot easily see where the piercing is located; therefore, the process is done mostly by feel. Since the channel is short, once you find the entrance, the exit is generally easy to locate.

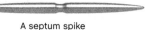

A septum spike

A *septum spike* is a fun and dramatic alternative jewelry style. It is straight piece with tapered ends that comes in many different lengths and materials. A notch or groove in the center will help the spike stay in position. This style is suitable for dress up but seldom practical or comfortable for full-time wear. The spike should be changed out for sleeping. Spike-style jewelry often causes pressure against the nostrils because of the shape of the nose and the placement of the piercing. This can cause your piercing to become tender. Pay attention to your body and don't wear jewelry that is uncomfortable or causes your piercing to regress in its healing.

Septum Piercing: Stretching

Septum piercings are significantly easier to stretch if the piercing isn't placed in the cartilage or too low, in the surface skin of the septum. With a little effort, they can usually be expanded several sizes over time. The septum can routinely be enlarged safely by one gauge as early as three months after the piercing.

Following a number of stretches, you may reach a point where the space between the cartilage and the surface tissue is filled. Subsequent expansion will become considerably more challenging. It is not uncommon for piercees to easily get to 6 or 4 gauge before running into this difficulty. When a septum piercing is stretched to these dimensions, your profile may be permanently altered by a visible hole. This is likely when you stretch too quickly and lose tissue elasticity.

If your piercing was improperly placed in the cartilage or the surface tissue of your nose, it will be very difficult to enlarge. If the piercing is low in the surface tissue, stretching can cause rejection and leave an unsightly split in your skin.

Septum Piercing: Retiring

The septum is one of few piercings that does not leave a visible mark if the piercing is abandoned, unless it was improperly placed or stretched to jumbo size. If your jewelry is removed after the piercing is healed, the channel is likely to remain open, though, as usual, there is a tendency for the hole to shrink somewhat. There is no harm in having a septum piercing that remains open but empty. Some people insert jewelry occasionally and are able to maintain the piercing without regularly wearing anything in it.

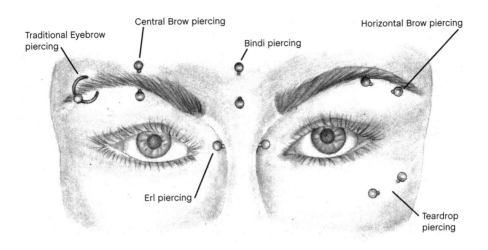

Traditional Eyebrow piercing

Central Brow piercing

Bindi piercing

Horizontal Brow piercing

Erl piercing

Teardrop piercing

The Eyebrow Piercing

- **Healing time:** 6 to 8 weeks
- **Initial jewelry style:** Ring-style, curved bar, or mini curved bar
- **Initial jewelry gauge:** 18 to 16 gauge, 14 gauge for fuller builds
- **Initial jewelry size:** Minimum diameter ³/₈ inch

Eyebrow piercings are no longer the sole province of punk rockers. Swapping safety pins for beautiful jeweled ornaments can elevate this exotic piercing to the status of an attractive, even classy, adornment. While this piercing lacks any known historical precedent, today it draws attention to the windows of the soul in a whole new way. The eyebrow piercing has lost its initial shock value over time, and now even mature individuals sometimes make a statement with this piercing.

Eyebrow piercings have an undeserved reputation for a high rejection rate. When appropriate jewelry is properly placed in pliable tissue, rejection is rare. Complications often occur if the brow is not sufficiently padded, which causes excessive pressure of jewelry against the bone. Wearing jewelry that is too heavy for the delicate tissue, or straight bars instead of curved ones, can also be problematic. If your skin does not seem ample or pinch up reasonably well in the area you would like to wear jewelry, you should consider a different piercing, especially if you are concerned about visible scarring.

Eyebrow piercings are sometimes rumored to cause facial paralysis. The main facial nerve in the general region is the *trigeminal nerve*, but the smaller branches nearby are responsible for sensation, not motion. To impact one of these nerves, a piercing would need to be placed far deeper than normal, or unusually close to the nose or temple. Even then, numbness would be a more likely consequence, not paralysis.

Eyebrow Piercing: Placement

There are many options for placing eyebrow piercings. The traditional modern spot is toward the outer third (or quarter) of the brow. While referred to as "vertical," it is usually most aesthetically pleasing when placed more perpendicular to the eyebrow with a slant mirroring the angle from the outer corner of the eye to the outer edge of the brow. When placed *too* vertically the piercing can look awkward; and, if a ring is worn, it will stick straight out. If the jewelry is positioned well, a ring rests flat against the face. Many piercees have eyebrows that are narrower than the channel, in which case, the piercing looks balanced when situated equidistant from the hair, above and below.

If you prefer a more central or vertical location, curved bars are the best jewelry. A horizontal alternative is less common but gaining in popularity. This piercing is placed slightly above or below the eyebrow hairs or directly within the brow, and may be angled to suit the anatomy. (The two basic forms are still referred to as "vertical" and "horizontal," even though a slant is common for either.) It can be placed anywhere from close to the center, to the outer portion of the eyebrow, *if* the tissue is plentiful and pliable.

Piercings at the inner edge of the brow, vertical or angled, are possible but fairly rare. One challenge is that this tissue is often tighter and more difficult to pinch, and therefore harder to pierce. Multiple eyebrow piercings are possible, and the variations are limited only by your anatomy, your imagination, and the skill of your piercer.

Eyebrow Piercing: Procedure

I use forceps for eyebrow piercings, though performing them freehand is also popular. The key to a comfortable experience is to prepare the area with tissue manipulation first, especially if your skin is at all taut.

When clamps are applied properly or not used at all, most piercees find the eyebrow to be a rather painless piercing. I've had plenty of piercees tell me that plucking or waxing the brows causes more severe or unpleasant sensations. When I had my eyebrow pierced, I described it as a "warm fuzzy" feeling (for a piercing).

Eyebrow Piercing: Healing and Troubleshooting

Eyebrow piercings are apt to bruise, bleed, or swell afterward, and this may persist for several days. Immediately following the procedure, a small percentage of eyebrow piercings swell considerably. Fresh eyebrow piercings are subject to the *new piercing salute*, in which ring-style jewelry stands straight out from your face, even if it is placed at an angle to lay flat once healed. This is temporary if the jewelry is sized properly, and when the tissue loosens around the jewelry, it will rest closer to your face. A ring will continue to protrude even after healing if it is too small in diameter or worn in a piercing that is placed too vertically.

You may be concerned about sweat getting into your eyebrow piercing, but this is not problematic when you clean your piercing regularly. If you need to mop your brow, pat the pierced area gently with clean, disposable paper products.

Eyebrow Piercing: Changing Jewelry

Once your eyebrow piercing is healed, it may be possible to change the jewelry yourself, but it is tricky: your hands obscure your view, you must manipulate jewelry above your eye, and your image is reversed in the mirror.

For concealment, a snug barbell with tiny $3/32$-inch (2.5 mm) balls work well. These mini balls can be painted with skin-tone nail polish as described under "DIY Retainers," on page 248.

Eyebrow Piercing: Stretching

This is not a good piercing for stretching. Only the meatiest of brows can support jewelry as large as 12 gauge. On some, 14 gauge proves too heavy. This is *not* a spot where bigger is better. I've seen piercees who attempted to enlarge eyebrow piercings and regretted it when the piercings rebelled and, in some cases, rejected.

Eyebrow Piercing: Retiring

Unsightly scarring is rare unless you experience healing complications or stretch up larger than average. If your piercing is placed within or close to the hairs, the marks may be somewhat concealed.

Other Facial Piercings: Teardrop/Anti-Eyebrow, Bridge/Erl, and Bindi

Several less common piercings are done in the region surrounding the eyes. They aren't considered traditional placements, and they are not as easy to heal as the more popular ones. Fewer people are anatomically suited to them; many simply have tissue that is too taut for success. If the idea of a visible mark on your face is unappealing, you should not attempt any of these variations because they are more prone to rejection and scarring. They are all essentially surface piercings, and some may do well with a surface bar. In this delicate tissue, small barbell ends are best.

Teardrop/Anti-Eyebrow Piercing

- **Description:** Placed in the tissue atop the highest crest of the cheekbone, toward the outer edge of the eye. It is like a traditional eyebrow piercing but flipped down below the eye instead of above. The angle may be diagonal, horizontal, or any orientation in which the tissue can be pinched and, therefore, pierced.
- **Differences:** This fine skin may do better with slightly smaller and thinner jewelry. I've had success with 18-gauge curved mini-barbells, and a slightly narrower piercing channel than that used for the bridge variations described next.
- **Healing time:** 3 to 4 months or longer
- **Initial jewelry style:** Mini curved bar or surface bar
- **Initial jewelry gauge:** 18 or 16 gauge; less often 14 gauge
- **Initial jewelry size:** Minimum ⅜ inch; average ⁷⁄₁₆ inch

The Bridge, Erl, or Mid-Brow Piercing

- **Description:** The bridge piercing gets its nickname from body art devotee Erl Van Aken, a Gauntlet customer who is believed to be the first to wear one. It is a horizontal piercing through the *glabella* (tissue between the brows above the nose) or on the *nasion* (between the eyes). It ranges from as high as the top of the brows to the bridge of the nose. Multiples are rare but sometimes possible.
- **Differences:** This tissue may respond better with jewelry that is a little thicker than some of these other areas, and healing time may be longer.
- **Healing time:** 4 to 6 months or longer
- **Initial jewelry style:** Straight or curved barbell

- **Initial jewelry gauge:** 14 or 12 gauge
- **Warning:** Even if the jewelry is in your field of vision, it won't make you go cross-eyed. But, there are other dangers, including a fairly high rate of rejection and scarring. Far more serious, however, is the effect of insufficient padding between your jewelry and the structures beneath. Direct pressure can cause diminished blood supply to the bone. This may lead to bone density loss and, in a worst-case scenario, bone *necrosis* (death).[1] If you don't have plenty of pliable tissue, a bridge piercing is not advisable.

Bindi/Vertical Bridge

- **Description:** A vertical surface piercing placed between the eyebrows or slightly above them. It is named after the mark traditionally worn by Hindu women. If the tissue is pliable enough, it may be placed a little higher, on the lower portion of the forehead.
- **Healing time:** 4 to 6 months
- **Initial jewelry style:** Curved barbell or surface bar
- **Initial jewelry gauge:** 16 or 14 gauge
- **Warning:** The same hazards of horizontal piercing in this region also apply (see warning for the bridge piercing, above).

The Point

Earlobe piercings are the most socially acceptable piercings, and they are also among the fastest and easiest to heal. The nearby cartilage of the ear presents more of a challenge; even so, many piercees find exotic ear piercings to be worthwhile. Facial anatomy is relatively welcoming to piercings when principles for appropriate placement are followed, but give careful consideration to facial piercings because, except for the nasal septum, they can leave visible scarring if abandoned later. An above-the-neck piercing can effectively customize the way you face the world.

Kiss of the Needle: Tongue and Oral Piercings

Before attempting to clean or care for any oral piercing, carefully review and follow the instructions in "Aftercare for Oral Piercings," page 193.

Oral Piercing Risks

You should be aware of the dangers before you decide to get an oral piercing. Once you know what they are, you can take precautions to minimize them, but these piercings are not risk-free. If you have a history of bad teeth or problem gums, a tongue or lip piercing may be inadvisable.

Contrary to what many people think, infection is not the most common risk from oral piercings. The human mouth is not prone to infection because the lymphatic system, mucus membranes, and saliva provide formidable defenses. The biggest danger is damage to teeth, gums, and oral structures from jewelry. The delicate enamel on your teeth can get cracked or chipped if you play with your jewelry. Biting or clicking jewelry often or hard—for fun or by accident—will result in *wrecking ball fractures* (small cracks in the teeth).[1] Continuous pressure from hard metal can diminish the density of the underlying bone over time. Gum recession is caused by jewelry that is too big or improperly placed, or from excessive rubbing of hard metal against the delicate soft tissue of the palate or gums. Enamel, bone, and gum tissue *do not* regenerate. Damage to these oral structures is serious and irreversible.

The likelihood of such complications is dramatically reduced when you adhere to accepted practices, wear properly sized jewelry that does not rub inside your mouth, and avoid playing with it. For more information, see the APP's brochure "Oral Piercing Risks and Safety Measures" (www.safepiercing.org).

The Tongue Piercing

- **Healing time:** 4 to 8 weeks
- **Initial jewelry style:** Straight barbell
- **Initial jewelry gauge:** Most commonly 14 and 12 gauge; sometimes 10 gauge
- **Initial jewelry size:** Bar length is anatomically dependent and must be long enough to allow for swelling. Initial jewelry lengths for centrally

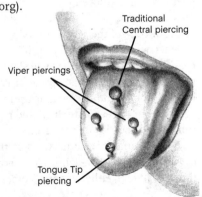

Traditional Central piercing

Viper piercings

Tongue Tip piercing

placed piercings range from 9/16 inch for slim tongues to 7/8 inch for thick ones; a 3/4-inch length is common. I find an 11/16-inch post is a better fit for many tongues, though not all piercers stock this in-between size.

The tongue is a unique and important body part because it is situated inside the mouth—the tool with which we express ourselves, a center for sensuality, and the way we ingest our sustenance. A tongue piercing can be private or public, and it can be fun alone or with a friend.

If asked whether tongue piercing is erotic, many piercees would proclaim an emphatic "Yes!" but an equal number would earnestly respond, "Absolutely not." None of these people would be insincere; they simply differ in their perspectives. A tongue piercing is what you make of it. For some, it is merely an ornament; for others, it is a useful sensual device. The wearing of tongue jewelry will not magically transform you into an oral Casanova, but it will provide you with an additional tool, should you desire to use it.

Tongue Piercing: Placement

The piercing can be positioned nearly anywhere along the tongue, from the tip to the back. Prior to marking, your piercer should evaluate the top and bottom of your tongue and discuss the issue of concealment, and whether you have thoughts regarding placement or future plans to stretch or add more piercings. Multiple piercings are not possible for all tongues.

A central position is popular because it minimizes visibility and keeps the jewelry well away from the teeth but still allows for fun and function. Piercing along the midline, top and bottom is absolutely fine. Due to a widely disseminated urban myth, many piercers mistakenly believe it is dangerous to pierce the midline of the tongue on the bottom. The major nerves and arteries in the tongue are clearly visible underneath, well off to the sides. A skilled piercer will have no problem avoiding these structures.

When anatomy under the tongue is normal, the piercing can rest right in the center, generally just in front of the attachment of the *lingual frenulum* (the thin band of tissue attaching the tongue to the floor of the mouth). If your web is exceptionally thick or connects farther forward than usual, the underside of the piercing can be placed just a little off to one side. However, if you physically cannot stick your tongue out, then piercing it will be difficult or impossible. When the lingual frenulum is tight and restricts tongue movement, this condition is called *tongue-tied* (or *ankyloglossia*, from the Greek for "crooked tongue"). A simple medical procedure can often correct this, but this is outside of the scope of services piercers are permitted to perform.

For safety and comfort, your piercing may be placed slightly farther forward underneath. The top of the barbell will slant back toward the highest part of the upper palate, where you have the most space for it in your oral cavity. This angle also prevents the jewelry from standing straight up in your mouth, which could jam the bottom ball against your lower palate. It should not have too steep an angle, or the bottom ball will rub behind your lower front teeth.

If concealment is a crucial factor, the piercing should be toward the middle or back of your tongue. However, it isn't necessary to place the piercing halfway down your throat to hide it, either. If your piercing goes back beyond a certain point, it will not be more obscured, but it *will* be less comfortable and fun. Let your piercer assist you with the best location.

Tongue Piercing: Anatomy and Choice of Jewelry

The initial barbell should be just long enough to accommodate the maximum size for expected swelling. An overly long barbell can cause serious damage to delicate intraoral structures, so wearing the correct size is vital. Your piercer must weigh a number of elements to figure the length that will be optimal for initial healing. The farther back the piercing is placed, the greater the expected swelling. Piercings at the tip are not inclined to swell much, so $1/16$ inch extra may be sufficient. Thick tongues are apt to swell more than slim ones. Offer your history of swelling from previous piercings or injuries to help pinpoint the measurement. Steer clear of any piercer who puts a "standard-length" barbell in every tongue piercing. Anatomy is variable and must be evaluated on an individual basis for a safe fit.

When you stick out your tongue, it might look slim and your new barbell might seem long. But the piercing heals with your tongue inside your mouth, where it thickens considerably. It may also appear that a proposed placement is close to the tip, but when your tongue rests inside, you will find that the mark is much farther back.

> **A Different Function**
> Nowadays everyone knows about tongue piercings, but this was not always the case. Back in the 1980s, before body piercing was in the public eye, I used to tell people that my tongue piercing was an acupuncture stud for weight control! I'd deliver a brief spiel about the way the metal stud diminished my appetite and satisfied my palate, and how it prevented me from eating quickly or thoughtlessly. Everyone believed me, and nobody *ever* asked me, "Didn't that hurt?" Instead, they would ask with interest, "Does it work?" Who knows? Depending on what you believe, it might. People who seemed open-minded about the other possibilities for tongue piercings would be let in on my secret: I did it for fun.

Acrylic barbell ends are softer than metal, and cheaper and easier to replace than a tooth. If you have veneers or caps, or wear dentures, bridges, or other oral appliances, acrylic is suggested. Acrylic is also a good choice if you are concerned about oral health or have a tendency to play with your jewelry. Some piercers do not use acrylic balls for initial jewelry, though I have suggested them for years and have found them to be safe and effective. Keep a spare ball handy, because acrylics are fairly fragile.

For safety and comfort, I insert initial jewelry that has a small ($3/16$-inch) ball underneath, where there is less room. I offer a choice of a matching size or slightly larger ($7/32$- or $1/4$-inch) ball on the top, where there is more space for jewelry.

Alternative Tongue Piercing Placement: Tongue Tip

A piercing within the first $1/2$ inch of the tongue is considered a *tongue tip* piercing. It can be worn as close as $5/16$ inch from the end of the tongue. Due to the distribution of nerve endings, this spot is more sensitive than a traditional placement. You can try out a ring after healing, but a barbell is better initially.

Speaking clearly with jewelry at the tip of your tongue is possible, but getting accustomed to it is more challenging than with a central placement. A ring or bar is also more apt to get caught between your teeth when the piercing is placed so close to them. You must be extremely careful to avoid biting the jewelry when you eat, especially at first.

Alternative Tongue Piercing Placement: Multiple Piercings

Piercees with the personal desire, appropriate anatomy, and an accomplished piercer can get multiple tongue piercings. Planning is needed to make the best use of the limited space, even on those with the longest of tongues. More than three along the midline is possible for the few who are lingually endowed. Two tongue piercings can be done in the same session if there is enough space between them and the first one does not swell significantly. Getting more than two at a time is not advisable due to the likelihood of excessive swelling and discomfort.

Because the surface area is greater on the top of the tongue, multiple piercings placed in a straight row down the center might rest in a cluster or alternate to either side of your web in the smaller space underneath.

Depending on anatomy, arrangements for multiple piercings include one (or more) along the midline plus a pair of piercings off to the sides. A few dedicated piercees wear piercings configured in triangle, diamond, and other shapes.

> **Helpful Hint**
> You may find your gag reflex kicks in when you stick your tongue out with your mouth open. If you can push it out of your mouth far enough for marking and piercing while keeping your lips closed, this usually solves the problem.

Alternative Tongue Piercing Placement: Snake Bites, Venoms, Vipers, or Viper Bites

These are terms for a pair of oral piercings placed off to either side of the midline. (Some of these names are also used to refer to lip piercings.) Before deciding to get this arrangement, take a close look at the underside of your tongue with a bright light to familiarize yourself with the obvious pathways of your blood supply. Your piercer must be extremely precise or you risk a punctured nerve or artery. Side-placement tongue piercings can be safe when properly placed, but they may take longer to heal and become accustomed to than a midline piercing. After the procedure, side-placement piercings are inclined to bleed more, even when a major vessel is not punctured. Depending on where you want them to be situated on the top, they usually need to angle inward or outward under the tongue to avoid the vital structures.

Tongue Piercing: Procedure

First your mouth should be cleaned with a germicidal oral rinse. Next your piercer will mark the top and bottom of your tongue using gentian violet on a sterile toothpick or a surgical pen (which should be discarded or given to you afterward).

Request a tissue or paper towel to hold during the procedure if you aren't provided with one. If you keep it at chest level your *drool patrol* will be poised for duty (to catch saliva) without being in your piercer's way. A swift piercer can get your jewelry in before you even have time to dribble, but it's good to have, just in case.

For the procedure, sitting is the safest position. Tipping your head back isn't helpful because it draws your tongue into your mouth; but, if you tilt your head forward slightly, moving your chin toward your chest, this helps you extend your tongue. If you are in a reclining position, your tongue must fight gravity; worse, jewelry (or, heaven forbid, the needle!) could be dropped into your throat. I advise against having a tongue piercing while you are lying supine.

Your tongue should be dried with sterile gauze to make it easier to grasp. I use forceps and make the piercing from the top, but it can be successfully done from either direction.

When you bite your tongue, you experience a painful crush injury, so most piercees are understandably concerned about the intensity of piercing this part of the body. But a traditional tongue piercing is placed where the nerves primarily get signals for taste and temperature. It is more painful to get pierced at the tip or edges of the tongue than in the center.

Tongue Piercing: Healing and Troubleshooting

Sipping cold water from a clean cup immediately after receiving an oral piercing can help minimize initial swelling, and it feels soothing, too.

During the first week, significant swelling, light bleeding, bruising, and tenderness are normal. After that, the swelling should diminish, but some often remains for several weeks. Don't panic if you see a whitish discharge coming from your tongue. All healing piercings secrete fluids; however, inside the wet environment of the mouth, the substance doesn't dry to form the crust you see in other areas.

Don't worry: you *can* eat with a new tongue piercing, but it isn't easy at first. You have the initial swelling to contend with, plus you have unfamiliar jewelry right in the middle of your mouth. Fasting or liquid diets are not required, though some piercees prefer to eat only soft or blended foods for the first few days. Piercings heal better if your body is well nourished, so eat whatever feels comfortable, and in a few days you should feel back to normal. Follow these tips for a safe, comfortable healing course:

Quick Trick

To assure the briefest procedure possible, I attach the jewelry and piercing needle together and I insert the bar as I create the piercing. When internally threaded jewelry is used, a small connector pin can be placed into the lumens of both jewelry and needle, creating a single unit that is easily disassembled once the piercing has been made. The needle and connector come away, the bottom ball gets screwed into place, and the piercing is done.

I've had more than one observer remark, "Wow! That was fast. I was watching, but I missed it." Some piercers work in a sequential fashion, piercing first, and then getting the jewelry and transferring it in, which takes slightly longer.

- Eat *slowly* and take small bites.
- Focus on keeping your tongue level. The jewelry can get between your teeth when it turns.
- Avoid foods like mashed potatoes or oatmeal; they may be soft, but they are hard to eat because they to stick to your mouth and jewelry.
- Smoothies, shakes, energy drinks, ice cream, soups, and the like are good menu mainstays.
- Use clean fingers or utensils to place small bites of solid food between your molars. The tongue moves food to the back of the mouth, so food that is already there requires less manipulation.
- Cold and frozen foods are soothing and help to minimize swelling.

- Chewing gum or sucking on candy may be injurious during healing.
- Salty, spicy, acidic, or hot foods and beverages may be irritating.
- A certain amount of speaking is unavoidable, but when your piercing is fresh, try to let your tongue rest as much as possible.
- Do not play with your tongue or jewelry!

Plaque can form on tongue jewelry just like it does on teeth. Most commonly it adheres under the tongue at the juncture of the ball and the post, and on the ball itself. You can use dental floss around the bottom of the post to help keep this area clean. See "Regular Maintenance: Oral Piercings," page 219, for additional cleaning measures you can take once the piercing has healed.

Tongue Piercing: Concealment

Many professionals successfully wear tongue jewelry in work environments where body modification is not acceptable. Clear or flesh-tone acrylic concealment balls or domes on the shortest post that fits will minimize jewelry visibility and safeguard your teeth and gums. If you avoid opening your mouth wide when you speak, your tongue piercing is apt to go unnoticed.

Tongue Piercing: Speech Problems

Your speech will probably be affected during a brief period of accommodation when your piercing is new. After the swelling has gone down (as quickly as three to five days) and you have had a little time to adjust, there is usually no impediment. If your piercing is placed correctly, speech is seldom altered after a shorter post is inserted.

Tongue Piercing: Scar Tissue

Scar tissue can appear as a pinkish or whitish raised ring of hardened skin that partially or completely surrounds one or both openings of your piercing. If it develops during healing—most commonly the result of the overuse of a harsh care product or too much talking, playing, or other activity—it is usually temporary. The oral cells regenerate very quickly, and they seem to go into overdrive if an oral piercing is traumatized during healing. Limiting tongue activity is very important, so even if your piercing feels fine, take it easy for the first month. See the tip about aspirin paste under "What to Do for Hypergranulation Tissue," on page 207, if you develop scar tissue. Sometimes the problem is caused by unknowingly playing with the jewelry in your sleep, and this can be difficult to resolve.

Tongue Piercing: Downsizing and Changing Jewelry

It is *absolutely vital* for your oral health that you wear the shortest post that fits once you are healed. In addition to harming teeth, long-term wear of an overly long barbell causes loss of jawbone density and gum recession.[2] These two structures play key roles in holding your teeth in your mouth. Your initial post—the one with extra length to allow for swelling—must be changed to a shorter one. It doesn't matter if you like the way the long bar feels or looks, or if everything seems okay in your mouth—downsize!

A professional piercer can put a new bar in as early as a week after piercing. If you cannot visit a professional for help and you are not experienced at switching your own jewelry, wait until after the four-week minimum healing time to avoid damaging the tissue with an inept jewelry change.

If externally threaded jewelry was used initially, wait the full four weeks before passing an externally threaded post through the channel. If your piercer has a taper to avoid exposing your new channel to the threaded post, she can change it for you once your swelling is gone.

Instead of a ball, some piercees prefer to wear a disc on the bottom. Experimentation may be needed to find the most comfortable size and shape for you. Once the piercing has healed, feel free to try some of the many different options. Large or heavy ornaments are seldom safe for extended periods of time. Think twice about vibrating tongue barbells or any jewelry that requires you to place a battery in a moist area.

Tongue Piercing: Stretching

The tongue piercing is often easy to enlarge by a gauge or two, but stretching tends to become more difficult as you expand to larger sizes. A general disadvantage of creating an oversized hole is that the jewelry becomes heavier and bigger, too, increasing your risk of oral damage. If you want to have a jumbo piercing in your tongue, consider wearing acrylic jewelry (it's lighter in weight), keep posts snug, and wear balls with a reasonable diameter.

> **Tongue Piercing: Downsize Policy**
>
> Anyone who pierces your tongue without educating you about the need to downsize the jewelry is remiss in her duties to safeguard your dental health. Does your piercer encourage downsizing by offering clear, detailed information and perhaps a discount on a shorter post? She will if she is knowledgeable and caring.

Tongue Piercing: Retiring

When you remove your jewelry, the hole may shrink or close right up, even if you have had it pierced for years. On the other hand, it is not uncommon for an established tongue piercing to remain viable without jewelry. If it seems to stay open, apply the principles described in "Resting," on page 229, to determine how long you can comfortably leave it out.

If you want to abandon your piercing, simply remove your jewelry. Unless it was stretched unusually large, the channel will shrink, so there is little likelihood of food working its way inside the hole. An abandoned large-gauge tongue piercing that remains open could benefit from a periodic spray through the channel with a Waterpik or similar water jet device.

The Labret Piercing

- **Healing time:** 6 to 8 weeks or longer.
- **Initial jewelry style:** Ring-style, disc-back labret stud, or fishtail labret.
- **Initial jewelry gauge:** 16 through 12 gauge, depending on placement and jewelry style. The 14 gauge is most common for labret studs.
- **Initial jewelry size:** Labret or fishtail posts from 5/16 to 7/16 inch. Ring diameters from 3/8 to 1/2 inch. To allow for swelling, rings should be one diameter larger than the size that will be worn in the healed piercing.

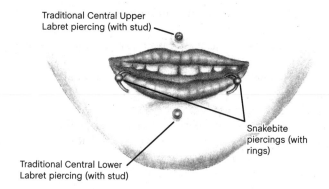

Traditional Central Upper
Labret piercing (with stud)

Snakebite
piercings (with
rings)

Traditional Central Lower
Labret piercing (with stud)

After the ear and nose, the lip is one of the most popular piercings in traditional cultures around the world. Throughout the ages, people have worn ornaments of horn, bone, gold, and other natural materials in piercings of the lips.

Labret Piercing: Placement

Labret derives from the Latin word *labrum*, meaning "lip." Any piercing in the region of the mouth is a labret, though some use the term only to denote the placement centered underneath the bottom lip. Within the limitations imposed by anatomy and aesthetic preferences, a piercing can go just about anywhere around the mouth.

The traditional labret placement is centered under the lower lip, below the *vermillion border* (the pigmented area). Labrets may be worn higher or lower, in pairs or in multiples. Situating the piercing so that the jewelry rests at a neutral angle is critical for comfort and safety. There is a maximum distance below the lip that can reasonably be pierced because the tissue connects to the gums. All labrets (including the variations described below) must be placed with this in mind. Excess pressure against teeth or gums—even from the slightest slant—can result in discomfort and damage.[3] The thin tissue inside the lip allows many of the blood vessels to be easily seen and avoided.

For accuracy, I mark both the inside and outside surfaces of the piercing. If you plan to switch back and forth between ring- and stud-style jewelry after healing, discuss this with your piercer, because the angle and depth of the piercing may be affected.

Labret Piercing Jewelry: The Labret Stud

A *labret stud* (see photo on page 79) is a short barbell with a slim disc that is worn inside the mouth. A ball, gem, spike, or other ornament shows on the facial surface. Some piercees prefer a slightly more domed backing design (like a flat M&M's candy). These backings are generally safer and more comfortable than a ball.

Some labret studs are made of two pieces: the disc-and-post combo is a single unit, and only the front end can be removed. Other labret studs are comprised of three separate pieces: disc, post, and the threaded end worn on the front. An advantage of the two-piece style is that you can't possibly lose the disc. A disadvantage is that you will need to replace this whole portion to downsize your jewelry after the initial swelling is gone. Two advantages to the three-piece style are that you can replace just the post portion once it is time to downsize, and it allows you to change both ends. The usual starting disc size is approximately 5 millimeters, but after healing you may wish to try a 3-millimeter disc instead. The disadvantage is that you have a slightly increased possibility of jewelry loss because both ends unscrew.

The length of the post is anatomy-dependent, and a good fit is imperative. The lip tissue is so soft and quick to regenerate that there is danger of the jewelry becoming embedded if it is too short. Once your piercing has fully healed and a shorter post has been inserted, you may see the disc *nesting* (sinking a millimeter or two into the inside surface of your lip). If you have no discomfort, this indentation is acceptable, and it may help to protect your teeth and gums by keeping the disc from directly pressing against them.

Labret Piercing Jewelry: The Fishtail

This is an L-shaped piece of metal with a ball or other ornament on the front. It is formed so the shorter leg of the *L* passes through your piercing, and the longer tail rests in the groove between your gum and lip. The fishtail is designed for lower lip piercings, and if worn in the upper lip, the tail would hang down.

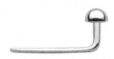

A fishtail labret with a half-ball (shown larger than actual size)

Fishtail labrets must be custom-bent (or at least adjusted) to fit each piercee. The inside portion must be contoured to your mouth or it will cause irritation. The front end is normally attached, but a threaded style with changeable ornaments is also made. On the best pieces, the metal stock that runs along the interior is flattened to minimize contact with the gums.

Experimentation may be needed to determine what works best for you. Labret studs are more common, and I prefer them, but opinion is divided among piercers as to which is superior.

Labret Piercing Jewelry: The Ring

Rings work best on lip piercings that are placed close to the vermillion border. If you have a full lip or your piercing is located far from its edge, the ring will need to be overly large. A set of lip piercings off to each side may be referred to as *snakebites* or *venoms*.

If you want to wear a ring to hug your lip, a tight fit must wait until after healing. A larger diameter ring must be worn to accommodate initial swelling. When a ring fights gravity (as with a lower lip piercing), it will rest over to one side. The ring will not sit straight up to frame the center of your lip unless it is snug. Drinking from a cup or glass can be a tad tricky when you first wear a lip ring. Clean dishware and a little patience and practice are required.

Labret Piercing Jewelry: The C-Ring or U-Ring

A custom-bent *C-ring* or *U-ring* is a safe and comfortable alternative for many piercees who wear labrets. This is a small-diameter circular barbell that is widened so that it is C-shaped (or U-shaped, depending on anatomy) rather than round. This will conform to your lip and help to avoid jewelry contact with your teeth or gums. There is a wide range of fit possibilities based on the way it is bent to accommodate individual anatomy. Sometimes an asymmetrical bend is used. This style may satisfy you if you like the look of a vertical lip (surface) piercing but don't want to face its risks of scarring and migration. The jewelry can give you the same appearance (one ball on top of your lip and the other right beneath it), but with the versatility of a traditional labret.

It sometimes takes a few attempts with different styles and sizes of jewelry to determine what works best for your labret piercing. The mouth is a dynamic area that moves and changes shape considerably when you speak, smile, and eat. No wonder comfortably accommodating a static piece of metal there is so challenging.

Labret Piercing: Procedure

I use forceps and generally pierce from the outside, but others work from the inside. A successful piercing can be done from either direction.

Men with facial hair need not trim or shave, even if the piercing will be placed within the whiskers. It will be more challenging for your piercer, but an adept technician will be able to do the job, even through a heavy beard.

Labret Piercing: Healing and Troubleshooting

Don't open your mouth too wide when you wear a labret stud because the disc on the inside can catch on your teeth.

Men may shave as normally as possible, given the obstacle of the jewelry. Avoid getting aftershave, especially alcohol-based products, into your healing piercing. See more tips under "Shaving," page 250.

Wearing lipstick or lip balm is fine, but keep the container clean and don't share it. The type you apply from a tube is safer than the kind you put on with your finger.

Plaque can accumulate on the part of labret jewelry that is inside your mouth, especially at the juncture of the disc and the post. It is difficult to access and scrub this area with a toothbrush, but dental floss can help to keep it clean.

Most of the tips in "Tongue Piercing: Healing and Troubleshooting," page 109, apply to lip piercings, too.

It is normal for jewelry to nest somewhat into your lip; however, if you suspect tissue is actually growing over it (inside or out), consult your piercer immediately. If you don't handle this problem in time, medical intervention will be needed. The facial surface of labret piercings has a tendency to discolor, usually pinkish or reddish, and to crust up throughout the healing period. Frequent mild saline soaks can be helpful.

A new ornament in your lip is hard to ignore, and you may be inclined to gnaw at the jewelry with your teeth or play with it with your tongue. There are many fun though potentially destructive ways to interact with a new lip piercing. Try to leave your piercing alone and let it heal. Once your labret is well healed, playing with the jewelry shouldn't irritate your piercing, but if the activity involves your teeth or gums, it can cause damage to those structures.

If you experience soreness inside your mouth as you adjust to the jewelry, dental or orthodontic wax can be applied inside to soften the impact. This harmless wax is inexpensive and can be obtained at drugstores. Problems are generally resolved by wearing smaller or shorter jewelry once healing is complete. If pressure on your teeth or irritation to your gums persists regardless of the jewelry size and style, the piercing will need to be abandoned.

Labret Piercing: Changing Jewelry

Caring, informed piercers offer a downsize policy for labret studs. Depending on your healing process and how long your initial post is, you might need to downsize the post more than once. Wait until healing is over before inserting tight-fitting jewelry.

The slippery nature of saliva makes changing your own jewelry in oral piercings tricky. Keep a clean paper towel or two handy, because you are probably going to need them. Disc-back labrets can be challenging to screw on without assistance because of their flat shape and small size. It may be easiest to insert a labret post from the inside and screw on the front. Small hemostats are very helpful for holding the post during this process. Or pay a visit to your piercer, as many piercees do.

Labret Piercing: Concealment

Even with the most discreet jewelry, unless you have a thick beard, total concealment of a healing labret is not possible. At least a trace of it is going to be visible, especially when it is new, because of the extra post length that is required to accommodate the swelling. After healing, concealment options improve, but this area is still challenging to hide completely. If you have facial hair, wearing a retainer in a color that blends with your whiskers may be best for camouflage, rather than the usual flesh-tone options.

To avoid the possibility of embedding, initial healing should be over before you wear small jewelry such as a ⅛-inch (3 mm) ball or disc, unless you have ¹⁄₁₆ inch of extra post length.

Labret Piercing: Stretching

Historically, lip piercings are among those most commonly stretched, and modern piercees wear impressive sizes. Do not stretch lip piercings beyond 10 gauge without due consideration. The tissue is relatively elastic, but the risks increase with the jewelry size. Larger and heavier adornments against teeth and gums compound oral health hazards. Depending on how big you enlarge, your hole might not shrink enough to prevent saliva from leaking if you abandon the hole. In fact, some individuals with large-gauge lip piercings experience saliva leakage while eating, even with their jewelry in place.

Labret Piercing: Retiring

Should you take out your jewelry, a small divot or spot that looks like an enlarged pore usually remains if healing was uneventful and the piercing was not stretched. If the piercing was placed under the curl of your lip, the natural crease might obscure the mark.

If tissue was expanded to a large gauge or stretched too quickly, a permanent void will likely remain, and it can be unsightly; surgery may be the only way to restore a normal appearance. Permanent damage to the lower front teeth or nearby gums is common with extreme lip enlargement.

Lip Piercing: Variations

The healing time and jewelry information are the same as for the labret piercing.

Lower Lip Side Placement

The self-explanatory *side lip piercing with ring* is commonly placed just below the vermillion border. There is usually space for the ring to rest at the juncture of the upper and lower lip, though some piercees prefer that the ring lie toward the center.

Because the tissue inside the lip is so soft, there is a tendency for the piercing to rise a millimeter or two from its original placement on the interior when you wear a ring. In anticipation of this, experienced piercers will cheat the initial mark down just a little on the inside so the jewelry will end up in the desired position (usually equidistant from the edge of the lip, inside and out) once healing is complete. Wearing a snug ring (after healing, of course) is less likely to cause gum damage, though there is still some risk of injuring your teeth by biting the jewelry.

Upper Lip Side Placement: Monroe, Madonna, or Chrome Crawford

This glamorous piercing is a beauty mark of metal worn off to one side above the upper lip. It is often embellished with a sparkling jewel. The names clearly derive from the ladies who bear an unpierced version near their own lips.

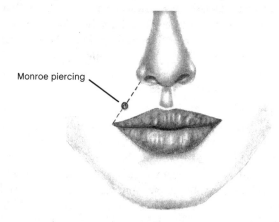

Monroe piercing

Other than a longer healing time of two to three months or longer, this piercing also shares many characteristics with the other lip area placements. Initial jewelry is usually a labret stud in 14 gauge, occasionally 16 or 12 gauge.

Upper Lip Placement

This style is placed toward the corner of the mouth, 5/16 to 1/2 inch above the lip line. This ornament is intended as a lip enhancement, but some piercers place them closer to the nose. While piercings often work best in the natural creases of the body, an upper lip piercing that sits in the *naso-labial fold* (smile line) is more difficult to heal.

When your piercer marks the interior she should take great care to see that the angle is neutral when your face is at rest. She should also consider how the area changes with different facial movements. On some anatomy the gums join the lip fairly low; a spot that seems reasonable from the outside sometimes sits above your gums on the inside. If your piercer is not meticulous and skillful, your piercing could end up at an awkward angle that is difficult or impossible to heal and potentially damaging to your teeth and gums.

Upper Lip Piercing: Healing and Troubleshooting

Some individuals heal this piercing rapidly, yet others find it takes commitment and patience over many months before it settles.

Regardless of how well upper lip piercings are placed, they can catch when you open your mouth wide. Be careful when eating burgers, big sandwiches, and the like.

Upper Lip Piercing: Changing Jewelry

Jewelry changes at home can be difficult, especially once the short post is in place or if you wear a tiny ball or gem. In fact, these can be challenging for even a piercer to change. Most piercees return to a professional for help.

Upper Lip Piercing: Retiring

The mark left after jewelry removal may be more obvious than one from a central lower labret. This is not a piercing to get as a temporary ornament; it may well leave a scar.

Upper Lip Center: Philtrum

This style may appeal to you if you like midline placements. Some alternative names for the anatomical term *philtrum* include *Medusa*, *divot*, and *upret*.

This piercing also takes an average of two to three months to heal and usually uses a 14-gauge labret stud.

Philtrum Placement

This piercing is placed in the center of the natural divot (also called the *infranasal depression*), between the mouth and the nose. It may be worn in conjunction with other lip piercings. Depending on personal preferences and available space inside and out, it may be situated closer to the lip, nearer the nose, or right at the midpoint.

During this procedure you may feel as if you're getting a strong bop on the nose rather than an oral piercing. Your eyes may water, too.

Philtrum Piercing: Retiring

Like all labrets other than the lower central placement, this is apt to leave a visible mark if the piercing is abandoned.

Changing Philtrum Jewelry

Some piercees opt to wear a ring in this location after healing. Depending on your anatomy, a D-ring with the flat side on the interior or a teardrop-shaped ring may be most comfortable.

Questionable Oral Piercings

Some oral piercings have a higher potential for complications than others. This isn't to suggest they never heal, but they do not have the same likelihood of success as more traditionally placed labrets. Before deciding on any of the following spots, weigh the risks.

The Lingual Frenulum Piercing

This is a piercing of the web under the tongue. This is not a viable option for people who do not possess tongue control for the procedure or sufficiently pronounced anatomy. For those who are well enough endowed, a small curved bar or 16-gauge ring (⁵/₁₆ or ³/₈ inch) is usually used. The piercing should be in the base of the web, but it must not be placed deep into the *sublingual* (under the tongue) tissues. There are vital structures and vessels there, including the *sublingual vein* and *sublingual gland* (a salivary gland). You must be able to cooperate by lifting up your tongue and holding it still for the procedure. When placed correctly, this piercing usually heals quickly and easily.

Good Dentist, Good Patient

I know most dentists aren't nearly as enthusiastic about my five tongue piercings as I am, but I was fortunate to find one with an open mind who treats me with all of my metal in place. I have had panoramic X-rays, regular teeth cleanings, and even a root canal, all without removing a single bar. My hygienist even spruces them up with a bit of polish on each ball. I visit the dentist every six months, floss daily, brush regularly, and avoid clacking jewelry against my teeth or chomping on the posts. My dentist reports that my oral health is "perfect," which demonstrates that it is possible to wear multiple oral piercings without causing damage.

Lip Surfaces: Upper or Lower, Vertical or Transverse

Many individuals do not have the full, pouty lips required to support a vertical surface piercing safely and with stability. There is a likelihood of migration or rejection and a high risk of scarring with any lip surface placement. The *transverse* (horizontal) lip piercing is subject to migration or scarring due to the softness of the tissue and motion of the area.

Smiley/Scrumper and Frowny

Smiley and *scrumper* are both names for a piercing of the upper frenulum that attaches the center of the lip to the gums. Most people have only a tiny web of flesh there that is insufficient to support a sturdy piercing. Migration and rejection are obvious risks. The proximity of jewelry to the teeth and gums can lead to irritation and erosion. For the same reasons, the *frowny* (piercing of the lower lip frenulum) is also questionable.

Nonrecommended Oral Piercings

There are several placements in the tongue and oral cavity that are not advisable, and I will not perform them, though other piercers do. I would suggest you avoid the following piercings:

Cheek Piercing/Dimple

Dimples are widely regarded as an attractive facial characteristic, and some people wish to enhance their natural indentations or create dimples via piercing. Unfortunately, that region of the face contains a host of significant structures, including blood vessels, nerves, and the *parotid duct* (a conduit for a component in saliva). Piercing into any of these can be disastrous. If abandoned, this piercing can cause permanent scars and excessive dimpling of the skin.

Mandible or Sprung Piercing

The mandible is a bone, but this term refers to a vertical piercing that passes under the tongue, through the floor of the mouth, to the underside of the jaw. Due to forces of gravity and the presence of saliva, there is potential for this to become a spit drain and funnel liquid out through the piercing.

The Worst Piercing Story

In all my experience as a professional piercer since the 1980s, this is the worst thing that ever happened to anyone I pierced—and it happened to me.

On November 13, 1998, I pierced my own cheeks to mark a significant personal milestone. I placed the piercings in the natural indentations that appeared when I smiled. I had fantasized about this for years; I imagined wearing dainty, sparkling diamonds in my dimples.

I carefully marked each side. I inspected the area with a strong flashlight, and squeezed and pressed the tissue between my fingers. I didn't see or feel any anatomical structures.

My dimples are pretty far back, so it was a bit of a challenge, but I was very pleased with how they turned out. (Honestly, it didn't hurt.) During the following week I had the interesting sensation of having been smiling too much, and that was about it for discomfort.

I followed the standard care and experienced normal swelling and no bleeding. My healing course was fairly lengthy, as is expected in this area, but entirely uneventful.

The piercings took about seven months to heal, but they didn't bother me in the least. On a daily basis, people admired my unique adornments and made complimentary remarks about them. I loved the way my fancy dimples looked, and I felt at least 33.3 percent cuter with them.

About a year and a half after I did the piercings, though, the right side started to leak and I couldn't figure out why. Every once in a while a drop of clear, odorless, tasteless liquid came from the piercing, wetting my cheek. It was lighter than water and not at all viscous like saliva. I thought I might have an allergy and changed my soap and detergent. I thought I might have a jewelry problem and tried larger discs. As time wore on, the leaking became worse and actually began to drip. My cheek became sore and chapped from the liquid, and from the friction of wiping it away. I went to my dentist for help. I saw an orofacial surgeon. My parotid glands and ducts were working fine, without obstruction. That was the good news. The bad news was that at some point a portion of the parotid gland or *duct* (the tube that delivers saliva from the gland to the mouth) opened into my piercing channel. Their advice: "Take those things out."

No way.

The leaking got progressively worse. The final straw was when the liquid from my cheek dripped from my face and landed right on someone I was about to pierce. Naturally, it is not at all appropriate for a piercer to deposit personal bodily fluids in the proximity of a fresh piercing. So, with extreme reluctance, I removed the jewelry and abandoned the piercings. I was devastated to be without my fancy dimples, so I figured out a way to glue small rhinestones into place where my jewelry used to shine.

My right cheek continued to leak off and on over the ensuing months, even after I took the jewelry out. I had to try something drastic. I used a medical tool called a cautery scalpel to burn the hole shut by generating scar tissue (not a service offered at piercing studios!). That worked for a few weeks, but then the leaking started yet again. It finally sealed completely after using the cautery scalpel for the third time, creating a deeper and more severe burn.

So, when people come to me requesting cheek piercing, I share this story with them, and obviously say, "No." I will not pierce the cheek area further back than the first molars. And, for obvious reasons, you shouldn't either.

Transverse Tongue Piercing

There are nerves, veins, and arteries inside that make piercing the tongue from side to side *extremely* dangerous. Another problem is that you are almost certain to bite the jewelry. Piercees risk uncontrolled bleeding and serious, permanent damage from this piercing. Shallow or surface transverse piercings are apt to reject and scar.

Peril Perspectives

Millions of people engage in hobbies and activities like skiing, motorcycling, scuba diving, and rock climbing. Though some of these interest me, they seem unacceptably perilous to me, so I don't do them. I find my oral piercings to be rewarding and enjoyable; to me, they are worth the risks.

Lowbret and Vertical Lowbret

These are both placed as low as possible inside the lip and pierce through to the surface of the face. The lowbret is perpendicular to the tissue like a regular labret, and the vertical placement exits closer to or at the jaw line. Gum and bone erosion are likely consequences due to the limited space for jewelry at this location inside the mouth.

The Point

Because oral piercings have certain risks, they deserve due consideration. However, when your anatomy is suitable, your piercer is qualified, and you adhere to all safety guidelines, the dangers are minimized. Each person must weigh the factors and decide for himself whether it is worth it.

12

Torso Piercings:
Nipple and Navel Piercings

The torso is a large region of the body, yet its surfaces proffer anatomy suitable for only a few piercing placements. These common piercings are extremely popular and rather complex.

The Navel Piercing

- **Healing time:** 6 to 9 months or longer
- **Initial jewelry style:** Curved bar or J-curve; in certain circumstances a ring
- **Initial jewelry gauge:** Minimum 14 gauge; sometimes 12 gauge and occasionally 10 gauge
- **Initial jewelry size:** Curved bar diameters ³/₈ to ½ inch, with ⁷/₁₆ inch most common; ring diameters ⁷/₁₆ or ½ inch.

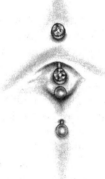

A navel with a jeweled navel curve in the traditional central placement and a curved bar on the bottom

Like the ear, the navel has become an acceptable place for adornment. Unlike the earlobe, however, navel piercings are not quick and easy to heal. Ironically this enormously popular piercing takes longer to heal than any other.

The abdomen is *avascular* (lacks blood supply), which causes slow healing.[1] It is also subject to stress from normal movement of the body and friction from clothing. Navel piercings have developed the reputation for being troublesome, in part because of their popularity with teens who lack the education or dedication to provide proper care during the extended healing time. They are also inclined to wear junk jewelry that can be disastrous for healing. Teenage girls have been the primary recipients of navel piercings, but women of all ages and men can—and do—get them.

Navel Piercing: Placement and Choice of Jewelry

A navel piercing frames the tissue surrounding the *umbilicus* (navel) at the epicenter of the body. Navel anatomy differs substantially from one individual to the next, but many piercers fail to take these differences into account. A superior piercer will carefully assess your structure and suggest placement and jewelry to suit your unique build.

Most people have a fold of tissue on the top of the navel, and a vertical piercing is placed through it, in the center. If your tissue is inflexible the procedure can be hard to perform, and the piercing will be more at risk for migration and rejection. If your navel area is flat, there is no lip, and the skin is not supple, pierce a different site.

Prior to the piercing, the size and configuration of your navel must be evaluated while you are standing and reclining. On some people the shape and dimensions of the area transform dramatically with the change in position, and this has to be considered when marking placement and selecting jewelry size. For success, the piercing must be situated so that your body will accommodate the jewelry in all common postures.

Many piercees want a skinny little belly ring. The problem is that the body seldom tolerates this splinterlike invasion for long. Plenty of piercers use jewelry that is inappropriately small and place it too close to the surface. These shallow piercings may remain viable for a time. However, there is a risk of the tissue cutting or tearing when thin rings are worn, and these will more frequently migrate and reject than piercings placed at the correct depth with appropriate jewelry.

Navel Piercing: Bar or Ring?

The piercing placement and initial jewelry style are more closely interrelated for navel piercings than for many others. Depending on your build, the shape of jewelry that is first inserted—whether ring or bar—could be the one you must always wear. Ring-style jewelry gained early favor as the navel ornament of choice simply because it was the design most readily available. The belly piercing craze preceded the availability of curved bars—and even the mass production of body jewelry. Nowadays, curved bars are the preferred initial jewelry style for most navels. If your abdomen is relatively flat or your navel is not deep, bar-style jewelry is best.

If your navel is deep and has a distinct lip, a ring may be used for a vertical piercing. On navels with this shape, a diameter of $7/16$ or $1/2$ inch is most common. A $3/8$-inch ring should be used only if you have a petite, but perfectly defined, lobe-shaped navel. When a ring is used as initial jewelry for a vertical navel piercing, the bottom must be pierced well away from the edge to keep the ring from protruding too much. But, if you change to a bar later, the bottom ball will be hidden inside your navel. This may be uncomfortable and not aesthetically pleasing.

If you are among the minority of people who have a flap only on the bottom of your navel, you must consult a piercer to see if you are a candidate for a piercing there. A bar is the preferred jewelry for lower-navel placement.

Bar-style jewelry must be long enough to accommodate the expansion of tissue when you recline. Generally an extra post length of $1/16$ to $1/8$ inch (added to the size needed when you're standing) is ample.

Navel Piercing: Jeweled Navel Bars and J-Curves

Curved barbells set with sparkly crystals, synthetic stones, or genuine gems are among the most popular styles of jewelry worn in vertical navel piercings. There are several basic varieties (curved bar, jeweled navel curve, and J-curve) and innumerable variations. See chapter 9, "Jeweled Navel Curve" (page 72) and "J-Curve" (page 73) for photos and more information.

The jut of the J-curve projects the bottom adornment forward to make it more visible and also prevents it from resting inside your navel. This reduces irritation and allows for better circulation and comfort. This style is excellent if your navel piercing is deep on the underside.

Navel Piercing: Weight and Weight Loss

Regardless of your weight, if your navel folds in and disappears when you sit down, this is a good reason to select a different piercing. Wearing jewelry on this type of build causes mechanical stresses that guarantee healing complications. If you have a horizontal crease across the area even when you are standing, you are unsuited to navel piercing for the same reason. Some heavy people are still able to get navel piercings because body size isn't as key a factor as your configuration in the area of the piercing. However, the diminished blood supply caused by excess abdominal fat does make healing more difficult. If you are diabetic and carry excess weight in this area, navel piercings are inadvisable because complications are to be expected and can be more serious.

If you are planning to lose weight, the overall shape of your navel area is still the primary consideration when deciding whether to postpone piercing. A protruding beer belly is generally suited to navel piercing because usually the area gets smaller with weight loss, but maintains the same basic contour.

Extremely rapid weight gain or loss during healing could cause irritation if the abdomen changes shape quickly enough to prevent the piercing from settling. It is unlikely that a weight fluctuation could impact a healed navel piercing, however, unless it is substantial enough to alter the shape or location of your navel.

Navel Piercing: Angled Navel Placement

You are unsuited to a traditional vertical navel piercing if your navel is formed with an asymmetrical or horizontal orientation, or if it has no pliable flap at the center. Placing a piercing at an angle is an alternative if you have acceptable anatomy with malleable tissue on the side. When the piercing is set at a distinct slant, a ring will rest against your abdomen and frame the area beautifully; it will feel comfortable, look integrated with your body, and rest flush to avoid friction and trauma. If it is only slightly offset from center, the piercing will end up looking crooked and awkward. Depending on build, bar-style jewelry may not be aesthetically pleasing in this type of placement.

An asymmetrical build with a ring in an angled navel placement

Many shapes and types of anatomy can be pierced safely and heal well using an angled placement. If you have a tiny navel, minimal tissue, or a scar or small hernia in the region, you might be able to take advantage of this variation. You may have a symmetrical build that can support a matching piercing on each side. Or, you might be able to wear multiple piercings on one side (though they should not be performed in the same session if they are close together). Unfortunately not all piercers are versed in this option.

Navel Piercing: "Outie" Anatomy

A protruding *outie* navel is fundamentally unsuited to piercing. I have never perforated one, but some piercers do, and this is referred to as a *true navel piercing*. A hardened outie that is scarlike may be a remnant of your umbilical cord. There is some chance it could be connected to the interior of your abdomen and internal organs. An infection of an outie piercing could travel rapidly to your *peritoneum* (membrane lining the abdominal cavity) or your internal organs, presenting serious health risks.[2] This tissue tends to be quite recessed on most people, but if you do have a protruding outie, consider carefully whether the risks are acceptable to you.

The outie that is softer and pushes in easily is probably an umbilical hernia. Some of your intestines can poke through this type of herniation, which is a weakness or hole in the abdominal lining near your navel.[3] If this tissue is pierced, there is a possibly of puncturing your small intestine, which could obviously be extremely serious. If there is a flap of skin above the protrusion, it could be pierceable, if it is distant enough from your hernia. A combination "innie-outie" structure is generally unsuited to vertical placement. An experienced piercer can determine if the tissue surrounding your outie presents any safe options for piercing.

Navel Piercing: Altered Anatomy

In today's body-conscious society, the *abdominoplasty* (tummy tuck) is more popular than ever. Unfortunately, post-surgical anatomy often can't or shouldn't be pierced. Incisions result in scar tissue, and these are not welcoming places for piercing. During a full abdominoplasty, the navel is cut free from its original position and then sutured into a new location.[4] The skin is often pulled so taut that it cannot possibly be pinched up, making piercing physically impossible. Even if the tissue has been formed into a lip-shaped fold, it is less vascular and much harder to heal. If you wish to show off an ornamented and surgically flattened midriff and find a piercer willing to attempt it, flexible plastic is preferable to metal jewelry.

Laparoscopy is another prevalent medical procedure involving small incisions created to insert instruments for exploratory and microsurgical purposes. The navel is a frequent site for these incisions. Most often, the cut is made on the bottom of the navel so it does not interfere with traditionally placed navel piercings. If an incision has been made on the portion of the navel you wish to have pierced, the scarring will need to be evaluated by a piercer. When there is a minimum of scar tissue, piercing is often possible. Occasionally a surgical scar does not heal correctly and continues to secrete fluid. Navels with weeping, active scars are potential passageways for bacteria to travel into the abdominal cavity; they should not be pierced.

Stretch marks are a form of scarring caused by stretching and tearing of the skin. They are frequently present in the region of the navel and they are weaker than other skin, so it is best to avoid them. Piercing near a stretch mark is preferable to going right through it because of the increased risk of migration or rejection.

Navel Piercing: Procedure

For navel piercing, pants are often unzipped and your shirt must be tucked up, but you should not have to remove your clothing and bare your entire torso unless you've worn a bodysuit. I perform navel piercings using the forceps method while you are in a supine or semireclining position. If your skin is especially taut, extra tissue manipulation can gently improve its suppleness. Also, having you sit up a little (rather than stretched out flat) can make it easier to grasp the tissue and apply the clamp.

Some people have sensitive navels, but many piercees experience nothing more intense than discomfort from the piercing. "It just felt like pressure," and, "It was a pinch," are common descriptions of the sensation. A few piercees report that cleaning is the worst part of the process because it tickles.

When compared to most other piercings, navels are less prone to bleeding, but the ones that do bleed might heal more rapidly. A superior blood supply makes it easier for your body to bring nutrients and oxygen to the region and process a wound.[5]

> **Painful Mistake**
> Before you are pierced, your piercer should check the marks while you are reclining *and* standing. An unfortunate man whose piercer skipped this important step once came to me for help. He was nearly doubled over by jewelry that constricted his abdomen. The width of his piercing required jewelry that was twice the diameter of the ring that his piercer had inserted!

Navel Piercing: Healing and Troubleshooting

Because the navel is challenging to heal, it is imperative that every aspect of this piercing is handled optimally. The navel is no more prone to infection than other piercings; however, it is more likely than many others to become irritated. It also has the longest healing period, so it has a wider window of time for potential infection.

Piercees and medical professionals alike frequently see a normal, healing navel that has become irritated and pronounce it infected. Some discoloration (pinkish, brownish, or purplish), secretion of clear or cloudy fluids, and *induration* (hardening of tissue) can all be present in a normal healing navel piercing. A misdiagnosis of infection is especially unproductive when you are prescribed a course of antibiotics: your irritation will not be resolved, and the real cause of the problem will not be addressed.

Wear low-rise pants or loose, breathable garments to prevent clothing from rubbing against the piercing and to allow for good air circulation. Sometimes a change as simple as switching to the fetal position for sleeping will help diminish irritation. The solutions aren't always complex.

Navel Piercing: Migration and Rejection

If your navel tissue is very taut you are more likely to suffer from these complications. See your piercer to check the fit of your jewelry, and consider trying a flexible plastic substitute. Sometimes, however, nothing will help, and all you can do is contemplate your navel with disappointment.

Navel Piercing: Bumps

Complications arise when you sleep on your stomach, wear clothing that is tight over the piercing, or have an abdomen that creases near the jewelry when you sit. Keeping the area dry is challenging, and this contributes to healing problems. Friction, pressure, and moisture can cause problems including a bump, lump, tenderness, swelling, redness, and delayed healing.

An unattractive, scary-looking growth can form at one or both openings of your piercing due to irritation. If it is dark red and resembles raw hamburger, you probably have a *granuloma*. It may not be as sore as it looks, but it might bleed easily or drain clear fluid. Navels are more prone to granulomas than most other body piercings. They are not always indicative of a need to give up on your piercing (though your doctor is apt to tell you otherwise); some piercings heal successfully following a bout or two with such growths. You must determine whether your irritation is from jewelry that is of poor quality or improperly sized or shaped, or perhaps from other external forces. That factor must be adjusted if you are to have any chance of healing.

Sometimes performing four to six saline soaks daily will result in an improvement of bumps, irritation, or troubled healing. See chapter 16, "Trouble and Troubleshooting," for more details on granulomas and other types of healing problems.

Navel Piercing: Ups and Downs

Throughout healing, all piercings tend to go through cycles of getting better and then regressing. These phases are especially characteristic of navel piercings and one of the reasons patience is vital for healing. Even if you experience some trouble-free periods during your healing, continue with the aftercare protocols for at least six months.

Navel Piercing: Exercise and Activity

Of all the body piercings, navels are most vulnerable to stresses caused by physical activity. Because the abdomen is so affected by the movement of the torso, this piercing is extremely challenging for active individuals to heal. During your entire healing period you should be cautious with movements that affect your upper body. To work out your abdominal muscles, especially during initial healing, avoid full sit-ups. Perform only controlled partial crunches or do exercises that simply contract the muscles with minimal movement of the body. Physical impact to the area must be limited for the piercing to heal. To prevent injury to your piercing during exercise or sports, wear a plastic eye patch over the piercing (see "Protective Patch," page 187).

Sexual activity can be perilous to your navel piercing due to friction on the wound and the potential for contamination from your partner's bodily fluids. Application of a waterproof bandage before sexual encounters is helpful for preventing problems.

Navel Piercing: Changing Jewelry

You should not change your own navel jewelry for about the first six months, though if you are wearing a style with removable beads or balls, those can be switched at any time. Should your initial jewelry be causing problems, visit your piercer to have it replaced as soon as possible. In as little as four months, a professional piercer might change the jewelry to another piece still suited for the healing phase, *if* the piercing appears to be doing well. You must avoid wearing elaborate body jewelry until the piercing is completely settled. Healing navels are touchy enough without the added weight, motion, and potential for catching that come with large or dangling jewelry.

Navel Piercing: Stretching

Once a navel piercing is seasoned (at least a year), it can be stretched up one gauge. After you wear the larger size for nine months or longer, if you have a substantial amount of tissue between the entry and exit holes, you may be able to stretch again. Enlarging beyond 14 gauge is not advisable if your piercing is close to the surface.

Navels are rarely sites for jumbo jewelry, but with an adequate amount of pierced tissue and very slow stretching, they can safely be enlarged up to 2 gauge or so.

Navel Piercing: Retiring

If you wish to abandon an unhealed navel piercing, it is best to do so when it is not irritated, infected, or needing to drain. Navel piercings frequently leave a fairly visible scar, and this tends to be amplified if you have difficulties healing. The residual mark may benefit from a scar-reduction product (see page 211). Refer to "Navel Piercings and Pregnancy," page 253, for questions about having a baby when your belly is pierced.

Your piercing might not seal up if it is abandoned after healing is over. The hole will tend to shrink, but full closure is not always dependent upon the duration a piercing was worn. Some navel piercings that are established for many years will shut after jewelry removal, and others that are in for a year or less may remain permanently viable. Navel piercings that are very shallow but fully healed have a tendency to remain open. There is no health risk or medical necessity to wear jewelry in the channel, even if it doesn't seal shut; the matter is purely aesthetic.

The Point

Despite the lengthy healing period, navel piercings can be very rewarding. They make a stunning accent to an attractive abdomen, and many women enjoy showing them off, to the delight of piercing fans. Ironically, they've become so popular that some people decide against getting one because of their prevalence. Piercing is a personal decision, and because they are widespread is no reason to deny yourself one if you want it.

The Nipple Piercing

While the piercings discussed so far are basically the same for either gender, male and female nipples serve different functions and are generally dissimilar in size. The aspects of nipple piercing that differ, therefore, will be described separately.

- **Healing times:**
  - Male nipples, 3 to 4 months or longer
  - Female nipples, 6 to 9 months or longer
- **Initial jewelry style:** Ring or straight barbell
- **Initial jewelry gauge:** 14 gauge minimum, 12 gauge for rougher play or larger anatomy, and 10 gauge only on highly developed anatomy
- **Initial jewelry size:** Highly anatomy-dependent. For barbells, 1/16 to 1/8 inch should be added to the post.
  - For men, minimum ring diameter usually 9/16 inch, but 1/2 inch may be suitable for small nipples that are not flat.
  - For women, minimum ring diameter 5/8 inch, 3/4 inch is common, and larger is sometimes used.

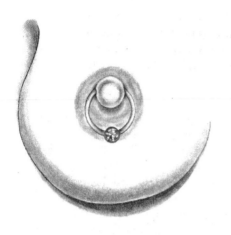

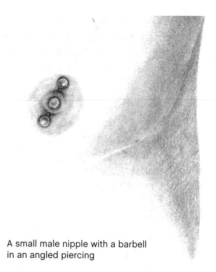

A well-developed female nipple with a ring in a horizontal piercing

A small male nipple with a barbell in an angled piercing

The contrast of metal jewelry through the flesh of a nipple is truly exotic and striking. Nipple piercing defines the region, frames the tissue, and makes the nipple stand at attention (though it doesn't necessarily cause the nipple to remain erect at all times). Prior to the early 1990s, when navel piercings became popular, nipples were the most prevalent location for body piercings.

Modern piercing enthusiasts—particularly in the gay and SM subcultures—explored the erotic potential of their bodies and started what has become the current style of nipple piercing. These days, people from all walks of life are experiencing the delights of this piercing. For some, it is simply an aesthetic preference or fashion statement; for others it reigns as a favorite in the realm of sexual and sensual pleasures.

Nipple Piercing: Placement and Choice of Jewelry

Virtually all adults' nipples—even tiny flat ones—are pierceable if they are pliable. Whether you prefer the angle of your piercing to be horizontal, vertical, or somewhere in between, it will work best if it is placed in the natural creases of your tissue. Depending on the shape of your chest, the "horizontal" placement may be more visually appealing if the outer side is placed just slightly higher than the inner side. This will barely tilt the ring up at a slant that frames the area nicely. A true horizontal placement can look a little droopy at the outer edge, depending on the angle and shape of the breasts or pectoral muscles.

If you have well-developed nipples, the piercing should be placed in the creases at the base of the nipple where it rises from the areola. If your nipple is defined with substantial height, the piercing can safely go in as little as 5/16 inch of tissue. If you have flat nipples, the piercing should encompass a minimum of 3/8 inch of tissue when the area is relaxed. If your nipples are relatively featureless, without an elevated tip, the tissue in the visual center of the nipple should be pierced so that the jewelry will rest evenly within your areola. (The piercing routinely extends into the areola, especially on men, but this is still considered a nipple piercing.) If you have elliptical or odd-shaped areolas, it is sometimes best to cheat one side of the piercing a little further from the tip of your nipple in order to have the ring appear more centered in the pigmented area. If you want a pair of piercings and you have large, protruding nipples that are uneven in size, is it sometimes best to pierce at the natural base of each nipple rather than making one piercing shallower (or deeper) in an attempt to make them match.

You may like the accent of a ring or bar in a single nipple piercing, or prefer the symmetrical appearance of adorning both sides. If you wish to have a pair of nipple piercings, you may wonder if it is preferable to do one and let it heal before adding the second, or to pierce both nipples during the same session. One advantage to having them done at once is that your piercings are complete after a single studio visit and healing period. Also, depending on the skill of your piercer and the amount of alteration in your tissue as a result of piercing, which can be substantial, it is easier to get more symmetrical results if you have them both marked and performed in the same session. Then again, an advantage to sequential piercings is that you will still have one nipple to play with while the other is mending.

Women may find that their nipples are more sensitive just prior to menstruating. Take this into consideration when scheduling a nipple piercing.

> **Tribal Nipple Piercing**
>
> The Karankawa, a now-extinct Native American tribe who lived along the Gulf Coast of Texas, widely practiced nipple piercing. Their healing abilities were impressive considering that they smeared their bodies with a mixture of dirt and alligator grease to repel mosquitoes.[6]

Nipple Piercing Jewelry: Rings or Bars?

Rings were the standard initial jewelry style for nipple piercings for many years. Over time they acquired a reputation as being bad for healing, but this is because piercers often insert jewelry that is too small in diameter. When you wear a hoop, the part of it that passes through your piercing must be relatively straight. If the ring is too snug, it will pinch your tissue at the entry and exit and cause irritation, discomfort, and healing problems. Piercees are frequently surprised that a safe diameter for a nipple ring is much larger than they had imagined. When properly sized, both bars and rings can be suitable options in traditionally placed nipple piercings. For nonhorizontal placements, barbells are superior.

Your jewelry, whether ring or bar, must have some extra space for the tissue to relax to its widest natural state, and to allow for swelling or tissue *development* (see "Nipple Piercing: Post-Piercing Nipple Development," page 131). To accommodate a piercing that measures just ³/₈ inch across, a ¹/₂-inch diameter ring will be too small if there is average development.

Multiple Nipple Piercings

A nipple can be pierced only once in a session; however, after healing, depending on its configuration and dimensions, it may be pierceable a second time. Few nipples are substantial enough to accommodate

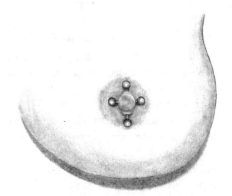

A double pierced nipple with barbells forming an *iron cross*

more than two piercings. Typical arrangements include two horizontal piercings (ordinarily moving closer toward the body for subsequent piercing), a cross shape (usually with a horizontal piercing in front and a vertical behind it), or an X shape formed by two diagonal piercings. Exceptional skill is required to accurately place additional holes in an already-pierced nipple.

Piercing Inverted Nipples

When performed on appropriate candidates, nipple piercing can be a revolutionary cure for inverted nipples. If the tissue can be coaxed out and pinched up, then it can probably be pierced. The jewelry blocks the nipple from returning to its retracted state. However, the tissue can fight against the jewelry. If this pressure is too forceful, migration is likely. Rings have a tendency to stand up and *salute* rather than rest flat against the chest, so barbells are superior. Because of the extra stress placed on the tissue, flexible plastic may be better for healing, and 12 gauge should be considered the minimum rather than 14 gauge, if the tissue is sufficient to accommodate it. The full alteration may not be seen until metal jewelry is inserted later.

Nipple Piercing: Procedure

All undergarments and clothing above the waist need to be removed for nipple piercings. You may be in a position anywhere from seated to reclining flat, depending on the preference of your piercer and the furniture in the piercing room. I use forceps to perform nipple piercings. For your comfort and to make the procedure easier, I do tissue manipulation prior to the application of the clamps, and provide more than usual for tight skin or underdeveloped nipples. If the forceps are especially difficult to apply, then more manipulation is in order.

Some studios offer *tandem piercings*, in which both nipples are pierced simultaneously by two synchronized piercers. This is an excellent method if you are planning to pierce both sides and you are concerned about being able to tolerate the procedure. One of the piercers may mark the placement for both nipples to assure symmetry. Nipple sensitivity is dramatically different from person to person. If you have tender nipples, it's all the more important to seek an accomplished technician; it will make a big impact on your comfort.

Nipple Piercing: Healing and Troubleshooting

Tenderness may come and go due to the fit of clothing, sleep habits, physical activities, and other factors. Women often find that nipple piercings experience a *flare-up* (secrete, swell, or become painful) just prior to and during menstruation, even well after the healing period.

Nipple piercings can take a long time to heal completely. They may regress for no apparent reason after many months of stability. Should your piercing take an excessively long time to settle, try different jewelry or change care regimens until you figure out what works best. This experimentation can require patience, but adjust at least one aspect before giving up. If you endured the procedure and some of the healing period, it is worth preserving the piercing.

You will probably find that the support of an undershirt for men or smooth-cup bra or sports bra for women is helpful for your comfort and protection, including while you sleep. A minute or two after settling into a tight garment, the piercing usually feels less tender. Men who are not partial to sleeping in a shirt can wrap a length of clean Ace bandage across the chest and around the body. This type of elastic bandage protects the area while still allowing it to breathe, and it avoids adhesives that could irritate skin or pull hair upon removal. A disposable nursing pad or cut-to-fit piece of panty liner worn inside a bra will absorb any blood or sweat and will also help to conceal your jewelry.

Nipple Piercing: Tightness Is Normal

Many piercees worry that something is wrong with a nipple piercing because the jewelry won't move easily. Nipple tissue is normally tight; the jewelry will seldom swing freely even in a piercing that is many years old. You must pay attention to your body; if the piercing feels too tight, go easy on it. See "Catching the Tube," page 214, for an explanation of the damage that can result from forcing your jewelry to move.

Nipple Piercing: Post-Piercing Nipple Development

Certain piercings are subject to swelling after the procedure. Nipples, however, are prone to *development* (a semipermanent or lasting change in the shape, dimensions, and texture of the localized nipple and areola tissue). This is often mistaken for swelling, though it is actually quite different. Development is most common in male nipples or underdeveloped female nipples, and the change can be relatively dramatic. In essence, the nipple grows in response to the stimulus of the jewelry and the piercing. When the piercing is placed in the natural creases of the body, this development is usually attractive and well formed. If the piercing is not made in the proper spot, however, the tissue can develop a blobby, awkward appearance. These changes may not dissipate even if the jewelry is removed; think about whether this is acceptable before getting a nipple piercing. While common, this is not a universal response to nipple piercing.

Nipple Piercing: Concealment

Male nipple piercings may be discernible under a lightweight white dress shirt, but adding an undershirt does a lot to diminish the visibility of average-sized jewelry. For women, wearing any but the sheerest bra will usually make it difficult to see nipple jewelry through clothing.

A captive cylinder or tube helps to diminish the visibility of nipple rings through clothing

Using a cylinder-shaped bead instead of a round one in your captive ring can eliminate the appearance of a second nipple protruding below your own. Snug-fitting barbells capped by small balls or discs are effective for concealment under clothing in most situations.

Nipple Piercing: Breast Health

There is no medical evidence that piercings increase the risk of cancer. Kelly Shanahan, MD, chair of the Department of Obstetrics and Gynecology at Barton Memorial Hospital in Lake Tahoe, states, "I am aware of no evidence that nipple piercing increases the risk of breast cancer."[7]

Nipple piercings will in no way interfere with breast exams or self-examinations. In fact, they may even remind you to pay attention to your breasts. They might also encourage a partner to assist you with regular breast exams.

Health-care personnel routinely require that all metal be removed from the area prior to a mammogram or other medical procedure. See your piercer for a nonmetallic jewelry alternative such as acrylic or inert plastic to keep your piercing open.

Nipple Piercing: Surgical Considerations

If you have undergone surgery such as breast reduction or augmentation, you still might be able to have your nipples pierced; however, it is essential to wait until you are thoroughly healed from an operation. You might experience gratifying results from nipple piercing if you have diminished sensation from breast surgery. If you have implants, use sound judgment when selecting a piercer and strictly comply with all post-piercing guidelines. The risks are more serious: an infection from the piercing can spread to your implant. This could require surgical intervention and may result in the loss of your augmentation.

If you have undergone radical breast surgery and reconstruction with nipple replacement using non-areolar tissue, you are generally not a good candidate. Piercing might be possible if the donor tissue is a type that heals easily, such as labial skin. An expert piercer and your surgeon should both be consulted. Under these circumstances, it is prudent to wait for a year following surgery before considering nipple piercing.

If you are scheduled to undergo surgery in which your nipples will be entirely or partially removed and repositioned, it is advisable to leave in a nonmetal jewelry alternative so the tissue can be reattached with the piercing at the appropriate angle. More than one piercee has awakened from surgery to find a previously horizontal piercing had become vertical. If necessary, have your surgeon discuss the matter with a trusted piercer.

Nipple Piercing: Breastfeeding

Nipple piercings do not ordinarily prevent breastfeeding. For detailed information, see "Nipple Piercing and Breastfeeding," page 253.

Nipple Piercing: Inflammation and Infection

Sometimes during initial healing a hardened lump will form behind the nipple or areola in conjunction with localized swelling. This is not unusual, and it does not always imply you're having a complication. If the bump exists in the absence of other signs of infection, there is little cause for alarm. Look for symptoms described on page 203, "Identifying Minor Localized Infection," and page 205, "Identifying an Abscess." If the bump is not accompanied by any of these other indications, keep watch over the area. This type of lump is often a temporary inflammatory process that resolves spontaneously. If saline soaks do not relieve it and it does not dissipate in two weeks—even if it does not worsen—visit your doctor. **If you have a health condition that would cause an infection to be of exceptional concern, see your doctor right away.**

Nipple Piercing: Migration and Rejection

When piercings migrate, they usually move directly outward from the body, but nipple piercings sometimes rise or twist instead. If you swap to inert plastic jewelry at the first sign of trouble, this may help stop the progression. If you are large-breasted, your bra may press against the lower portion of ring-style jewelry. This can result in the ring being forced away from your body, causing irritation and migration. A simple solution is to wear your ring flipped up inside your bra instead of hanging down. This maneuver changes the stresses on the area and can make all the difference for your comfort and healing. Wearing barbells is a good alternative.

Nipple Piercing: Changing Jewelry

Some piercees are comfortable changing their own nipple jewelry once the piercing has healed. This is not particularly challenging for the deft, though the tightness of the skin can make moving your existing jewelry difficult. Try a warm water soak or compress to loosen the tissue first, and use sterile jelly or emu oil for lubrication.

Don't dally in the middle of a jewelry change; nipple piercings are notorious for being among the quickest to shrink and the most difficult to reinsert once left empty, even momentarily. If you run into trouble, an insertion taper can help you to open the channel and stretch the piercing enough to reinsert jewelry. Unless you feel sure about what you're doing, it is best to visit your piercer for help.

Nipple Piercing: Stretching

Nipple piercings are not easy to stretch, and the tissue responds irritably if you attempt to expand too quickly. Wait a minimum of nine months to a year from the initial piercing, and don't force it or you are more likely to end up with a rejected piercing than a larger gauge. An enlarging schedule of one gauge per year is a steady pace. A double stretch (from 14 to 10 gauge, for example) is seldom possible, even if the piercing has been healed for many years. Unless the next size slides right in without pushing and the thicker one does not need to be forced, keep to the one-size-at-a-time plan. With time and patience, however, nipples can be stretched to very large sizes.

Nipple Piercing: Retiring

Expect some permanent modification to the area from piercing your nipple. If you have had tissue development, much or all of it may remain, even if you abandon the piercing. A divot at the entry and exit may be the only lasting marks if you do not experience tissue changes.

Do not impulsively remove nipple jewelry. Many a piercee has returned to me over a closed nipple piercing they wished they'd left in place. It is much easier to keep in an existing nipple piercing than to get a reinsertion or repiercing later.

The Point

Nipple piercing is a favorite among many well-adorned body art fans. Healing this area sometimes requires patience, but you will probably find it well worth the effort. A piercing in your nipple can highlight the area in an enticing way and may add a whole new dimension of sensation and enjoyment. The subject of physical pleasure leads us right into the next chapter.

Below the Belt:
Female and Male Genital Piercings

Disclaimer: This chapter openly discusses adult matters including male and female genital anatomy and sexual function. Intimate piercings are not available to minors; these sections are thus not intended for individuals under eighteen years of age.

The first section in this chapter covers introductory information relevant to both male and female genital piercings. The next section covers female genital piercing, followed by male genital piercing. For more information about genital piercings, see chapter 20, "Sex!"

Our Western culture does not foster genital pride, so many people feel disconnected from their nether regions. Intimate piercings encourage self-awareness and often educate piercees about their own bodies. Countless women have come to me saying, "I want my clit pierced." When I show them a photograph of a clitoris piercing, they shout, "Oh, no! Not *there*." What they actually want is a piercing of the *clitoral hood* (tissue above the clitoris), but they are not sufficiently acquainted with the territory or terminology to know the difference.

If you don't comprehend the attraction to below-the-waist piercings, don't ridicule them or underestimate their pleasures; learn about them instead. If they are of interest, there is much to know, so read on.

Genital Piercing: Selecting the Right Piercer

Genital piercing is special because there is the potential to affect your sexual pleasure. A poorly placed piercing can result in a missed opportunity for enhancement or even a temporary or permanent loss of sensation. Because of variations in genital anatomy and personal preferences for sexual stimulation, each piercee must be evaluated (and even counseled) on an individual basis before deciding on a genital piercing.

Locate an experienced professional who has had specific training in placing and performing genital piercings, and who can communicate with you openly. The right piercer will have a professional manner that helps you feel comfortable and safe.

Your piercer must be able to undertake her role with sensitivity, and you must be prepared to honestly describe what you expect from your piercing. Many piercers simply do not have enough knowledge to guide you and cannot determine, for instance, whether a certain placement is more simulating or ornamental. A good piercer will have an in-depth conversation with you to be sure that you have all the education you need to make an informed decision about your piercing. Don't settle for a piercer who does not impress you with her vast knowledge and outstanding qualifications.

In order to place piercings properly, your piercer must scrutinize your genitals and may need to do some stretching, tugging, and pinching of your tissue to take a close look for veins or other vital structures. For accurate placement, the area must be marked, and then the skin may need to be moved. For men, the tissue may have to be pulled taut (as it is when you are erect), and if you have a foreskin, it may need to be retracted. If you are a novice piercee you might misconstrue these activities as being sexual in nature, but these procedures are invaluable for accurate placement. Nonetheless, always listen to your intuition. It is appropriate to call off your piercing if you believe your piercer is behaving unprofessionally.

Genital Piercing: How Much Does It Hurt?

Simply the thought of genital piercings is enough to cause many people to reflexively slam their knees together, but—contrary to what the uninitiated usually think—intimate piercings are not especially painful. You should anticipate feeling well; however, you probably won't want to wriggle into your tightest pair of jeans that day.

Many of my clients have compared the intensity of getting a genital piercing as similar to that of getting an earlobe piercing. Exceptions include ampallangs, apadravyas, dydoes, and the serious (though rare) clitoris piercing. These are more intense spots, but getting them pierced can also be very rewarding.

Genital Piercing: Bleeding

Just like any other piercing or break in the skin, a new genital piercing may bleed, off and on, for a few minutes to a few days. Certain placements have a tendency to flow, which is addressed in the sections covering each piercing.

Following any genital piercing, men and women are advised to either get bandaged (men see "Male Genital Piercings: Bleeding," page 155) or wear a panty liner or sanitary pad to protect clothing, car seats, and home furnishings. You may not bleed immediately, but once you stand and the force of gravity takes effect, it often begins. Men and women can both use panty liners or sanitary pads throughout healing. Initially, they absorb blood and help to cushion the piercing; later, they also help to keep it clean and dry.

Placed opposite your jewelry inside your underwear, napkins or liners can be helpful for any genital piercing. They come in a wide variety of thicknesses, sizes, and designs. To maintain hygiene, keep dirty fingers away from the surface that will rest against your body; handle it only from the back or the edges. First pull up your underwear to your knees, and then stick the pad or liner into place to avoid contaminating it with your feet or shoes.

If you experience heavy bleeding, you may benefit from a potentially embarrassing purchase: disposable adult diapers. They are extremely absorbent and can help prevent messy accidents, especially overnight, because they can handle a much large volume of blood than any pad.

Genital Piercing: Underwear and Hygiene

Tighter undergarments help to hold your jewelry in place, thereby reducing discomfort and tissue trauma. The extra layer of fabric is helpful for maintaining cleanliness, and, of course, it is hard to wear a sanitary pad or liner without some underwear to which you can attach it. Cotton fabric is more absorbent and permits better air circulation than synthetics. Make sure your underwear has no holes or loose threads to snag your jewelry. Yanking your skivvies down when they are caught on your ring or bar can damage—or even tear out—a genital piercing.

If you accidentally step on the crotch of your underwear and then pull them up against your piercing, this is about as filthy as putting your open wound on the floor! When you don your undies, make plenty of room for your feet, especially if you are already wearing shoes.

During healing, always wear underwear or clothing, or put down a clean towel before you sit on a questionable surface. See "Safer Sex," page 255, for important information about maintaining hygiene while healing a genital piercing.

Genital Piercing: Urinating

Bodily fluids are apt to get on certain genital piercings, which is not a problem—*if* they are your own. Urine is one of man's first antiseptics and, if you are healthy, your own liquid waste will not harm your piercing. The regular passage of urine over the jewelry helps to minimize crusting, too. Urine can sting during the first few days of healing, so drink lots of water. This dilutes the urine and lowers the acidity, which minimizes discomfort. Cranberry juice or large quantities of orange juice or vitamin C will make your urine acidic,[1] which may cause excess discomfort. Additionally, you can pour a clean cup of water—warm or cool, as you prefer—over the area as you urinate. This rinses off the urine so it doesn't linger uncomfortably, and the water feels soothing.

Shaving and Trimming

Shaving or trimming your pubic hair before visiting a studio for a genital piercing is a good idea. Not only will it help your piercer by making it easier for her to see what she is doing, but it might also make the experience easier on yourself, since having your pubic hair accidentally pulled during a procedure can be more uncomfortable than getting the piercing itself.

Shaving with a new genital piercing in place can prove a little tricky at first. Let the piercing heal for several weeks before shaving close to it. Once the piercing is healed, some jewelry (such as outer labia or scrotum rings) can actually be used as handles to hold the tissue taut while you shave. See "Shaving," page 250, for more tips.

Female Genital Piercings

Below is general information about female genital piercings, followed by a detailed discussion of each of the most common placements.

Female Genital Piercing: Anatomy

Female genitals are formed with tremendous—though sometimes subtle—variations. Not all women are able to get every genital piercing placement. In fact, some women with small hoods and inner labia are built only for outer labia piercings. Most women are not configured for a triangle piercing, and many are poorly shaped for a horizontal hood piercing. Everyone is different; heed the advice of an expert, and don't take it personally if the piercing you want doesn't anatomically suit you.

Female Genital Piercing: Hills and Valleys

This terminology helps us to identify and discuss two basic shapes of female genital anatomy. These builds could also be described as *innie* and *outie*, but I'll reserve those terms for navels. If you are built with a *valley*, you have outer labia that are higher than your hood. You have a very vertical shape and are poorly suited to horizontal piercings; the jewelry would twist when you close your legs. You lack sufficient hood tissue to support a horizontal piercing or have too much outer labia and surrounding skin, which would interfere with horizontal jewelry.

If you are built with a *hill*, you have a hood that is substantial, and higher than your outer labia. You may be a better candidate for horizontal piercings, depending on the configuration of your hood. Even though women with hills are better suited to horizontal piercings than those with valleys, some still opt for vertical placement, or both.

Female Genital Piercing: The Startle of the Stick

Even if your piercer guides you to breathe deeply and you know a piercing is about to happen, the stick may startle you, causing you to jump or move. An experienced piercer will anticipate this, but it is also good for *you* to prepare yourself by being aware that this is a common response. Try to keep your knees apart so your piercer can put in your jewelry and finish the job.

Female Genital Piercing: Hypersensitivity

In the event you ultimately feel your genital piercing is too intense, you can change the jewelry to a different size or style. This is not a frequent problem, but if you still have discomfort, the jewelry can be removed with no permanent changes to your sensation. See "Overstimulation, Sensation, and Desensitization," page 257, for related information.

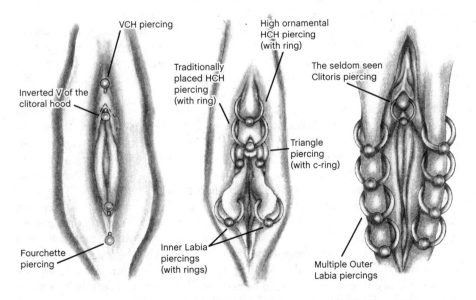

Female anatomy with a valley Female anatomy with a hill

The Vertical Clitoral Hood (VCH) Piercing

- **Healing time:** 4 to 8 weeks
- **Initial jewelry style:** Straight or curved barbell, or ring-style jewelry
- **Initial jewelry gauge:** Commonly 14 or 12 gauge; maximum 10 gauge
- **Initial jewelry size:** Average length or diameter 3/8 to 1/2 inch

Many women like the idea of making their genitals more functional and attractive at the same time. They don't mind having an extra spot to wear a diamond or ruby, either. These are some of the driving forces behind the growing popularity of the vertical clitoral hood piercing. Women of all types, from sorority sisters to empty-nest retirees, are getting VCH piercings. This is not only for alternative individuals. Numerous women who have no other body art wear the VCH piercing. It is suited to any woman who wants to explore new avenues of erotic sensation, if she is anatomically built for it. It is liberating and stimulating as well as appealing and inspiring. The momentary pinch and quick, easy healing period are a small price to pay for the pleasure you can derive.

Dr. Vaughn Millner and associates at the University of South Alabama conducted a research study on VCH piercings as they relate to female sexual satisfaction. The results led to the following statement: "In this exploratory study, we identify a positive relationship between vertical clitoral hood piercing and desire, frequency of intercourse and arousal." These encouraging findings have been published in the prestigious (and conservative) *American Journal of Obstetrics and Gynecology*.[2]

"I even wonder if it is delaying menopause because I am almost 46 and sexually so much younger and wetter than my age! So exciting . . . I love it." S.

VCH Piercing: Placement and Choice of Jewelry

The VCH is the most popular of the female genital piercings for several reasons. As the name describes, the piercing is placed in the same direction that women's genitals are formed, so the jewelry rests comfortably between the legs and is not subject to stress or irritation. Approximately 90 percent of women are built with a *prepuce* (the protective fold of hood tissue above the clitoris), in which jewelry can be placed for a comfortable and stimulating piercing.

This hood is normally configured like a tiny one-ended tunnel, and the VCH pierces through just the thin membrane of skin above your clitoris, not through the clitoris itself. Most of the jewelry rests under the hood. When the piercing is properly placed, your clitoris receives direct action from contact with the jewelry during sex. Many women enjoy this a great deal, but if you would describe your clitoris as hypersensitive, you will probably not want to wear jewelry in this location.

To determine if you have sufficient depth for the piercing, try to slide a lubricated cotton swab underneath your hood. If most of the cottony end fits under the tunnel, then you are built for a VCH (presuming you lack a visible vein along the midline). If the swab is too wide, you can remove some of the fluff; the concern is depth, not width. If you have a shallow tunnel and only part of the tip fits under your hood, you are probably a poor candidate for the VCH. In some cases, an expert can cheat the piercing a little further up for safety, a minimum of 5/16 inch from the edge.

Traditional placement for the VCH is at the *apex* (the deepest part) underneath the hood, along the midline. The piercing should be situated ³/₈ to ¹/₂ inch up from the edge of the hood. The jewelry has the appearance of passing through the whole length of tissue from the piercing to the bottom of the hood. However, because of the tunnel shape, only a small amount of skin is pierced, and most of the jewelry simply rests under the hood against the clitoris. I can usually see through this thin flesh during the piercing. On the deepest of hoods, the piercing may be placed lower than the apex to moderate the jewelry size. If you have a deep hood but don't care to add much sensation, you might want to have the piercing placed a few millimeters below the apex.

Most frequently, I put a curved bar in a fresh VCH piercing. This style helps to minimize friction and prevent irritation during healing, especially if you are built with a hill. The curve allows the jewelry to rest a little closer to the clitoris and provides a small amount of extra room without added length. If you prefer a little less stimulation, you can use a straight barbell. If you are seeking maximum sensation or have a recessed clitoris, then a J-curve is a good option. The shaped post underneath your hood increases contact between the jewelry and your clitoris. If you have a deep valley, the ring and bar are both suitable styles for initial jewelry.

If you are overweight, you may still be suited to a VCH piercing if you have sufficient hood tissue and your piercer can access the area to perform the procedure. Sometimes an assistant is needed to help expose the area (either you or a studio employee, wearing clean gloves). Even if your jewelry will be entirely tucked in and hidden by full outer labia, once it is in place, the VCH generally heals well.

Inexpert piercers frequently place the VCH too close to the edge of the hood. Shallow piercings result in less pleasure because the jewelry is too far from the clitoris. Also, if too little tissue is pierced, you have a greater risk of tearing, migration, and rejection.

Women need to wear initial VCH jewelry that has some room for growth. When a bar is used for healing, the bottom ball should show below the inverted V that forms the peak of the hood; it should not be hidden under the hood (though this is a popular option once healing is concluded, since many find it pleasurable). If a ring is used for initial jewelry, it must be large enough so it does not constrict the hood tissue.

VCH Piercing: Procedure

Before you sign up, ask the piercer how she performs the piercing. If she replies, "With forceps," turn around and leave! Clamping with forceps endangers your clitoris, and it could be intensely—and unnecessarily—painful. Further, using forceps for the VCH seldom, if ever, results in proper placement. The piercing gets positioned too shallow, or just through surface skin on top of the hood, and the jewelry does not touch the clitoris at all. Unfortunately, this blunder is very common.

Standard procedure is to use a needle receiving tube (NRT) under the hood. Some tissue manipulation makes placing it easier and more comfortable if you have a small hood or if it fits tightly to your body. I simply lift your hood and gently pull it away from your body to loosen the tissue. The piercing is done through the dot that has been marked for placement and into the tube, which protects your clitoris underneath. The skin that is pierced is considerably thinner than that of an earlobe. A small percentage of women have thicker hoods; these are usually a little more sensitive to have pierced and take a bit longer to heal.

You might find that the cleaning under your hood with a swab or the pressure from the receiving tube is the most uncomfortable part of the procedure. When performed properly, the sensation of the piercing itself is very brief, and afterward there is seldom lingering discomfort. By the time you are dressed, you're likely to find that your VCH piercing feels good already, or simply that you notice something is there. It is also normal to feel nothing different at all.

VCH Piercing: Healing and Troubleshooting

The VCH piercing has a *very* quick healing time. Some women swear theirs is healed in a week or even less. To be on the safe side, you should care for yours during the entire four-week minimum healing time, even if it feels fine sooner.

If you have a hill with an exposed hood, you may find healing more challenging and the first week or so a little more sensitive. Wearing the smallest jewelry that is safe will help minimize any discomfort. If your initial jewelry is still uncomfortable or irritating after the early accommodation period, its size or style will need to be changed by a professional as soon as possible.

A traditionally placed VCH piercing does not pierce near any major nerves, so there is no basis for a loss of sensation under ordinary circumstances.

VCH Piercing: Physical Activity

Engaging in physical activities after getting a VCH piercing is fine, though a one- or two-week break from bicycling or horseback riding is surely advisable. With the exception of these activities, you will probably find that your new piercing doesn't cause any discomfort while exercising; in fact, you may not even notice it. Then again, it may inspire you to work out. More than a few women have discovered that the stair-stepper or other gym equipment holds new interest for them after genital piercing!

VCH Piercing: Changing Jewelry

The VCH piercing can feel quite different when you change the style or dimensions of your jewelry. Consider experimenting with other sizes of bars, rings, and balls after you have healed. You might enjoy the feeling of a short post with a ball resting under your hood, touching your clitoris, or you might enjoy a longer bar. Then again, you could favor the feeling of a ring, or the way it can be looped onto your partner's tongue barbell during oral sex. Personal preferences vary, but the research can be fun.

VCH Piercing: Stretching

Most women find the VCH rather easy to stretch at least a size or two and have sufficient anatomy to wear gauges thicker than the initial size. Heavier jewelry may produce different sensations. After two to three months or so, the piercing should be ready to enlarge one gauge.

VCH Piercing: Retiring

The VCH has a tendency to shrink and close quickly on many women, though a few find they can easily take the jewelry in and out after healing. Since the clitoral hood is not a public area, any residual mark is unlikely to go unnoticed. Only an expert who is looking for the spot would be able to tell you had ever been pierced.

"How funny it sounds to say that a piercing has changed my life, but it has. Not only did I find a lifelong friendship with someone special (Elayne Angel), I got a VCH piercing that has freed me. In the past, I'd had a few multiple orgasms, but the norm was one, and I was done. Well, now I have multiples often, and very strong, too. I never knew it could be this good.

I had been molested as a child, so my genital area was something I looked at in shame. . . . This piercing has freed me from the bonds of the molestation. I can look at my genitals with pride and joy. . . . I look at my piercing every day and love it more and more. I didn't think a piercing could have this effect on me, but surprisingly, it has. No amount of therapy could have healed me the way this piercing has—by taking ownership of my body and choosing to have the VCH—by a piercer who is loving, kind, and very knowledgeable." J.

The Princess Diana Piercing

- **Healing time:** 4 to 8 weeks
- **Initial jewelry style:** Straight or curved barbell
- **Initial jewelry gauge:** Minimum (and most common) 14 gauge; maximum 10 gauge
- **Initial jewelry size:** Average length or diameter ³/₈ to ¹/₂ inch

Princess Diana (or simply Diana) piercings are identical to VCH piercings, except that they are located off to the side of the hood instead of being placed in the center. Ordinarily they are done in pairs; however, if you are asymmetrically built, with more tissue on one side of your hood than the other, a single Diana could be a good option. Dianas are generally angled at about ten and two o'clock or at nine and three o'clock. Many women do not have a wide enough hood to allow for this placement, so the Dianas are not nearly as popular as the VCH. A number of amply built gals have both: one VCH and two Princess Dianas.

The piercing is named after the first woman I performed them on, and Princess Diana had been in the news at the time, so we added "Princess" to give female royalty some exposure in the piercing world (the Prince Albert male genital piercing, of course, has had so much of it).

The Horizontal Clitoral Hood (HCH) Piercing

- **Healing time:** 6 to 8 weeks
- **Initial jewelry style:** Ring-style
- **Initial jewelry gauge:** Minimum 14 gauge; maximum 10 gauge
- **Initial jewelry size:** Ring diameter ³/₈ to ¹/₂ inch

The HCH piercing is generally better at looking good than feeling good. This piercing, which traverses the hood tissue above the clitoris, is aesthetically appealing to many women. A genital piercing can be visually delightful and bolster self-image, even if it is not placed for action. But most women who seek a genital piercing desire to physically enhance their erotic pleasure. Unfortunately, because of the way most women are built, the HCH won't be able to deliver.

HCH Piercing: Placement and Choice of Jewelry

You need sufficient tissue in the configuration of a hill to get an HCH piercing. If you are built with a valley and a deeply recessed hood, you are not a candidate. Most women are formed with a hood that nearly—or completely—covers the clitoral glans. Therefore, the ring in an HCH simply rests atop the hood. For an HCH piercing to be stimulating, your clitoral glans needs to be somewhat exposed, the piercing must be perfectly placed, and the jewelry accurately sized. Only when all of these conditions are met can the bead of the ring touch your clitoris to add sensation.

The piercing should be placed in the natural creases at the base of the hood tissue where it forms from your body. Your piercer should carefully check for blood vessels in the region, because they are sometimes visible where the piercing should be made. If apparent veins cannot be avoided, then the HCH piercing should not be attempted. Your piercer must also be certain that your hood tissue is pliable enough to pinch up and lift away from the nerve bundle of your clitoris below, so she doesn't give you an unintentional clitoris piercing.

If you are not built symmetrically, which is common, the ring will usually twist or lean to one side. This type of pressure causes discomfort and migration or other healing difficulties. If you want this piercing solely for adornment rather than sexual enhancement, you may prefer it to be positioned for visibility toward the top of your hood.

The correct diameter ring will encompass the tissue without pinching and it will be situated so the ball rests on the desired spot. A bar is seldom comfortable or safe: if it is short enough to avoid twisting, it may embed or pinch. If it is long enough to accommodate your hood, it will be prone to shifting and causing problems when you close your legs.

HCH Piercing: Multiple Piercings

If you have a long enough hood, multiple horizontal piercings (among other options) may be possible. Two or three are not unheard of, but more than that is rare. Rings are usually positioned so that they overlap to some extent, but there has to be enough space between them so the jewelry does not pinch your sensitive tissue. You must have highly symmetrical, well-developed anatomy and a skilled piercer for multiple hood piercings. It is best to get them one at a time, unless they will be located relatively far apart. More than two hood piercings per session could be excessively traumatic to the area.

HCH Piercing: Procedure

The tunnel-like shape of the hood makes the receiving tube an ideal tool to simultaneously protect the clitoris and support the tissue for the VCH procedure. However, for the HCH piercing through the skin atop the clitoris, forceps are very well suited to hold the tissue of the hood. Forceps not only secure the skin, they also help to assure that only the hood tissue is clamped and pierced, and not the nerve bundle just underneath. I find that tissue manipulation helps to separate the hood from the clitoral shaft before clamping. Most women do not describe this piercing as particularly intense since it passes through only the relatively thin, pliable flesh of the hood.

To be safe and sturdy, the HCH must pierce through a solid section of hood tissue, so I am careful to pinch up the skin from the midline in anticipation of its tendency to fold in on itself. Otherwise you can end up with a channel that is too shallow in the middle and wears through over time, or an unsafe double piercing that misses the center completely and just pierces through an unstable sliver of skin on each side of your hood. If the tissue of your hood cannot be lifted up and kept elevated in the center, do not attempt this piercing.

HCH Piercing: Healing and Troubleshooting

The most common complaint during healing is that the jewelry twists. Prevention is key: if your anatomy is not well suited, don't get an HCH piercing. Depending on your build and piercing placement, the twisting might be minimized by wearing a *C-ring* or *U-ring* (widened circular barbell), which I suggest for triangle piercings. See "Triangle Piercing: Placement and Choice of Jewelry," page 144, for details. This alternate style may help you get through the healing period, but it will not be as stimulating as a complete ring, due to the gap between the balls.

HCH Piercing: Changing Jewelry

Sometimes a smaller ring can be worn after you are healed, which may improve your comfort by reducing the tendency toward twisting. Changing the diameter of the ring will alter the way the piercing feels, however, since the bead will rest in a different spot. A shaped ring such as an oval or inverted teardrop may be more comfortable and also functional. Bar-style jewelry cannot be expected to improve sensation since it will not touch the clitoris at all.

HCH Piercing: Stretching

This skin is somewhat stretchable on most women. If you have a substantial amount of tissue in the piercing, over time you can safely enlarge to rather large sizes. You may find the HCH more stimulating when you wear heavier jewelry. After four to six months it should be ready to expand one size.

HCH Piercing: Retiring

Your piercing can shrink or close quickly when the jewelry is removed. Because the piercing is placed in the natural creases at the base of your hood, if you abandon an HCH, even your gynecologist may not notice any remaining marks. There is no physiological basis for a lasting change in sensation from getting this piercing and later retiring it.

The Triangle Piercing

- **Healing time:** 3 to 4 months
- **Initial jewelry style:** C-ring or U-ring, fit to the anatomy (customized circular barbell)
- **Initial jewelry gauge:** Commonly 12 gauge, also 10 gauge, and rarely 14 gauge
- **Initial jewelry size:** Circular barbell ³/₈- to ¹/₂-inch diameter before widening

The triangle is a modern innovation. According to *PFIQ Magazine,* Gauntlet piercer Lou Duff first performed one in the early 1990s (see "The Inventor," page 146). The triangle is a horizontal piercing underneath (not through!) the shaft of the clitoris, at the base of the hood tissue. The stimulation from this piercing comes from added sensation behind your clitoris. This is quite unlike the other genital piercings, which only contact the clitoris from the front.

The triangle is a very advanced piercing because it is placed largely by feel in an area where unfortunate and unacceptable damage could be done if a mishap occurs. Scrutinize the qualifications of any piercer who is under consideration to perform your triangle. Find out exactly where and how she learned to do this particular piercing and how many she has done. If you aren't thoroughly impressed with her training and experience, keep looking.

Triangle Piercing: Placement and Choice of Jewelry

You must be able to pinch behind your hood and raise your clitoral shaft (the cordlike nerve bundle) away from your body for a triangle to be possible. Optimal anatomy is symmetrical with a protruding hood. If your anatomy in that area is very narrow or small, or if you have a valley shape, then you are not a candidate for this piercing. Most women are not anatomically suited to the triangle piercing.

A triangle and an HCH both pierce through the same type—and even a similar amount—of hood tissue. However, for most women the triangle is far more pleasurable than the HCH piercing. Many women ask whether a VCH or a triangle is the most stimulating piercing, but the answer is that they are completely different. Lots of women get one of each. If you are built for and interested in both, the VCH is an excellent introduction to genital piercing because it is fast and easy to heal as well as rewarding. The triangle is a more intense piercing with a longer healing time, so previous experience with genital piercing is helpful but in no way mandatory. Wearing both a VCH and a triangle creates a titillating sandwich: your sensitive clitoris is surrounded by jewelry, front and back.

Due to the recessed location of the piercing and the vertical orientation of the vulva, the safest and most comfortable jewelry for a healing triangle piercing is a custom-fit circular barbell. The base jewelry should be a diameter or two smaller than you need to accommodate your tissue. Your piercer will then widen the gap between the balls by spreading out the ring. This can be done very easily with ring expanding pliers. She will make it C-shaped or (almost) U-shaped, depending on your build. The gap between the circular barbell balls must be wide enough to accommodate your hood so the jewelry tucks down flat, to cradle your inner labia. The surrounding structures hold the jewelry securely in place. The portion of the ring that passes through your tissue fits properly in the limited space between your legs without twisting like circular ring-style jewelry, nor shifting like bar-style jewelry.

Triangle Piercing: Procedure

I use forceps to perform triangle piercings. First I perform tissue manipulation to lift and isolate the clitoral shaft. This is essential to assure correct placement, and it makes it safer and easier to apply the forceps. It is crucial that your piercer maintain a constant hold that keeps your clitoral shaft elevated while she applies the forceps and does the piercing. If she lets go, the cordlike structure will drop down and the piercing will not be in the correct position. Your clitoral shaft itself might get pierced, or you will end up with a low or deep hood piercing, but not a triangle. If your piercer does not seem concerned with keeping your clitoral shaft lifted, she probably does not know where a triangle is supposed to be placed.

I've had piercees comment that the triangle was easier than a nipple or hood piercing; but others find the experience more intense and draining. Still, when skillfully executed, the piercing should be brief.

Failed Geometry

Unfortunately, many of the so-called "triangle" piercings I see are not properly placed because they are not located behind the clitoral shaft. Fortunately, most of these failed triangles have not resulted in damage or dysfunction; but they can cause grave disappointments and lost opportunities for enjoyment. These misplaced triangle piercings often cause uncalled-for pain and discomfort and must frequently be abandoned. I have also seen more than one incorrectly placed piercing that accidentally pierced through the clitoral glans or shaft (and these were performed by piercers who claimed to be skilled in triangle piercings).

Triangle Piercing: Healing and Troubleshooting

The triangle is the female genital piercing most likely to be a heavy bleeder, so don't be surprised if you spot, or even flow, for several days afterward.

If you have an asymmetrical build or your jewelry is too wide to rest evenly between your legs, migration is to be expected. It may move just a little and then stop, or you may need to abandon the piercing. Wearing the proper jewelry type and size is imperative for healing. If your C-ring or U-ring does not comfortably tuck close to your body, the ring, ball, or gap size may need to be adjusted. If your piercing is not healing well and you are not wearing a custom-fitted circular barbell, then you should have one inserted.

Triangle Piercing: Changing Jewelry

After healing, you can wear a captive ring, bead ring, teardrop, D-ring, curved or straight barbell, or other jewelry style. Because the anatomy is manipulated (the clitoral shaft is lifted) to put in the piercing, removing the jewelry occasionally results in a total loss of your triangle, instantaneously. The channel can be very hard to locate immediately following jewelry removal. I suggest you always use insertion tapers for jewelry changes, keeping something in the piercing at all times.

Success!

I have had more than one client confide that she had never experienced an orgasm until after I performed her triangle piercing. Their partners and sexual activities were the same as before, so it must have been the piercings that caused the desired effect.

Triangle Piercing: Stretching

The triangle is a sturdy piercing and, although not always easy to stretch, it can be expanded to hefty sizes with time and patience. Some women enjoy the way heavier or thicker jewelry looks and feels after enlarging a healed triangle to a larger gauge.

Triangle Piercing: Retiring

Consider carefully a decision to remove triangle jewelry; reinserting it later is often impossible. Because the piercing is tucked back against the body at the natural folds, evidence of an abandoned triangle is hardly visible.

Outer Labia (Labia Majora) Piercings

- **Healing time:** 3 to 4 months
- **Initial jewelry style:** Ring or curved bar
- **Initial jewelry gauge:** Most commonly 14 or 12 gauge; 10 gauge for well-developed anatomy
- **Initial jewelry size:** ¹/₂- to ⁵/₈-inch diameter ring-style jewelry; ⁷/₁₆- or ¹/₂-inch diameter curved bar

These piercings are situated on the sides of the *vulva* (external female genitalia) in the thick, fleshy folds of tissue where hair grows. *Labia* mean "lips" in Latin; the awkward singular form of the word is *labium*.[3] Outer labia piercings are often done in pairs, with one on each side, or in multiples, to form a *ladder*. You are not expected to experience erotic sensation of the sort that is often derived from wearing jewelry in your hood; piercing here is apt to be primarily visually pleasing.

The Inventor

I didn't conceive of the triangle piercing myself, but I performed one on Lou Duff, the San Francisco piercer who did invent it. She originally called it the "Triangle of Submission," after the basic shape of the area through which the jewelry runs (a triangle formed by the pubic bone, the clitoral shaft, and the edge of the clitoral hood), and for the bottom (the submissive partner in a BDSM relationship) on whom she first performed it. Since she felt that such a name wouldn't be popular with the general public, she shortened it to the "the triangle" when she brought it to Gauntlet, and thereby the world.

Outer Labia Piercings: Placement and Choice of Jewelry

These piercings can be situated nearly anywhere along the pliable rim of the outer lips. They pass through denser tissue and take longer to heal than hood and inner labia piercings. If placed next to the clitoris, they might provide clitoral stimulation from the sides. Some wear them higher up on the lips, to make them more visible, or lower, adjacent to their vaginal opening, where a male partner might feel them during intercourse.

The size and shape of your anatomy should be considered—both when your legs are together and when they are apart—to determine the most comfortable spot for your piercing. If you have large thighs and the space between your legs is more crowded, a curved bar is a better choice. The diameter of the jewelry is dependent on the size and the shape of the area. If your labia are more defined and convex-shaped, then a smaller diameter can be used because it will encompass sufficient tissue. When the area is flatter, a larger diameter is needed to safely include the optimal width between entry and exit. If you have undefined lips or large thighs, you might find outer labia piercings hard to heal.

Outer labia piercings can be placed to frame the most exposed part of your lip (the surface that faces the floor when you are standing), or they can be tucked inward, to frame the edge of the labia—half on the smooth, hairless part, and half on the surface where hair grows.

You can make a statement with multiple labia piercings—inner and outer—depending on your build. Wearing six or eight is not unheard of, and some women have even more. If you plan to wear a single ring to join both sides together after healing, let your piercer know so she can line them up accordingly. Women are sometimes concerned that placing matched piercings directly opposite one another will be troublesome, but because the tissue is so malleable, pairs need not be purposely offset.

> **Putting the *Fun* Back in *Function***
> Labia piercings have *some* potential for function. At least one inventive piercee I know has used multiple outer labia rings to hold up her stockings on occasion.

Outer Labia Piercings: Procedure

I use a forceps technique to perform outer labia piercings. Even when a pair is done directly across from one another, they are pierced one at a time. Many women describe the feeling of getting outer labia piercings as "biting and pinchy." Once the procedure is over, you may experience some tenderness or bleeding afterward. When you receive a pair of outer labia piercings, it is normal if one side bleeds and the other doesn't.

Outer Labia Piercings: Healing and Troubleshooting

Your bleeding may continue for a week or so, and swelling may remain for longer. Snug underwear helps to support the jewelry, but tight pants will cause discomfort and irritation, so wear loose or stretchy clothing at first.

You may experience thickened or hardened tissue, excess scarring, or other problems around the openings during healing; don't panic. This is generally caused by the unavoidable trauma of walking and sitting. It has a tendency to come and go throughout healing. Saline soaks may help; if not, try other troubleshooting techniques that are suggested in chapter 16. If your problem is persistent, a change in the size or style of your jewelry is warranted. This type of complication frequently resolves over time, and the piercings heal without ill effects.

Outer Labia Piercings: Changing Jewelry

Unless you are very flexible or your piercings are located closer to the front than usual, it may be necessary to get assistance to change your jewelry. After healing, adding weights, bells, or charms on your piercings could be pleasurable. Some women also like the feel of tugging on labia piercings during sexual activity. These are the types of erotic sensations you can expect to derive from outer labia piercings.

Outer Labia Piercings: Stretching

Wait six to nine months from the initial piercing before stretching larger. If you have had troubled healing, wait a year or longer. This is a sturdy piercing, and if the channel is reasonably wide, you can safely wear jumbo jewelry. If you have especially pliable tissue, or wear weights (or attach your stockings to your jewelry), you might be able to skip a gauge.

Outer Labia Piercings: Retiring

Outer labia piercings may not close completely upon removal, but they do shrink. Because the area is not in public view and may be masked by hair, these piercings will not leave much of a mark. If you are shaved and had healing problems, more obvious signs of your piercings may be visible to your doctor or lover.

Labia Minora (Inner Labia) Piercings

- **Healing time:** 4 to 8 weeks
- **Initial jewelry style:** Ring-style
- **Initial jewelry gauge:** Most commonly 14 and 12 gauge
- **Initial jewelry size:** Minimum diameter $^3/_8$ inch; commonly $^7/_{16}$ and $^1/_2$ inch

The inner labia are the delicate, hairless folds of flesh situated between the outer labia. This tissue is nearly identical to that of the clitoral hood; it is quick and easy to heal. Some women's inner lips are not large enough to pierce, but this is not all that common. A single ring on either side is popular, and they can be pierced in pairs or multiples.

Inner Labia Piercings: Placement and Choice of Jewelry

This area is frequently shaped much like an earlobe, and a traditional placement for a single piercing is at the visual center of the lobe. However, any spot along the lip is acceptable as long as the piercing is located at least $^3/_8$ inch from the edge of your tissue. Your piercing should be equidistant from the edge on both sides to frame the area aesthetically and comfortably. Unlike most other piercings, this skin is so slim that a ring without any added diameter won't constrict the tissue. If you wear jewelry that is too thin, it can cut your skin or stretch it unintentionally. Even short ($^1/_4$-inch) barbell posts are generally too long for inner labia piercings because the tissue is so slender. When a post is too long, the bar doesn't sit evenly, and one ball rests too heavily against the fresh piercing. Rings are best for initial jewelry; bars are acceptable later.

Few women report experiencing pleasurable sensations from inner labia piercings, so normally they are worn for their visual appeal. If jewelry is placed quite high on the lip, there is some chance it may contact and stimulate your clitoris. Jewelry situated midway across your vaginal opening may be felt by a male partner during intercourse.

Inner Labia Piercings: Procedure

I use forceps to secure the tissue for piercing. Most women feel a brief pinch or sting, but few describe inner labia piercings as intense. Afterward you can expect minimal discomfort, though there may be some bleeding.

Inner Labia Piercings: Healing and Troubleshooting

Inner labia piercings are generally trouble-free to heal, thanks to a good blood supply and fine tissue. The main concern is to avoid excessive trauma during healing from rough sex or physical activity. This is one of the female genital piercings that urine has a tendency to sting, so follow the suggestions on page 136, "Genital Piercing: Urinating."

Inner Labia Piercings: Changing Jewelry and Stretching

The subjects of changing jewelry and stretching are usually discussed separately in this book, but inner labia piercings stretch so easily that the two must be covered as a single subject.

You may enjoy the sensation of tugging on healed inner labia piercings or wearing weights, bells, or charms; however, these activities usually result in stretching because the tissue is so thin. Twelve-gauge jewelry is a safe minimum if you want to wear extra weight or play with your jewelry in this way.

Inner labia piercings are the female genital piercings most frequently expanded to oversized gauges: some determined women stretch to ¾ inch or larger! This tissue is thin, but it is also resilient and strong. Large holes tend to be stable if they are sufficiently set back from the edge.

Inner Labia Piercings: Retiring

If you abandon inner labia piercings, they will leave small marks that are not readily visible—unless you have stretched them or hold an unusual job. The holes may shrink, but even when they are left empty for an extended period of time, this is one of the few areas of the body that routinely remains open once healed.

The Fourchette Piercing

- **Healing time:** 6 to 8 weeks
- **Initial jewelry style:** Curved bar
- **Initial jewelry gauge:** 12 or 10 gauge
- **Initial jewelry size:** 7/16 inch or longer

The mellifluous anatomical term for the site of this piercing is the *frenulum labiorum pudenda*, also known as the *fourchette* (French for "little fork"). This piercing is located in the perineum. It is similar to the guiche piercing in a male, but it is more practical and comfortable for a woman because it is oriented vertically.

Fourchette Piercing: Placement and Choice of Jewelry

The fourchette piercing frames the border of tissue at the back perimeter of the vagina. The lower portion of the piercing is positioned between the vagina and the anus, and it should be situated no closer than ½ inch from the anus. If you have had a midline *episiotomy* (incision to facilitate childbirth), you are not a good candidate due to localized scarring. Because this tissue is so fine, the jewelry must be thick enough to prevent tearing or cutting. A 12 gauge is a safe minimum size. If you don't have a defined lip of skin in this location, then you are a poor candidate. Cheating the fourchette in deeper is not successful; there is a strong tendency for the piercing to migrate and reject if it is not seated in a natural fold of pliable tissue.

Fourchette Piercing: Procedure

The procedure is rather tricky for your piercer because of the piercing's almost internal placement. I generally use forceps, but I have also performed it using a receiving tube, depending on the piercee's build. For this procedure, you may be positioned on your back or on your hands and knees. Most women do not find this to be a particularly intense piercing, though the procedure can be a little awkward. These don't tend to be heavy bleeders, but some bleeding is always possible.

Fourchette Piercing: Healing and Troubleshooting

You basically sit on this piercing, so you must be careful not to seat yourself on unclean surfaces during healing, unless you are wearing underwear or clothing. To increase your comfort throughout healing, sanitary pads or panty liners can provide extra padding and wick away moisture. Maintain excellent hygiene due to the proximity of the piercing to the anus: shower regularly, and be careful when wiping after visiting the toilet.

Fourchette Piercing: Changing Jewelry and Stretching

This spot is all but impossible to access yourself, so expect to require assistance for jewelry changes. Similar to the inner labia, this fine, elastic tissue easily accommodates larger sizes, but it does not withstand heavy jewelry well because of a propensity to stretch larger than desired. You may find it stretches so much with normal wear that an ordinary barbell ball ($3/16$ inch, or 5 mm) can pass right through the piercing! To avoid losing your jewelry, if the channel appears to be stretching on its own, avoid wearing balls that are too small. If your fourchette piercing continues to stretch, you may need to switch to a ring to avoid losing jewelry—unless you wear balls that are significantly larger than average. The catch-22 is that large balls may cause unintentional stretching, yet wearing a ring might make penetration difficult. Most women find a curved bar is the most comfortable jewelry style.

Fourchette Piercing: Retiring

The area is not subject to public view, and the piercing is placed within natural creases, so it will not leave a visible mark. A divot or slight pit may be observable on the outside surface, but the inner portion will be invisible. Once the piercing is well established, it is fairly likely to remain open without jewelry in place.

The Christina Piercing

- **Healing time:** 6 to 9 months or longer
- **Initial jewelry style:** Tygon, PTFE, or other inert, flexible plastic; or, surface bar
- **Initial jewelry gauge:** 12 or 10 gauge
- **Initial jewelry size:** 1 inch or longer

The Christina (or Venus) piercing is a comparatively recent innovation. It is a surface piercing that is placed vertically at the top of the *cleft of Venus* (top of the *vulva*), optimally extending about an inch up the *pubic mound* (soft mound of flesh just above the genitals).

It takes significantly longer to heal than any other female genital piercing. The jewelry does not contact the clitoris, so this placement is ornamental in nature. The Christina is not one of the most popular piercings because it is not expected to add erotic sensation and takes a long period of time to heal. However, if you are a motivated piercee and you are attracted to this adornment, these aspects may not prove to be barriers.

Christina Piercing: Placement and Choice of Jewelry

You are suited to a Christina piercing if you have plenty of pliable tissue on your pubic mound and also a defined valley or divot at the very top of your hood (where the vulva separates into two sides), because this is where the bottom ball will rest. It is much less prone to migration or rejection when a significant amount of tissue (one inch or longer) is placed between the entry and exit. The Christina does not ordinarily heal as well or remain for a long time when the piercing passes through less tissue or a regular style of metal body jewelry is used initially.

Flexible, nonmetallic jewelry is very forgiving and comfortable in this region, which is subject to considerable stress from clothing and missionary-position sex. My clients have had success healing Christinas wearing Tygon. A specialized surface bar is the only metal jewelry that should be worn for healing. To conform to your anatomy, the top is angled and the bottom end is left straight.

Christina Piercing: Procedure

It is best to shave before visiting the studio for a Christina piercing. If you fail to do so, your piercer will usually have to trim your hair. I prepare the area using tissue manipulation and use a forceps procedure.

Like many other surface piercings, this one is not apt to feel as sensitive as it might seem. Bleeding is fairly common afterward. Place your pad or liner farther forward than usual and cover the piercing.

Christina Piercing: Healing and Troubleshooting

For a Christina piercing to be successful, you must avoid trauma. Sanitary pads can help to protect and cushion the piercing throughout healing. Direct, frontal sexual contact is unadvisable during the entire lengthy healing course. Consider your lovemaking preferences before deciding to get this piercing, because even after healing, this type of friction may prove uncomfortable and irritating.

The Rigors of Research: The Fourchette

The fourchette piercing is an innovation of the 1990s. I got the first three of them on different occasions, each in a slightly different spot. I tried diligently to identify the optimal placement. My investigation, while enjoyable, revealed that the best place for a fourchette is on a woman who has a defined flap or fold of tissue in the region. I—most unfortunately—do not. The research was worthwhile, though, because many of the women who wear them find that the fourchette piercing produces unique and enjoyable sensations. Mine did, too, while they lasted.

Christina Piercing: Changing Jewelry

This area is a little more accessible for home jewelry changes, but because the piercing channel is long, a taper should always be used. If you wear Tygon, a few millimeters of extra length should be left to accommodate initial swelling. You can have the jewelry shortened after the first week or two of healing. Tygon must be changed out every few months because it stiffens and may degrade over time.

Christina Piercing: Stretching

Large gauges are not usually desirable because the Christina is a surface piercing. If you do want to stretch, wait for a year or more following the piercing.

Christina Piercing: Retiring

Abandoning a Christina piercing will leave a mark on your pubic mound. However, if you grow your pubic hair, it may not be visible. If you object to scars and plan to be depilated on a long-term basis, the Christina is not a good piercing for you.

The Clitoris Piercing

- **Healing time:** 4 to 8 weeks
- **Initial jewelry style:** Ring- or bar-style for horizontal placement, bar-style for vertical
- **Initial jewelry gauge:** Usually 16 gauge, rarely 14 gauge
- **Initial jewelry size:** 3/8-inch minimum diameter, up to 1/2-inch for well-endowed women

If you're like most women, the thought of piercing your clitoris (rather than your clitoral hood) is likely to make you slam your knees tightly together and exclaim, "Ow!" You probably comprehend that the clitoris is a profoundly sensitive part of your anatomy. This small but significant structure contains approximately 8,000 nerve endings, which is twice the number found in the average penis.[4]

Piercing of the *clitoral glans* (visible beneath the hood) is rare, and it is serious business. A piercing mishap can result in the loss of your clitoral sensation and the termination of your erotic pleasure if your sexual activities are clitorally focused. Only a highly experienced master should perform this piercing, and only on candidates who are ideally suited to it. Exercise extreme caution before embarking upon a clitoris piercing; this is not an area with which to take risks.

Out of the very small number of women who genuinely desire a clitoris piercing (rather than the much more common hood piercing), approximately 90 to 95 percent are not suitably built to accommodate jewelry through the clitoral head.

Women who are suitably endowed and properly pierced usually find that a clitoris piercing does increase the sensitivity of the area. However, you could lose sensation if the piercer is not masterful enough to carry out the job perfectly, if you are anatomically unsuited, or if you experience healing complications. Sensation sometimes returns upon removal of the jewelry.

Clitoris Piercing: Placement and Choice of Jewelry

Chances are, your clitoris is simply too small to withstand a piercing; the average one is no bigger than a pencil eraser.[5] Even when you have a well-developed clitoris, 16-gauge jewelry is the usual starting size. This is the only below-the-neck piercing that I normally start that thin. To preserve the sensitivity of your diminutive but precious organ, jewelry must not comprise too great a proportion of the clitoris.

A number of women are built with a clitoris that is large enough to pierce, but their hood tissue fits too tightly or heavily over it, and this would interfere with the jewelry. To be safe to pierce and have a chance to heal well, your clitoris must be relatively large (at least a full ¼ inch wide) and be easily exposed beneath a short or loose hood. Most women are simply not formed this way.

The proper placement is always at the base of the glans of the clitoris. For a horizontal piercing, when the head is oval, the piercing is placed at the midpoint, and when the glans is teardrop shaped, it goes a small distance below that. For a vertical piercing, it goes at the top and bottom of the clitoris. Some women cannot comfortably retract the hood enough to expose the upper part of the clitoris for the procedure or to accommodate a barbell ball.

A perfect jewelry fit is critical. If a ring or bar is even slightly too large, it can interfere with the way your hood naturally rests. Pressure against the jewelry will be painful and can lead to scarring, migration, and healing problems.

Clitoris Piercing: Procedure

If your clitoris can't be clamped because your anatomy is too small, your hood is in the way, or the process is too intense for you, then you aren't a good candidate for clitoris piercing. Even if clamps aren't used, these remain reasonable criteria for would-be piercees. Slow, deep breathing is especially important to help keep you as relaxed as possible. Moving during the procedure can be ruinous. Most of the brave, determined women who do receive a clitoris piercing find that it is a very intense (though ultimately rewarding) experience.

Give yourself some extra time to recover before arising. You may want to take a day or two off from work and physical activities. Always wear a pad or liner following the procedure. Due to the vascular nature of this area, bleeding is normal. It can be fairly heavy and may last for several days. The trade-off is the same as other spots with a good blood supply: the clitoris usually heals quickly.

Clitoris Piercing: Healing and Troubleshooting

You can expect intense discomfort or actual pain for several days after piercing this exquisitely sensitive area. Excessive pain or discomfort beyond the first week or two may indicate that your jewelry isn't resting properly and that you have too much pressure against it from your hood or labia. See your piercer for an evaluation and possible jewelry change. If you cannot find a jewelry size or style that situates comfortably, your piercing will need to be abandoned. Do not persist in trying to heal. Scarring from this problem is to be expected, can be permanent, and may cause diminished sensation.

Hypersensitivity is also normal during the initial phase, and it may continue after you are healed. If you are left with an undesirable level of intensity, removing your jewelry should resolve the problem.

Clitoris Piercing: Changing Jewelry

You will probably want some help with jewelry changes. Once you are fully healed, altering the jewelry style and size can have an impact on the mechanics of your sexual activities and satisfaction, so consider experimenting with different options to find your favorite.

Clitoris Piercing: Stretching

You can stretch a clitoris piercing if your anatomy is of sufficient dimensions to support larger jewelry. Increasing one or two sizes is usually possible if you allow plenty of time between stretches. After that, the tissue may be more challenging to enlarge. A few hardy women have expanded their clitoral piercings to 6 gauge and even larger.

If you have your mind set on a large-size clitoris piercing, put in the heaviest jewelry you can wear comfortably. Try adding light charms or bells as tolerated to help it stretch over time. Never endure discomfort for the stretching process; if your piercing will not enlarge easily, do not force it. Even after healing, this can cause complications such as migration and scarring.

Clitoris Piercing: Retiring

When you leave jewelry out of a well-healed clitoris piercing, it may stay open. However, if the channel shrinks much, this spot could be too tender to stretch up for jewelry reinsertion. The piercing is recessed at the base of natural folds, so there will not be any visible mark left if you abandon the piercing, unless there was scarring. A clitoris piercing often causes some enlargement of the area, and this can be permanent, but other evidence of piercing will be difficult or impossible to see.

Male Genital Piercings

Introductory information common to both male and female genital piercings is located at the beginning of this chapter. A few additional points are covered below, followed by detailed discussions on of each of the standard male genital piercings. For more information about genital piercings, see chapter 20, "Sex!" See also "Safer Sex," page 255, for important facts about maintaining hygiene while healing a genital piercing.

Male Genital Piercings: Urinating

Urine will run directly over certain piercings, including the Prince Albert and foreskin. To soothe stinging, follow the suggestions under "Genital Piercing: Urinating," page 136. Alternatively, put some water in a big, clean cup, submerge the piercing, and urinate underwater.

Putting unwashed hands anywhere near your piercing poses some risk of infection, even if you don't touch it when you use the bathroom. To avoid contamination from dirty fingers, wash your hands before you urinate, use a tissue or toilet paper to handle yourself, or sit down, but make sure your piercing never touches the inside surface of the toilet bowl.

Male Genital Piercings: Bleeding

I always apply the amusingly named "rubber chicken" wrapping for piercings on the head or shaft to help you avoid an embarrassing mess. This dressing consists of sterile gauze around the piercing plus tissues for extra absorbency, covered by a medical glove (the drooping fingers look like a chicken comb). I secure it with a rubber band that is snug enough to keep the bandage in place, but not so tight as to diminish your circulation. Prince Albert, ampallang, and apadravya piercings regularly bleed enough to fill a whole glove multiple times. Keep the rubber chicken on until it is full and needs to be changed or until you must urinate. Reapply a leak-proof wrapping if there is any sign of bleeding, and for a day or two longer.

Male Genital Piercings: Sensation

You need not be concerned about feeling continuously aroused and distracted by your new genital piercing. Unless a piercing is being handled or moved, it will produce almost no physical sensations. This is true even for a fresh piercing once the procedure is over and your nerve endings settle down. It is possible, however, that the idea or the appearance of your new ornament will result in an excited state. Because of the much wider distribution of nerve endings throughout the penis and scrotum, desensitization and hypersensitivity are seldom issues with male genital piercings.

Male Genital Piercings: Cock Rings

If you wish to wear a cock ring with a male genital piercing, discuss this openly with your piercer if it ordinarily rests near the pathway of the piercing. This can be of concern for pubic, guiche, and high scrotum piercings. You may need to put on your favorite model so your piercer can see if there is room for both. Even if you have space for a cock ring, you'll probably need to forgo wearing it for a while to avoid excessive pressure on your new piercing.

Male Genital Piercings: Erections

It is natural to get an erection during the cleaning or marking phase of a genital piercing, and this will not surprise an experienced piercer. In fact, this can allow him to obtain an accurate jewelry measurement, which is advantageous for certain piercings. If you are still erect when the time comes for your piercing, the procedure will be more difficult or impossible for your piercer, and you will surely bleed more. Try to think about baseball or dinner at Grandma's house for a few minutes to alleviate your condition. Getting an erection from seeing your piercing with the jewelry in place is also a frequent occurrence. Again, bleeding is a common consequence.

The jewelry you wear in genital piercings must accommodate your largest engorgement. If your jewelry is too tight when you are erect, return to your piercer as soon as possible for a larger piece. Jewelry that is too small can cause discomfort, migration, and healing problems.

When your piercing is new and tender, you may want to keep a glass of ice water by the bedside to douse any nighttime or morning erections. If there is dried matter on your jewelry, getting an erection can be painful, as the crust gets pulled into your piercing. This rough material can also be injurious to the delicate tissue. Frequent saline soaks will help to keep your jewelry smooth, safe, and comfortable.

The Prince Albert (PA) Piercing

- **Healing time:** 4 to 8 weeks or longer
- **Initial jewelry style:** Ring—circular barbell preferred, or a curved bar
- **Initial jewelry gauge:** 12 or 10 gauge
- **Initial jewelry size:** Minimum ⅝ inch, but anatomically dependent

In the world of modern body piercing, the Prince Albert is a historic piercing, not because Queen Victoria's consort wore one—he didn't. It is because during the early years of modern body piercing, the PA was the most popular male genital piercing. Many heavily pierced men describe the Prince Albert as their favorite.

The PA looks like a severe puncture of the male organ. However, the piercing traverses only a very small amount of tissue, encompassing much less skin than the average earlobe piercing. In fact, it goes through some of the thinnest pierceable tissue on the body. Because it goes through the urethra, men are often concerned about whether the Prince Albert piercing is more dangerous, harder to heal, or more susceptible to infections. To the surprise of many, it is an easy piercing both to receive and to heal. Your own urine is not harmful to the piercing. In fact, it functions much like the saltwater treatments that are suggested to promote healing.

Prince Albert Piercing: Placement and Choice of Jewelry

The piercing is made on the underside of the penis at the juncture of the head and shaft; the jewelry rests within the urethra and is worn out the tip of the *urinary meatus* (urethral opening). Many men greatly enjoy the sensation of jewelry inside the urethra, though it may take a short time to become accustomed to its presence. The urethra is not in the center of the penis—it runs along the bottom—so the piercing passes through a membrane of skin.

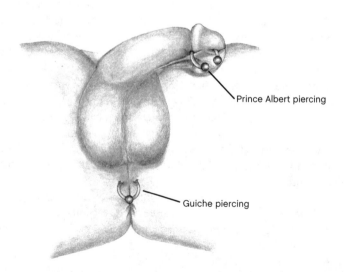

Prince Albert piercing

Guiche piercing

The 10 gauge is a reasonable maximum starting thickness; the 12 gauge is less apt to bleed and can easily be stretched later. Let your piercer know if you have plans to stretch to jumbo gauges, because this should be factored in when marking the placement. If you don't have a large penis or a high urethra (allowing for a substantial distance between the piercing and the lower edge of the urethral opening), the piercer can mark the placement a little further down the shaft to cheat some extra tissue into the piercing. The skin it pierces through won't be any thicker—it will just be a little further from the tip of your penis. You should have no less than ½ inch of tissue between the piercing and the edge of your urethra when your penis is flaccid. If you want to stretch up to large gauges, the piercing should encompass at least ⅝ inch.

You need not become erect during the procedure because your piercer can get a measurement for the jewelry diameter by simply pulling on the skin near the end of your penis between the spot for the piercing and the tip of your urethra.

Circular barbells are versatile for PAs because you can modify the ring diameter for a precise fit by spreading or narrowing the gap between the balls. You can make adjustments (or have your piercer help) even when your piercing is new.

Instead of a flat, pierceable surface, many men have a cordlike web in the center of the area where the Prince Albert is worn. In this case, the piercing can sometimes be set a little further down the shaft, or, more commonly, slightly off to one side. The web should be avoided because penetrating it makes an unstable, uncomfortable PA and tends to result in little flaps of cut tissue. If the skin is not webbed, then the piercing can safely go right in the center (if no visible blood vessels are present). Sometimes PAs are placed unnecessarily off to the side, probably for the same reason that a lot of so-called "pros" don't pierce the midline under the tongue: poor training.

Several factors can help you and your piercer decide whether the piercing should be placed to the left or right of the web if it can't go in the center. The piercer should look for visible blood vessels and, obviously, select the other side. He can also see if one side lines up better with your urethra; the jewelry will sit straighter when the piercing aligns with it.

If you are uncircumcised, you may still be built for a PA piercing. You must be able to comfortably retract your foreskin far enough for the piercing to be placed in an appropriate location. The piercer must check your tissue with your foreskin in both positions to be certain the jewelry will fit properly. If your foreskin fits snugly over your head, a curved bar may be needed for healing. You must not wear a ring so large that it prevents your foreskin from resting in its natural position. The ball at the tip of your penis must not be so small that a curved or circular barbell easily slips into your urethra. This will cause the remainder of the ring or bar to hang down from your piercing, which can irritate your tissue and might feel unpleasant inside.

Prince Albert Piercing: Anatomy/Hypospadias

Approximately one in every three hundred male children is born with a form of *hypospadias*, a birth defect in which the opening of the urethra is not located at the tip of the penis.[6] The Prince Albert piercing is inadvisable in severe cases. In milder cases, the urinary meatus is still on the head of the penis (sometimes in the spot where a PA would traditionally be placed). A piercing might still be possible by situating it further down the shaft. You must consult an expert piercer if you have hypospadias.

Prince Albert Piercing: Procedure

This procedure may be difficult for you mentally, but it is not terribly challenging physically. Many men compare it favorably to an earlobe piercing.

I perform the Prince Albert using a needle receiving tube. For your comfort, I warm the tube between my gloved fingers and lubricate it before inserting it a short distance into your urinary meatus. The NRT is not overly large, but many men still find its presence inside to be the most unpleasant part of the procedure, so I leave it there as briefly as possible. My technique is to just slightly overshoot the dot when I insert the tube, so when I draw it back into position underneath the mark, I am certain the tissue inside the urethra is taut and flat. In most cases, I can see right through the skin to the tube inside. I make the piercing from the outside, through the mark, into the protective tube, which safely guides the sharp tip of the needle out your urethra. I transfer in the jewelry following the direction of the needle.

Prince Albert Piercing: Healing and Troubleshooting

The amount of post-PA bleeding that frequently occurs can be alarming even if you think you are prepared for it. It is cruel and unprofessional for a piercer to perform your Prince Albert without educating you about what to expect during the aftermath. Rest assured, intermittent blood flow for several days is absolutely normal. After that, it can continue to bleed off and on for a few more days. Keep bandaged up for a while longer than you think you need to, even if it seems that your bleeding has stopped.

Healing of Prince Albert piercings is usually quick and trouble-free, unless you are overzealous with sexual activity before healing is complete.

Prince Albert Piercing: Urination

Many men are apprehensive about being able to urinate standing up after getting this piercing. A few easy maneuvers can help you to normalize the act once you have healed. When a ring sits in the middle of your urethra it can split the flow and cause a splashy mess. Also, many Prince Albert piercings stretch on their own, leaving extra room around the jewelry, which results in leakage from the piercing hole. A simple solution is to manually plug the hole on the bottom when you urinate. Place a finger on the underside of your penis just at the front of the jewelry. If you wear a ring, put your fingertip within the ring. This draws the jewelry to the lower edge of your urinary meatus so it doesn't interrupt the flow. Or, rotate your penis so that the ring faces the ceiling. This helps to merge urine leaking from the piercing hole back into the main stream.

Prince Albert Piercing: Changing Jewelry and Stretching

It is usually easy to change your own Prince Albert jewelry, especially if you insert it from the outside, rather than trying to feed it inside your urethra. Sometimes the PA stretches so readily that you may be able to skip several sizes. However, once it is expanded, the tissue may not shrink back much if you remove your jewelry later. This is the most popular body piercing for jumbo expansion; jewelry of 0 to 00 gauge (8 or 9 mm) is not unusual. Many men and their partners enjoy the sensations of a Prince Albert piercing with big, heavy jewelry in it. Sizable rings do not prohibit urination, because when thicker jewelry is added, the urethra stretches, too. Caution: hefty rings or bars can be dangerous to your partner's teeth during oral sex.

Prince Albert Piercing: Retiring

Unlike most piercings, once the Prince Albert is healed, it is usually there to stay. Even if you abandon it, you can probably reinsert jewelry later. Depending on how large the piercing was stretched, the hole could remain open enough to leak after you remove the jewelry. Simply covering the hole with your finger during urination is an acceptable resolution for most men. If not, consult an understanding urologist or surgeon to learn about the pros and cons of a procedure to excise and stitch up your unwanted aperture.

Prince Albert Piercing: Alternate Placement—Deep Prince Albert

When the piercing is made further down the shaft, this is called a *deep Prince Albert*. This is sometimes performed as a result of mild hypospadias; other times it is just a personal preference, especially for those who want to wear large jewelry. The tissue is just as thin and pierceable as in the traditional location, but the tube needs to be inserted further into the urethra for the procedure. These tend to heal quickly, and other aspects are the same as a traditionally placed PA.

Prince Albert Piercing: Alternate Placement—Dolphin Piercing

When a deep PA piercing is made (farther down the shaft) and jewelry is threaded between it and a traditionally placed PA, this is called a *dolphin piercing*. I usually start these with Tygon passed out the tip of the urethra for comfort and ease of healing. Men who have a large difference in size between flaccid and erect states may never find metal jewelry comfortable in a dolphin piercing.

The Frenum Piercing

- **Healing time:** 3 to 4 months or longer
- **Initial jewelry style:** Straight barbell
- **Initial jewelry gauge:** 12 or 10 gauge
- **Initial jewelry size:** Anatomically dependent; commonly ⅝ inch, though sometimes ⁹⁄₁₆ to ¾ inch or more

The frenum is a versatile genital piercing that is second in popularity only to the Prince Albert. The name is derived from shortening the anatomical terms *frenulum* or *fraenum* (a fibrous cord of connecting tissue, in this case on the underside of the penis), in which the piercing is placed. It joins the glans to the foreskin, and the bulk of it is commonly removed during circumcision.[7] The remaining tissue is what is pierced on those who have been circumcised.

Frenum Placement

A traditional frenum piercing is placed horizontally on the underside of the penis about ½ inch down the shaft from the usual location of a Prince Albert. Poorly trained piercers frequently place the frenum too close to the head of the penis, so there is not enough room for the PA. The classic frenum is situated on the bottom of the penis, opposite the groove where the corona joins the shaft on the top. After healing, if you wear a large ring through the piercing and around the shaft, the hoop rests level on the penis. A ring wide enough to encompass the optimal width of tissue for this piercing is too large and cumbersome for healing. The barbell is superior initial jewelry for safety and comfort.

The frenum piercing does not penetrate into the shaft or the urethra; it simply goes through the fine, pliable tissue. If the skin can be pinched up, it can be pierced. The term "frenum" initially referred only to the traditional spot on the underside, but it is now used to describe any piercing along the surface of the shaft, including the top, sides, and in between. Success rates vary for frenum piercings placed in nontraditional spots. Some men can heal anywhere along the shaft, but others find that alternative placements are more apt to migrate or reject.

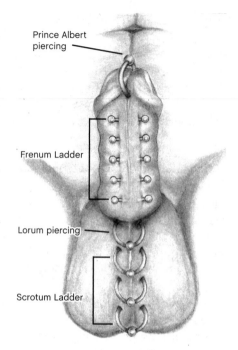

Prince Albert piercing

Frenum Ladder

Lorum piercing

Scrotum Ladder

Frenum Ladders

Multiple frenums are common, and when placed in a row they are referred to as a *frenum ladder*. You can wear a ladder on the underside, on the top, and the sides of the shaft. The piercings, however, need to be an adequate distance apart to avoid pinching. Depending on how many you ultimately desire, one option is to put several evenly spaced piercings wide apart and add more between them over time. Each piercer has his own policy regarding how many he will perform in one session; I seldom do more than four. The more piercings you get at once, the longer they may all take to heal. When your body is taxed beyond its ability to repair, rejection is sometimes a consequence, so patience and planning are required for ladders.

The Frenum Piercing: Procedure

I use the forceps method for frenum piercing. If your tissue is tight, you may find the forceps somewhat uncomfortable. Illumination is very effective to locate veins in the area. Most men don't find the piercing to be intense. Any man who has ever had a zipper accident will probably say that it was considerably worse than a frenum piercing.

Frenum Piercing: Healing and Troubleshooting

Because frenum piercings have a tendency to experience a lot of friction during sexual activity, you must modify your behavior if you experience discomfort. Pleasure Plus condoms have extra room in the traditional frenum area.

Frenum piercings frequently migrate a small amount during healing, and those placed in nontraditional spots often move even more. A barbell that fits well at first can end up a little long. Downsizing to a snug bar after healing makes your piercing more comfortable and less prone to irritation. Frenum (and several other genital) piercings could result in thickening of the tissue, which becomes harder and denser around the jewelry. This does not indicate a complication. These tissue changes can be permanent, or they may diminish over time.

Frenum Piercing: Changing Jewelry

After a traditionally placed frenum piercing heals, you may want to replace your jewelry with a large ring or add a *frenum loop* (band of metal that encircles the shaft) by attaching it to your barbell. The tissue is sometimes malleable enough that the frenum loop can be added onto your existing barbell. If your post is too snug you will need a longer one to accommodate the attachment ends of the loop. A functional style variation has several balls around the outside of the loop for your partner's pleasure.

> **Tribal Frenum Piercing**
> A documented reference shows that a tribe in Southeast Asia practiced frenum piercing for sexual enjoyment long ago. According to an ethnology publication dated 1884, "Amongst the Timorese of Indonesia, the Frenulum beneath the glans penis is pierced with brass rings, the function of the ring is to enhance stimulation during sex."[8] Lacking other historical precedents, the frenum piercing appears to be primarily a modern innovation, intended for the pleasure of the wearer and possibly his partner.

Determine the diameter you need for an around-the-head jewelry style while you are erect. Measure using a draftsman's circle template (available at office and art supply stores). The frenum loop or ring should be snug when you are erect. If you have a substantial size difference between flaccid and rigid states, these jewelry styles will stay up behind your glans only when you are erect.

Ring-style jewelry is not sturdy enough for this usage in 12 gauge unless it is less than an inch in diameter; 10 gauge or thicker is preferable. A circular barbell is a good option because the two balls on the top of your penis provide extra stimulation for your partner, and you can alter the diameter of a circular barbell to your exact size by spreading or narrowing the gap between the balls. If two balls are good, a third is often better; add an extra one to create a captive circular barbell. It will be harder to find a bead that fits in a wide gap if you have spread the ring diameter.

Frenum Piercing: Stretching

If your frenum piercing is placed in very loose excess skin, it will be a better candidate for stretching to a large size. A frenum piercing through taut tissue or a nontraditionally placed frenum will be less likely to respond well to attempts at stretching.

Frenum Piercing: Retiring

Removing jewelry from a healed piercing often results in complete closure of the channel. Some permanent changes in the appearance of the area are common. Once hardened scar tissue forms, it generally remains fairly obvious because this skin is fine. Dimpling or pitting of the skin might also be evidence of an abandoned piercing.

The Lorum Piercing

- **Healing time:** 3 to 4 months or longer
- **Initial jewelry style:** Ring-style or curved bar

- **Initial jewelry gauge:** 12 or 10 gauge
- **Initial jewelry size:** Minimum bar diameter ⅝ inch; minimum ring diameter ¾ inch

The lorum is located at the natural fold that divides the penis shaft from the scrotal sack (see illustration, page 160). The name was coined in the late 1980s as I was performing a genital piercing on the late Dan Kopka, my former coworker at Gauntlet, Los Angeles. He wanted a frenum, he said, only lower.

"Not a frenum, a lower-um," Dan declared, pinching the tissue at the desired spot.

"Oh, that would be a good spot. Yeah, a 'lorum,'" was my reply, and thus it was named. Piercing in that particular location has been called a lorum ever since.

Lorum Piercing: Placement and Choice of Jewelry

The lorum is a horizontal piercing on the underside of the penis at the juncture of the penis and the scrotum. It can be cheated slightly toward the shaft for functionality: in this spot, the jewelry helps to anchor a condom in place—though this would be uncomfortable and traumatic during healing.

This stretchy tissue changes substantially depending on factors including temperature and arousal. Your piercer should carefully check the spacing of proposed marks before piercing you, because the skin can expand dramatically.

Lorum Piercing: Procedure

I perform the lorum with forceps, as I do other piercings in this area. Your piercer may request that you wash your hands or don a glove to help hold your penis out of the way. Some piercers will make use of a Prince Albert piercing, if you have one, by attaching a cord to your jewelry and tying it around your neck to keep your penis from obstructing the area. Your piercer may, however, manage to access the area without assistance.

If you have failed to trim or shave, the pulling of some hair may end up being the most uncomfortable part of your piercing experience; men do not usually find the lorum to be an intense piercing. This area seldom bleeds heavily.

Lorum Piercing: Healing and Troubleshooting

The piercing is protected because it is sandwiched between the scrotum and the shaft of the penis; healing tends to be easy and comfortable. Like other genital piercings, this one sometimes develops lumpy or hardened tissue around the openings as a normal part of healing.

Because the lorum rests just inside the open end of a condom, during healing a waterproof bandage should be used to seal off and protect your piercing and the surrounding area before sexual activities.

Lorum Piercing: Changing Jewelry

Once you are healed, it is not particularly difficult to change your jewelry. A minor challenge is that your penis needs to be kept out of the way in order to access the area.

Much like a frenum loop, a large ring can be worn around the shaft at base of the penis through the healed piercing. To make an even more effective pierced cock ring arrangement, wear this in conjunction with a pubic piercing and thread a single ring through both healed channels. Accurate placement is imperative for this to be workable; even so, it can be uncomfortable for daily wear. If you have a large size differential between flaccid and erect states, this combination will not be possible.

Lorum Piercing: Stretching

The lorum is a sturdy piercing that can be stretched to large gauges. It is not particularly challenging to enlarge, but you must have sufficient tissue in the initial piercing and wait long enough (six months or more) between stretches.

Lorum Piercing: Retiring

Because the lorum rests in a natural fold under the penis, evidence of the piercing will not be obvious upon removal. Residual scarring will not be noticeable even on a nudist.

Lorum piercings tend to shrink and close quickly. Once jewelry is removed from a well-healed lorum piercing, it cannot ordinarily be reinserted easily later.

The Scrotum Piercing (Hafada)

- **Healing time:** 3 to 4 months or longer
- **Initial jewelry style:** Ring-style or curved bar
- **Initial jewelry gauge:** 12 or 10 gauge
- **Initial jewelry size:** Minimum bar diameter ⅝ inch; minimum ring diameter ¾ inch

If you prefer a piercing that is ornamental and not inserted during intercourse, a scrotum piercing may appeal to you (see illustrations, pages 160 and 175). The general location of a scrotum piercing is evident in its name, but the particulars are limited only by the imagination. They can be placed pretty much anywhere the skin can be pinched. The piercing is sometimes called a *hafada*, especially when placed on one or both sides in the upper portion of the natural fold. Scrotum piercings can go along the midline, from lorum to guiche, and in its most plentiful expression, multiple piercings can form a chain mail pouch surrounding the entire sack.

Scrotum Piercing: Placement and Choice of Jewelry

The piercing traverses only the surface tissue and does not penetrate the interior of the scrotal sack. To help you decide on placement, imagine the way jewelry will rest in your skin and how clothing and motion from your activities will affect the healing wound. The orientation of the piercing is not a limiting factor when you wear bar-style jewelry; vertical, diagonal, or otherwise, it will rest close to your body. A ring is suitable as initial jewelry only when the piercing is set at a horizontal angle.

Be patient with your piercer, because the scrotum can be tricky to mark. This tissue expands, contracts, and changes drastically and rapidly. Your piercer may require you to stand and sit several times to check the placement. A set of marks represents a baseline for the way the tissue rests at that particular time. A pair of dots can appear level and then rise, fall, or spread to change position by as much as an inch. Asymmetry of the scrotum is standard, so marking matching pairs can be challenging. If you are uncertain about the marks, ask your piercer to let you wait for a few minutes to see if any tissue changes require adjustments. If you plan to have a scrotum ladder, getting several piercings in one session can lead to more accurate alignment and spacing.

Scrotum Piercing: Procedure

This procedure is essentially the same as the lorum piercing.

Scrotum Piercing: Healing and Troubleshooting

As far as sexual activity is concerned, it could be considered either a pro or a con that the piercing is not on your penis. It won't be tender during penetration, but the healing wound still needs to be protected from bodily fluids, even though it doesn't go inside a condom. Therefore, you must use a waterproof wound-sealant bandage to cover the piercing and surrounding area during sexual activities.

Scrotum Piercing: Changing Jewelry

If you are comfortable changing your own jewelry, the frontal placements can be swapped out on your own. Further toward the back of the scrotum, they may be more difficult to handle on your own. You might experience pleasurable sensations from adding weight to your scrotum piercing.

Scrotum Piercing: Stretching

Scrotum piercings can be expanded to relatively large sizes after healing. To safeguard your piercing, wait at least six to nine months from the initial piercing before attempting your first stretch, and the same amount of time between subsequent enlargements. Unless you wear weights, the one-gauge-at-a-time schedule is standard.

Scrotum Piercing: Retiring

Once you take the jewelry out, there is a tendency for the piercing to shrink and close; it can be difficult or impossible to reinsert if you change your mind later. If you had substantial tissue changes during healing, some lumpiness or thickening may be visible. If you do not depilate your hair and the piercing is placed within the natural folds of the scrotum, these changes may not be obvious.

The Guiche Piercing

- **Healing time:** 3 to 4 months or longer
- **Initial jewelry style:** Ring-style or curved bar; also PTFE or Tygon barbell
- **Initial jewelry gauge:** 12 or 10 gauge
- **Initial jewelry size:** 9/16-inch minimum bar diameter; 5/8-inch minimum ing diameter

The term *guiche* (pronounced "geesh") refers to a piercing behind the scrotum that straddles the *perineal raphe* or *perineum*, the faint ridge of tissue that runs from the scrotum to the anus (see illustration, page 156). This piercing is specifically for the pleasure of the wearer, and jewelry creates various possibilities for erotic stimulation. Ornamenting the perineum with a piercing calls attention to the region in addition to making it more sensitive. Folklore has it that South Pacific Islanders pierced this area during puberty as a rite of passage into adulthood. They reportedly wore a leather thong through the piercing with a shell dangling from it. Although this story is quaint, this is another colorful fabrication, courtesy of Doug Malloy. The guiche appears to be a modern innovation, originating in the gay leather community.

Guiche Piercing: Placement and Choice of Jewelry

The guiche is a horizontal piercing between the scrotum and the anus, near the meeting point of the center seam and inseam of your pants. The piercing should be placed at least ⅝ inch from your anus. You might have limited space, with only a single location where a guiche can be situated. If you are more generously built in that region, you may have a range of options. Your piercer may point out (by gently pinching and prodding) the traditional central placement and then offer sites slightly north and south so you can select the one that feels the best to you. Multiple guiches are possible if you have a long perineum, but more than one is not usually performed in the same session. I have done a few vertical perineum piercings, but they are not common.

> **Gigantic Guiche**
>
> The largest guiche piercing I've ever seen was at least 00 gauge (9 or 10 mm). It was the ever-present companion of a long-distance truck driver who attributed his patience for his job to the enjoyment he experienced while riding on his impressive guiche piercing.

You are suited to the guiche piercing if you have loose, pliable skin in this region. If you have a flat build, you will need to wear jewelry that is a little wider in diameter to encompass sufficient tissue. If you are built with a pouchy, convex-shaped perineum, then a ⅝-inch diameter ring or 9/16-inch curved bar usually works well. The size and shape of your thighs also affect the placement, and this should be factored in during marking. A small amount of migration is normal during healing, so if your piercing is started with too little tissue, you can end up with a shallow piercing that might reject.

Guiche Piercing: Procedure

Your piercer will find it easier to mark and pierce your guiche if you have trimmed or shaved. Depending on the thickness of your hair, he will probably need to do this for you if you have failed to do so yourself. Some piercers position you on your back with your feet on the table or in stirrups. Others place you on your hands and knees. Both are valid options, and your piercer may use one to mark and the other to double-check the placement and/or to pierce you.

As when performing all male genital piercings that are not on the glans, I use forceps.

Guiche Piercing: Healing and Troubleshooting

You may want to wear sanitary pads or liners throughout healing to help the area stay dry and provide protective padding. Keep the piercing as free from moisture as possible and maintain good air circulation.

Due to the wound's proximity to the anus, you must be careful to avoid contact with waste during healing and to shower once or twice a day. Following bowel movements, wipe away from the piercing to uphold good hygiene practices. If you use wet-wipe products after visiting the toilet, do not allow the towelettes to touch your piercing if they contain detergents, fragrances, chemicals, or preservatives. The ingredients may be suitable for feminine freshening or post-potty cleanup, but they aren't meant for use on open wounds like piercings. Protect the piercing with a waterproof bandage before engaging in receptive anal sex during healing.

This region is subject to considerable friction from daily activities, which can cause the piercing to become irritated. A healing guiche doesn't prohibit exercise, though it is certainly best to avoid biking and horseback riding for the first few weeks. Lumpy, protruding scar tissue sometimes temporarily forms at the openings of the piercing during healing. You may need to change your jewelry style or size to resolve this problem.

Guiche Piercing: Changing Jewelry

You will need to get a piercer or a capable friend to help you because it is very tricky to access a guiche by yourself unless you are extraordinarily flexible. The added sensation of wearing weights on your guiche could be enjoyable.

Guiche Piercing: Stretching

Some men like the look and feel of wearing large guiche jewelry after the piercing has healed. If you have sufficient tissue, your guiche can slowly be stretched to substantial gauges. A solid guiche piercing in this sturdy and resilient area can support relatively heavy weight. You should be ready to stretch up one gauge approximately six to nine months after piercing.

Guiche Piercing: Retiring

Guiche piercings tend to shrink quickly, though occasionally they will remain open without jewelry in place. The guiche generally leaves two divots that are not highly visible. An abandoned piercing is unlikely to be noticed.

The Pubic Piercing

- **Healing time:** 3 to 4 months or longer
- **Initial jewelry style:** Curved bar, ring-style, or PTFE or Tygon barbell
- **Initial jewelry gauge:** 12 gauge minimum, but 10 gauge preferred
- **Initial jewelry size:** 7/8-inch minimum diameter ring or 3/4-inch minimum curved bar

There is no apparent historical precedent for the pubic piercing, but it has been making a showing in recent years. Rock star Lenny Kravitz has displayed his pubic piercing in a few of his more risqué photos. This is a good choice if you desire a genital piercing that is easily visible when you are undressed, or one that does not actually pierce the penis. The pubic piercing is not involved in penetration, but it still has the potential to be sexually functional. A ring in your pubic piercing can stimulate your partner's clitoris when you are face-to-face during intercourse.

Pubic Piercing: Placement and Choice of Jewelry

The pubic piercing should be located in the natural fold where the top of your penile shaft meets your body (see illustration, page 175). It is frequently placed—incorrectly—on the flat portion of the pubic mound. This too-high pubic piercing is significantly harder to heal than one that is properly positioned. Because so many piercers put them in the wrong area and in skin that is too taut, this piercing has developed an undeserved reputation for high rejection rates. For the pubic piercing to be successful, the initial placement needs to be wider than that of most body piercings: I encompass a minimum of almost ¾ inch of tissue. When the piercing is set wide enough in pliable tissue at that juncture, healing is seldom eventful.

> **Instant Gratification**
>
> So many piercees find that the guiche piercing feels good as soon as the jewelry is in place that I became a little envious. Their immediate enjoyment—and my resulting guiche envy—was my inspiration for researching the female *fourchette* piercing.

If you are marked while you are seated, the piercer should also check the placement while you are standing, because the angle may change with the position of your body.

The curved bar is the safest, most comfortable style for initial jewelry; it is subject to less friction and stress than a ring.

Pubic Piercing: Procedure

Prepare by trimming or shaving the area before you go in for a pubic piercing. Following tissue manipulation to prepare the area, I use forceps to perform the pubic piercing.

A pubic piercing may bleed, swell, or bruise afterward, but it is not among the most vascular or tender of the male genital piercings. Most men do not find the pubic piercing to be particularly sensitive or intense.

Pubic Piercing: Healing and Troubleshooting

You might find it comfortable to wear a panty liner to protect the area with a layer of absorbent padding for the first few weeks.

Like the lorum, the pubic piercing may be able to help hold a condom in place. But a prophylactic won't cover this area, so you must wear a waterproof bandage to avoid sharing bodily fluids during sexual activity throughout healing.

Pubic Piercing: Changing Jewelry

If you begin with a bar, you may want to change to a ring later, especially if the sexual pleasure of your female partner is among your motivations for getting this piercing. The captive circular barbell is one of the best options for that purpose, as the three balls provide the best chance of connecting with the right spot for her enjoyment. Keeping your pubic hair trimmed will help make home jewelry changes easier. Because the channel is wider than most, you should use an insertion taper during swaps.

Pubic Piercing: Stretching

Because pubic piercings are essentially surface piercings, it is not common practice to stretch them to large sizes. A sturdy 8 or even 6 gauge is not unheard of, but jumbo jewelry is seldom worn here.

Pubic Piercing: Retiring

Only if you depilate the region will residual marks be noticeable. Pubic piercings are not likely to stay open well without jewelry in place because of the long channel and relative density of the tissue.

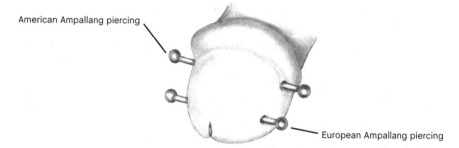

American Ampallang piercing

European Ampallang piercing

Getting the Shaft: Ampallang and Apadravya Piercings

In the West, we have come to call the vertical placement an *apadravya*, although it is uncertain if this term was used the same way in ancient times. The name *ampallang* (pronounced "am puh lang"), used for the horizontal placement, is said to derive from the Dyaks in Borneo. Traditionally, when Dyak boys reached manhood, their rite of passage would be celebrated with the placement of the *palang* (cross bar) horizontally through the head of the penis; no woman of quality would marry a man without it.[9] Ampallangs are now more popular in modern culture than they are among tribal peoples; today the men in Borneo seldom get them.

A bar worn vertically through the head of the penis may be capable of stimulating a woman's *G-spot* (a sexually sensitive spot on the front wall of the vagina) and increasing sensation and pleasure for both partners. Sexual motivations remain an inspiration for most modern men who seek these piercings. An *iron cross* or *magic cross* is made when the same piercee wears both horizontal and vertical piercings.

The Ampallang Piercing

- **Healing time:** 6 to 9 months or longer
- **Initial jewelry style:** Straight barbell
- **Initial jewelry gauge:** 14, 12, or 10 gauge
- **Initial jewelry size:** Anatomically dependent; bar length must fit your erect size

The piercing, healing course, and aftercare concerns are very similar for both piercings through the glans. Therefore, the ampallang will be described in detail first, followed by a section to highlight the differences and specific considerations of the apadravya piercing.

Ampallang: Placement and Choice of Jewelry

What I refer to as the *American ampallang* goes horizontally through the head of the penis above the urethra. It is generally set back closer to the corona than to the tip of the penis. The *European ampallang* is placed considerably lower and more forward on the penis head, and it passes through the urethra. The European version will probably heal faster because it is located where the penis is narrower, so it pierces less tissue; and, because it traverses the urethra, urine may help promote healing. This will not interfere with urination unless the gauge is excessively large. Whether American or European placement is best is a matter of personal opinion.

A 14-gauge ampallang bar can bend with heavy use (after healing, of course). The 12 gauge is a more serviceable size. Jewelry over an inch long (and sometimes 1 ½ inches or more) is frequently used. The barbell must comfortably accommodate your maximum girth across the penis head when you are fully erect.

If you can measure yourself for post length before coming in to be pierced, this will help your piercer. However, it is important to take your measurement at the spot where the piercing will be placed. If you have not premeasured and you do not get an erection during the course of cleaning and marking, your piercer may step out of the room to have you assess your maximum size. Having to achieve an erection and measure it in the studio right before a piercing is not easy for most men, but accuracy is crucial. If your bar is too short, it will pinch painfully when you are erect; if it is overly long, it will snag. In a worst-case scenario, you have to estimate bar length. Regardless of your piercer's expertise, you are more familiar with your own penis and you will need to help select the diameter. Strive for precision rather than to impress.

Ampallang Piercing: Procedure

Most men find the ampallang rather daunting because of the lengthy piercing channel, though plenty of my clients have said that their nipple piercings were more sensitive. The ampallang goes through the spongy tissue of the glans, where most nerve endings are capable of conveying the sensation of pressure. You will feel the greatest intensity as the needle exits, where the nerve endings inform you, "This stings!" Even so, piercees routinely say that it wasn't as bad as they thought it would be.

Because the area is large enough to support well in my fingers, I favor a freehand technique for the ampallang and apadravya. A skilled piercer can accomplish the piercing in just a few moments. The larger the initial gauge, the harder it can be to push through the dense tissue. The 10 gauge can be difficult and take longer to complete.

Some ampallang piercings do not bleed at all, though many bleed freely but intermittently for several days.

Ampallang Piercing: Healing and Troubleshooting

If your initial jewelry is uncomfortable because it is shorter or longer than you need, have a professional piercer swap it out as soon as possible. It is generally more damaging to leave an ill-fitting barbell in place than to change it early.

You may find that the correct post length catches and causes soreness if you have a large size differential between your flaccid and erect states. A telescoping bar that widens and shrinks with your changing anatomy would be perfect but has yet to be produced. Loosely wrap the head and jewelry in a figure-eight bandage with roll gauze to support and stabilize the exposed portion of the post and prevent excess movement.

Ampallang Piercing: Changing Jewelry

After the piercing is healed, it could be pleasurable to wear a barbell that is short enough to pinch slightly when you are erect. The fit between intimate partners is unique; some couples enjoy large balls, while others prefer minimal jewelry such as flat discs or small balls. Because the channel is so long, an insertion taper should always be used to help with jewelry changes for this piercing.

Ampallang Piercing: Stretching

Patience is needed to stretch piercings that have a long channel or dense tissue, and the ampallang has both. Making a full jump to the next gauge can be difficult. The shrink tubing method (see "Tape Wrap and Heat-Shrink Tubing," page 227) can facilitate the process by using intermediate sizes to enlarge the bar a small amount at a time.

Another challenge with piercings that have a long channel is that an average insertion taper is about 2 1/2 inches long, so the entrance side of the piercing may be stretched to the desired gauge before the far side has even been tapered up in size at all. To keep advancing the taper through, maintain constant pressure on it and support the tissue around the exit side. You can have a professional piercer help you with a stretch in the studio, or you can purchase a taper and do it over a more prolonged session at home.

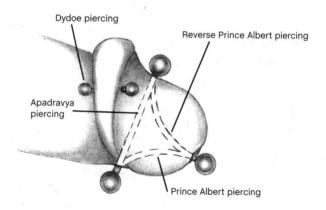

Dydoe piercing

Reverse Prince Albert piercing

Apadravya piercing

Prince Albert piercing

Ampallang Piercing: Retiring

Abandoning the piercing usually results in some pitting or scarring on the glans. If the piercing was no larger than 14 or 12 gauge, the marks may be minimal. Once jewelry is removed for any length of time, it is rare to be able to reinsert it. The interior of the channel has a tendency to shrink quickly, and it usually closes completely.

The Apadravya Piercing

The information below describes the placement of this piercing and highlights its few differences from the ampallang, described above.

Apadravya Piercing: Placement and Choice of Jewelry

The apadravya is pierced vertically through the penis head. It may rest in the center of the glans on the top or be placed closer to the coronal ridge. Because it passes through the urethra, it usually heals faster than an American ampallang.

The apadravya is unique because this single placement encompasses multiple piercings: it is comprised of a Prince Albert on the lower portion and a reverse Prince Albert on the upper.

The apadravya is usually started with a barbell from bottom to top. Later, separate jewelry can be worn in various combinations: a ring in the PA, plus a barbell through the entire head; or, separate jewelry in the PA and reverse PA segments, for example.

When you have the entire piercing performed in one session, advantages include a single healing period and the assurance that the upper and lower parts of the piercing line up nicely. The apadravya can also be performed in any sequence to work with previous piercings: most common is to extend an existing PA up through the top.

If you already have a Prince Albert piercing that is set well off to one side of your midline, it may be possible to make an apadravya on the other side and keep your PA as a separate piercing, if desired. However, the jewelry will pinch the sensitive tissue underneath if there is not enough space between the two piercings.

Apadravya Piercing: Procedure

I perform the apadravya piercing using a freehand technique from the bottom up through the top, though different scenarios are possible. If you already have the upper or lower portion of the apadravya, I carefully place the needle into the existing hole (sometimes with the assistance of a guidance tube that is like a short NRT) and pierce through the opposite side.

Depending on placement, jewelry choice, and previous Prince Albert size, some men elect to heal for a few days or weeks before reinserting PA jewelry. The channel may shrink but it can't close—your new apadravya jewelry occupies the hole. If you have an enlarged PA, you might have room to put your jewelry back right away. Alternatively, you can drop to a thinner gauge in your PA or stretch up to reinsert your usual jewelry.

Apadravya Piercing: Stretching

A notable feature of the adaptable apadravya is that once it has healed you have multiple piercings and the freedom to treat each section differently. For example, you can add a ring or other jewelry to stretch only the lower part of the piercing, leaving the top as is. In fact, you might want to do just that, because enlarging the upper side of the piercing is like stretching an ampallang: difficult. The bottom portion, however, is an easy-to-enlarge Prince Albert.

Apadravya Piercing: Retiring

As with stretching, you have the same flexibility to keep part of the piercing and not the other. If you abandon it, the top may leave a divot or scar. The bottom may remain open, as a PA tends to, especially if it was stretched. Once you heal an apadravya, you probably have a permanent Prince Albert opening.

The Reverse Prince Albert Piercing

- **Healing time:** 4 to 6 months or longer
- **Initial jewelry style:** Curved barbell; if extending a PA, a straight barbell
- **Initial jewelry gauge:** 14, 12, or 10 gauge
- **Initial jewelry size:** Length or diameter anatomically dependent; 7/16-inch minimum curved barbell

This is a midline vertical placement that passes from the urethra to the top of the glans (see illustration, page 170). In essence, the reverse PA is the upper part of an apadravya. The piercing procedure and initial jewelry for the reverse PA depend on whether it is performed as a single piercing or as an extension of an existing Prince Albert piercing.

Reverse PA Piercing: Placement and Choice of Jewelry

Like the apadravya, the top may be positioned closer to the corona than to the urethral opening. It should span a minimum of a ½ inch of tissue from the top edge of the urethral opening when the penis is flaccid.

The jewelry style for a new reverse PA is a curved bar that you wear from the piercing on the top of your glans, through your urethra, and out the urinary meatus. If you already have a regular PA, it is best for healing to extend it through the top using a straight barbell in the apadravya position, even if you plan to wear separate jewelry in the reverse Prince Albert position later.

Reverse PA Piercing: Procedure

If you will wear a curved bar, then the urethra is the avenue for piercing. A needle may be introduced gently into the urethral opening (a guidance tube can help). The piercing is made up through the glans. Alternatively, an NRT may be placed inside the urethra, and the piercing made into it from the top. This skin is thick and tough, so this is a lot more challenging than performing a Prince Albert with the same technique. Regardless of method, your piercing must be angled as vertically as possible for the jewelry to rest correctly.

When a Prince Albert is present, the piercing is the same as described for extending an existing piercing on page 171, "Apadravya Piercing: Procedure." During healing, you wear a barbell through the entire head even though only the upper portion is new.

Reverse PA Piercing: Healing and Troubleshooting

The tissue of the reverse PA is much denser than that of the Prince Albert. You won't leak or drip urine because the tissue remains tight around the jewelry and doesn't stretch on its own, as the PA does. Also, because the piercing is on the top of the penis, above the urethra, gravity works in your favor.

Reverse PA Piercing: Changing Jewelry

You will find it easier to insert new jewelry from the outer surface of the piercing, rather than trying to feed it in through your urethra. After healing, one common jewelry option is to wear a ring. Another possibility is to wear a ball or other ornament on the top of the glans as the only visible part of the jewelry. This is somewhat challenging to insert: a post passes through your reverse PA piercing channel, and a small ball or disc rests inside your urethra. A ³/₁₆-inch ball or a 5 mm disc generally fits comfortably in the interior without blocking the flow of urine. You must attach a threaded taper to the jewelry to help feed the post (and firmly secured ball or disc) in through your urethra and out the piercing. Use hemostats to hold onto your post so you can remove the taper and screw the top ornament into place. Obviously, you must be careful to maintain a solid grasp on the post until the end is affixed to avoid releasing jewelry inside your urethra. Should this happen, it is improbable that you will lose the jewelry inside your urethra. Urinating forcefully will probably drive it out. You can reverse the process with the threaded taper and hemostats to remove or change the jewelry.

Reverse PA Piercing: Stretching

Wait nine months or longer before you attempt to stretch your reverse PA. Do not expect the tissue to be anything like the easy-to-stretch Prince Albert for which it is named. Stretching a reverse PA is much more akin to enlarging an ampallang or apadravya. Measures to create and wear in-between sizes, as described in "Tape Wrap and Heat-Shrink Tubing," page 227, are helpful for stretching this dense tissue.

Reverse PA Piercing: Retiring

If you remove a reverse PA piercing, you will be left with a mark where the jewelry was worn. It should not be disfiguring if it was not stretched to a large gauge. Because the channel is relatively long compared to a PA, and the tissue is solid, there is a strong likelihood that the piercing will close completely upon removal.

The Dydoe Piercing

- **Healing time:** 3 to 4 months or longer
- **Initial jewelry style:** Curved bar
- **Initial jewelry gauge:** 14 gauge; occasionally 12 gauge for men with a full build
- **Initial jewelry size:** Diameter anatomically dependent, with a ³/₈-inch minimum

The dydoe piercing frames the rim of the corona (see illustration, page 170). It appears to be a modern innovation. Many men are not built with enough defined flare to the glans to comfortably or safely accommodate jewelry in this location. Therefore, the dydoe isn't the most popular of the male genital piercings.

Dydoe Piercing: Placement and Choice of Jewelry

Those suited to a dydoe piercing will have a substantial mushroom-shaped ridge at the rim of the glans. If the piercing is made too close to the surface, migration and rejection are usual consequences. Dydoes are traditionally done in pairs off to the sides, near three and nine o'clock or two and ten. Some men are formed to wear a single piercing at the center. A suitably contoured corona is worthy of a being crowned with multiple studs around the upper perimeter. You may be able to heal this piercing if you are uncircumcised, but you must have a fairly loose-fitting foreskin. If your head is sheathed too tightly, the excess pressure on the jewelry will cause trauma and healing difficulties.

A curved bar conforms well to the area to reduce catching and irritation. The ³/₈-inch minimum jewelry diameter will accommodate enough tissue for a safe and enduring piercing when the corona is well defined. Jewelry may be ⁷/₁₆ inch or longer, depending on individual structure. Enough room must be left on the post to allow for growth during erections.

The Cyprian Society

The dydoe was ostensibly invented to increase the sensitivity diminished by foreskin removal in circumcision. The term was coined by piercing pioneer Doug Malloy as a free association for the word *doodad* (an added decoration). Doug claimed that after World War I, a group of men who called themselves the Cyprian Society opposed the indiscriminate circumcision of babies. Malloy reported that they carried out dydoe piercings to "heighten sexual pleasure . . . to offset the less sensitive skin which came with the loss of the foreskin." No evidence beyond Doug's claims has been found to confirm this tale.

Dydoe Piercing: Procedure

Forceps can be used to secure the tissue if the area is pronounced enough. They do, however, feel very pinchy in this spot. I generally use a freehand procedure for dydoes. An NRT may also be used.

Because the dydoe doesn't encompass a wide span of tissue, you might mistakenly believe that this is not a very intense piercing. Most nerve endings, however, are located close to the surface, as anyone who has had a scrape or rug burn that stings like mad will understand. You may be surprised to learn that a single ampallang is probably easier to receive than a pair of dydoes.

Dydoe Piercing: Healing and Troubleshooting

You must be very gentle during sexual activities while you are healing because the dydoe generally frames the widest part of the anatomy. Using a sterile gauze wrap around the jewelry when the piercing is fresh can diminish jewelry movement.

Dydoe Piercing: Changing Jewelry

The channel is short from entry to exit, so it shouldn't be difficult to change the jewelry on your own dydoes once you are healed. Just don't leave it empty for long, because this type of tissue has a tendency to shrink quickly.

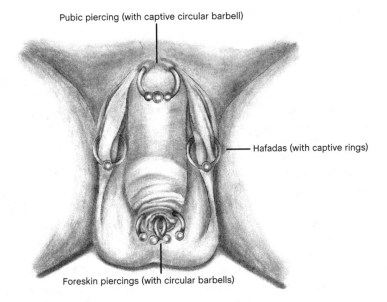

Pubic piercing (with captive circular barbell)

Hafadas (with captive rings)

Foreskin piercings (with circular barbells)

Dydoe Piercing: Stretching

The dydoe is situated in a minimal amount of tissue close to the edge of the penis, so large sizes are not desirable. These are seldom stretched beyond 12 or 10 gauge.

Dydoe Piercing: Retiring

When you remove a dydoe piercing you can expect to have some visible marks left on your glans. Even if a dydoe doesn't close entirely when you abandon it, the channel usually shrinks, and you will probably find it difficult and tender to reinsert jewelry.

The Foreskin Piercing

- **Healing time:** 2 to 3 months or longer
- **Initial jewelry style:** Ring, barbell, or curved bar
- **Initial jewelry gauge:** 12 or 10 gauge
- **Initial jewelry size:** Minimum length or diameter ½ inch or larger; commonly ⅝ inch

Foreskin piercing is obviously reserved for men who are uncircumcised. Therefore, this placement is not especially popular in the United States, where most men have been deprived of this opportunity. However, men who engage in successful foreskin restoration[10] may be able to rebuild enough tissue to pierce. In turn, the piercing (once healed) can assist in the process by providing greater purchase on the area for further tissue expansion.

The foreskin is one of the genital piercings with significant historical precedent, mostly for *infibulation* (the enforcement of chastity through mechanical means). Some contemporary piercees engage in consensual infibulation using multiple foreskin piercings (see "Infibulation," page 258), but nowadays this piercing is mostly used to enhance sensation.

Foreskin Piercing: Placement and Choice of Jewelry

Because the tissue is fine, jewelry that is not thick enough can cause cutting or tearing. To withstand rougher friction and for durability, 12-gauge jewelry is a suitable minimum. Jewelry with a length or diameter of ⅝ inch will encompass sufficient tissue for a safe piercing. Let your piercer know during marking if you plan to stretch up later or use them for infibulation so he can place them a little farther back.

When the foreskin is fully retracted, this piercing rests like a vertical frenum, generally near the mid-shaft of the penis. This impressive tissue change must be scrutinized during marking. Even though your foreskin will remain over the head most of the time, jewelry must not pinch excessively when the foreskin is retracted.

Standard procedure is to mark a reference line at the edge of the foreskin as it hangs down naturally, and to pierce to either side of that border so that the jewelry frames the rim. Marking for the piercing when your foreskin is in the retracted position assures placement that will fit with the size of your chosen jewelry. When the foreskin is in its flaccid position it may appear that the piercing will be through only a small amount of skin near the edge of the rim. (If your piercer were to mark placement while your foreskin is down, the marks would probably spread to over an inch apart when it is retracted. It is not practical to wear jewelry that would accommodate this placement.)

You can wear a single piercing, a pair, or multiples, depending on your personal preference. Pairs of piercings positioned at three and nine o'clock, or at twelve and six o'clock, are popular. Anywhere around the perimeter of your foreskin is acceptable as long as you have enough space between the piercings. Depending on your anatomy and the jewelry size and style, you might be able to wear four or more piercings in your foreskin, though certainly no more than that should be performed in a single session.

Foreskin Piercing: Procedure

I use forceps to clamp the foreskin because the tissue rolls and slides. Illumination easily demonstrates where your veins are located so they can be avoided. Bleeding in this region is usually minor. For comfort and ease of healing, I perform the piercing when your tissue is in the flaccid position to straddle the fold naturally. This procedure is very similar to a frenum piercing, and most men describe the sensation as fairly minor. Bear in mind that this tissue is routinely removed from infants sans anesthetic.

Foreskin Piercing: Healing and Troubleshooting

Try to be gentle and to retract your foreskin as little as possible while maintaining sound hygiene during initial healing. Do a saline soak or other maintenance to remove crusty matter beforehand. Since urine will pass over the area, you can use the measures suggested under "Genital Piercing: Urinating," page 136, and "Male Genital Piercings: Urinating," page 154.

Foreskin Piercing: Changing Jewelry

Later you can wear a ring or bar smaller than the initial diameter, but jewelry must be large enough to allow you to comfortably retract your foreskin. Because of the membranous nature of the tissue, you might want assistance with changes. If you plan to swap it yourself, use an insertion taper, at least initially. Changing jewelry will be easiest when your foreskin is down and the piercing is at its most compact.

Foreskin Piercing: Stretching

Foreskin piercings can be stretched to larger sizes, even though the tissue is relatively fine. If you engage in heavy play or wear weights, it might be possible to safely skip a gauge, as these activities help you stretch. Wait six months or more after piercing before stretching.

Foreskin Piercing: Retiring

This piercing frames the edge of a natural fold, so evidence from only one of the marks will be visible if you remove the jewelry from a foreskin piercing. The second mark will be exposed only when your foreskin is retracted. It can be difficult to find the channel if you want to reinsert jewelry in an abandoned piercing due to the mobile nature of the tissue.

The Point

Because of the private nature of the area, intimate piercings are a viable option for adults who do not have the freedom or desire to wear visible piercings. Many men and women derive intense enjoyment and satisfaction from genital piercings. If you are attracted to one, take the plunge. Genital piercing can provide an extraordinary way of celebrating the beauty of your body and the freedom to enjoy your sexuality to its fullest.

PART 5

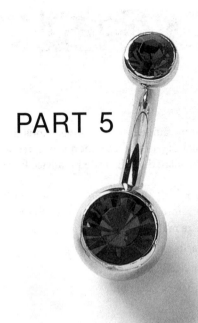

Healing and Aftercare

Healing 101: Standard Aftercare

Disclaimer: These care guidelines and suggestions are based on a combination of extensive professional experience, common sense, research, and vast clinical practice; they are not to be considered a substitute for advice from a medical professional.

A piercing is a wound, albeit a unique one, because it is created intentionally and meant to heal with a foreign object present in the body. Even so, when we refer to "aftercare," what we're really discussing is *wound care*,[1] which includes:

- Minimizing factors that inhibit healing
- Enhancing the healing process
- Reducing the risk of infection

The Evolution of Aftercare

Years ago, the usual treatment for a healing piercing involved applying alcohol twice daily and frequently turning the jewelry so it wouldn't get stuck. This antiquated method is now viewed as a rather brutal abuse of a piercing.

Most over-the-counter wound care remedies are not appropriate because they are not intended for the long-term care piercings require, nor are they meant for use on puncture wounds. Piercers and piercees had to improvise because products specifically designed for the purpose of healing body piercings had yet to be introduced. Over the past few decades, piercers advocated an assortment of products, including Betadine, Hibiclens, alcohol, hydrogen peroxide, Neosporin, and Dial soap. Yet, today, these are all considered potentially detrimental to healing piercings. Bactine and other pierced ear solutions were also commonly suggested, but they, too, have fallen out of favor. See details in "What Not to Use on Your Piercings," page 191.

The methods of cleaning and caring for piercings have developed over time through trial and error. New regimens have come about through a better understanding of how piercings heal and access to more suitable products.

Consider the experience of an unfortunate man who got his nipple pierced in 1986:

"That piercing took six or seven years (yes, years) to properly heal. . . . I would attribute that to the 'aftercare' we practiced back then. The usual choices were washing with Betadine (iodine scrub) or Hibiclens, a (possibly carcinogenic) surgical scrub. Yup, way too harsh. I cut the Hibiclens to half-strength a few years into it. See, aftercare was evolving even then. . . ." C.

Countless piercees have healed well using the commonsense aftercare guidelines offered below. That said, there is one fundamental principle about healing: *human bodies vary*. Not all piercees respond in the same way to the same products and procedures. Effort and patience are sometimes needed to figure out what works best to heal your piercing. You may even find that what worked well in the past does not have the same effect on a subsequent piercing. Variations in climate, water quality, your health, and many other factors impact the healing course.

Aftercare Advice: The Good, the Bad, and the Ugly

Understandably, you may feel confused by conflicting aftercare advice advocated by different piercers, friends, and medical professionals. Some methods are obsolete, others are too new, and still others are bizarre or downright harmful. Individuals on Internet forums may swear by off-the-wall products like rum or meat tenderizer, but beware of wacky care regimes such as these, or a strict no-cleaning approach.

Products designed for piercing care have inundated the market in recent years. Many are touted as "the best" or "the only" thing to use, so it can be confusing to decide which, if any, to buy. In general, it is prudent to follow a straightforward healing regimen that emphasizes health and hygiene rather than miracle products.

Your primary resource for care instructions should be a competent piercer. Most professionals will provide information that is similar to what is advised below, though in less detail than is described here. (No piercer has the time to go into this amount of depth!) Other care regimens might work, but if your piercer's advice differs radically from everything discussed in this book, use caution and common sense.

The aftercare guidelines should be conveyed to you at the piercing studio both verbally and in writing. Some laws governing piercing mandate this dual approach because the information is so important. A piercer who does not take the time to thoroughly explain the required care and cleaning is doing an unprofessional job, regardless of whether her implements are sterile and her piercings well placed.

The Wound-Healing Process

In order for you to care for your piercings properly, it helps if you understand the basic process your body goes through as it heals. The piercing follows a progression from a new wound to a healed piercing, during which the *fistula* (flesh tunnel) that holds the jewelry forms, seals up, and toughens. The stages described below overlap during the healing process.

During stage 1, or the *inflammatory phase*, a piercing is a fresh, open wound. Bleeding, swelling, and tenderness are all normal. Over the first few days, the blood clots and platelets and plasma infiltrate the wound to achieve *hemostasis* (stoppage of bleeding). As the wound begins to heal, the body forms and lays down *basal* (base) cells—the foundation layer of the *epidermis*.

Stage 2, or the *growth* or *proliferative phase*, lasts several weeks for most wounds. However, this stage routinely takes several more weeks, months, or even longer when you get a piercing, because these processes must take place around the jewelry present in the wound. This phase includes both *granulation*, during which your body produces cells, including *collagen* (proteins), to heal and strengthen the wound, and *contraction*, during which the edges of the wound usually pull together (contraction, however, is impeded in piercing because of the jewelry). This is the stage when *"crusties"* regularly form (see "Normal Piercing Secretions," below).

During this phase, new skin cells, called *epithelials*, begin to grow from the edges of the wound inward, building upon the base layer. In a process called *epithelialization*, these cells grow together and thicken, and finally they completely line the wound, merging from end to end across the piercing, creating a sealed channel. The new skin is delicate and can still be torn quite easily at this stage. By the end of this phase, initial healing is considered complete.

Stage 3 is called *maturation* or *remodeling*. During this phase, the collagen becomes more organized. For a piercing, it takes months to years for the cells that have lined the interior of the channel—essentially, scar tissue—to strengthen and stabilize after the fistula has formed from end to end. Piercings commonly go through a series of cycles between the second and third stages.[2]

When one or more of these stages is disrupted or delayed, complications frequently occur. This is why healing piercings can be so challenging: keeping a foreign object inside a wound predisposes each stage to take longer than usual.

Normal Piercing Secretions

During stage one, as a response to the injury just hours after piercing, an *inflammatory serous exudate* (red and white blood cells, blood proteins, and other components) fills the wound to help with clotting, prevent infection, and begin the repair process.

During much of the healing course, it is normal to experience *"crusties,"* a nonmedical term used to describe the dried discharge of *serous exudates* (lymph, dead cells, and *interstitial fluid* [liquid from between cells]) that comes from a healing piercing. A small amount of clear or straw-colored fluid seeps from the channel, dries, and forms a bit of crust on your jewelry and the tissue around the openings of your piercing. Never pick at it with dirty fingers!

This secretion is distinguished from *pus*, which is a yellowish-white, thick, often foul-smelling fluid. It is made up primarily of white blood cells, bacteria, and dead cells. Pus is secreted in response to inflammation or infection. You may see a small amount early in the initial stage due to inflammation; after that, this is not a normal piercing secretion. Compounds produced by certain microbes cause it to have a yellowish, grayish, or greenish appearance. Colored pus is indicative of infection.

Sebum is a substance from your oil glands that collects in healed piercing channels. It is a naturally occurring product of the body, containing fat, *keratin* (a fibrous protein), and cellular material.[3] The purpose of sebum is to protect your skin and hair, keep it moisturized, and to inhibit the growth of microorganisms on the skin. People sometimes mistake it for pus, but it is more solid and cheeselike and has a distinctive rotten odor that reflects the dead cellular debris it contains.

What to Expect

Immediately after being pierced, some bleeding, swelling, and tenderness or pain are standard consequences. Bleeding may continue—usually intermittently—for a few days. Localized bruising is normal, though not typical for most piercings. Heavy blood flow or bleeding that continues for longer than a few days may be cause for concern, and you should contact your piercer or a physician. The placements that routinely bleed freely are discussed in chapters 10–13.

If a piercing bleeds or swells substantially right after the piercing, an ice pack should be applied as soon as possible. Prepared piercers keep disposable instant cold packs ready for use. They can be wrapped in a clean dental bib or paper towel to maintain hygiene. Occasionally, a piercing will swell so much that your piercer needs to swap out your jewelry for a larger piece before you leave the studio. An adept technician will use an insertion taper to change it for you without causing pain or trauma to the area. Internally threaded jewelry is safer and easier to deal with in these situations.

Piercings that bleed under the surface can leave a colorful bruise. *Arnica montana* (a natural herb) may help to diminish the discoloration. Arnica is available in cream or gel form at health food stores. Apply it on the bruise, but do not put it directly into the wound.[4]

On occasion, some localized swelling of a fresh piercing can impinge upon a nerve, causing temporary numbness or tingling, loss of taste in oral piercings, or diminished hearing in ear piercings (rare). However, barring an unusual placement or healing complications, these are transient troubles.

You can expect slight swelling, redness, and oozing of fluid to persist for a prolonged period of time. You might not have bleeding or tenderness immediately afterward, but a few weeks or months later it might happen. This is normal, and in the absence of other problems, there is no cause for concern. Any time a piercing has a flare-up, treat it as if it were new by resuming or accelerating your aftercare regimen.

Healing vs. Healed

Your piercing has passed through the first two stages of healing when there is no tenderness, no secretions forming a crust, and no discoloration. The openings look smooth and sealed, not raw or ragged. If there is sebum present in your piercing, this is a good indication that you no longer have an open wound. Your piercing has passed through the initial healing and entered the final stage, maturation.

After the channel forms and seals, you are still in the third stage, as the scar matures over a long period of time. A piercing that has only recently healed is more delicate than a seasoned one. The skin can be broken, turning your piercing into an open wound again. Just because a piercing has made it through initial healing doesn't mean that it can't regress if it is mistreated.

Minimum Healing Times

The healing time ranges listed in this book are only estimates. They represent the typical amount of time you can expect your piercing to take to reach the end of the second stage of healing and begin the final stage. It varies considerably from person to person, and yours may take longer. You should keep up with your care routine for the entire minimum healing time, even if you believe you have healed faster than usual. You must also continue being gentle with your piercing for longer than that. Wait until your piercing has been settled and stable for months before you attempt any heavy play or stretching.

Basic Aftercare

The sensible suggestions in this chapter are the result of years of informal research and clinical experience; they reflect and expand upon the current industry standard. Safe and appropriate piercing aftercare consists of the following:

- Upholding hygiene
- Maintaining good health habits
- Avoiding trauma
- Soaking in saline
- Cleaning your piercing

You may have noticed that the act of cleaning a wound is only one of several aspects. Caring for your healing piercing is not mysterious or difficult, but you must be consistent and committed. In-depth details are included here so you will be well equipped to ensure that your piercing enjoys a smooth passage through each healing phase.

Hygiene

Hygiene involves keeping your piercing and your environment clean. If you go to a reputable piercer who uses sterile implements and follows proper aseptic techniques, your chances of contracting an infection at the studio are extremely slim. However, if you expose the wound to bacteria by playing with it, swimming in dirty water, or not washing your clothes or body, you risk contracting an infection.

The Golden Rule of Piercing Hygiene that all piercees must follow to avoid infection is this: *do not touch your piercing with dirty hands.* If your hands aren't freshly washed, you should keep them far away from the jewelry. Many bacteria exhibit *motility*, which means they can move on their own.[5] Therefore, you could deposit disease-causing microorganisms simply by touching your body *near* the piercing. I suggest keeping a distance of two hand-widths away from the piercing in every direction. That's about six full inches (15–20 cm) away. Of course, the same goes for anybody else's hands.

These hygiene precautions minimize your risk of infection during healing:

- *Properly* wash your hands before touching your jewelry and the surrounding area (see "Hand Washing Technique," opposite page).
- Change your bedding and towels at least once a week.
- Don't let pets sleep in your bed unless the piercing is well protected.
- Regularly *disinfect* (clean with an antimicrobial product) objects that rest in close proximity to your piercing, such as telephones, earphones, or eyeglasses.
- Avoid the exchange of bodily fluids, even with a monogamous partner: no oral contact, kissing, or sexual contact without barrier protection (i.e., condoms, dental dams, or waterproof bandages) through the third stage of healing. Details are in "Safer Sex," page 255.
- Do not allow personal care products such as sprays and lotions to get into your piercing. Keep these at least a fingertip's distance away from facial piercings—and make sure applicators such as makeup sponges are clean.
- Disposable paper products are safer and more hygienic for drying all piercings.

- Your own sweat and bodily fluids won't harm your piercing if you clean according to instructions (but avoid everyone else's).
- Follow these rules for bathing in a tub to avoid hygiene risks:
  - Before bathing, wash the tub with a 10 percent bleach solution and rinse well.
  - After a bath, rinse your piercing with running water under a faucet, or douse with several clean, large cupfuls of water.
  - Follow this process every time you take a bath during healing.

Be aware of your piercing as a vulnerable open wound, and assess your environment and lifestyle for threats to the cleanliness of your piercing. Take all steps necessary to preserve hygiene at home, work, and play.

The T-Shirt Trick

Before you go to sleep the first night after you get an above-the-neck piercing, put a fresh pillowcase on your pillow, and then dress it in a clean t-shirt. If you have concerns about bleeding, use a black shirt or an old one. This gives you a soft surface and avoids staining your pillowcases.

The following night, flip the pillow over and use the second clean surface. The third night, turn the T-shirt inside out; the fourth night, flip it again. Replace the shirt every four nights. If you're a pillow flipper, you may want to change the shirt every other night.

Health Habits for Rapid Healing

Healthy people heal faster than those who are stressed or run-down; therefore, your first line of defense during the healing period is to take care of yourself. Here are some things you can do to encourage a speedy and smooth healing experience.

- Get plenty of rest.
- Eat a balanced diet of nutritious foods, including complex carbohydrates, plenty of protein, and fresh fruits and vegetables plus healthy fats such as nuts.

Hand Washing Technique

Hand washing has long been recognized as one of the simplest and most helpful practices to prevent the spread of germs and disease. According to the Centers for Disease Control (CDC), "Hand washing is the single most effective way of preventing the spread of infection."

Always wash your hands before and after handling a piercing. The proper method is easy:

- Wet your hands with warm running water, add soap, and rub your hands together to create lather. The friction is crucial to dislodge dirt and germs.
- Keep it up for at least twenty seconds. Wash every part of your hands thoroughly, including wrists, palms, between your fingers, and fingernails.
- Liquid soaps are more hygienic than bar soaps.[6] Antibacterial products may be uncalled for. This is explained in "The Antibacterial Controversy," page 191.
- Rinse well, and dry your hands with a paper towel; the friction of the towel also removes dirt and bacteria.[7]
- After washing your hands, it is vital to avoid touching anything that may harbor bacteria until after you have dealt with your piercing. Use paper towels to turn off the faucet that you just turned on with dirty hands.

For more information on the importance of hand washing, visit www.cleanhandscoalition.org.

- To help healing and bolster your ability to fight infection, take nutritional supplements daily, including iron, B vitamins, 1,000–5,000 mg of vitamin C (divided into a few equal doses throughout the day), and 30 mg of zinc for women (50 mg for men).
- Drink lots of water every day.
- Avoid emotional stress. Stress can increase healing times by 40 percent.[8]
- Don't ingest excessive alcohol or caffeine, and don't use recreational drugs.
- Don't smoke! The carbon monoxide causes *vasoconstriction* (narrowing of the blood vessels), which inhibits oxygen circulation in the blood and negatively impacts healing ability. Smoking also suppresses immune function. These are a few of the reasons doctors advise patients to cut down or quit smoking before surgery. Try not to smoke for a week before you get pierced. At the very least, avoid smoking for ninety minutes before your piercing; a single cigarette can cause vasoconstriction for that long.

These suggestions may sound so basic that you fail to give them more than a passing glance, but don't underestimate the power of healthful habits to boost your immune system and healing capacity. Taking good care of your body is one of the most effective treatments, whether you are healing normally or experiencing complications.

Rubbing You the Wrong Way: Friction and Trauma

Physical trauma is one of the biggest dangers to your new piercing, whether it is caused by mechanical stress from the movement of your body, accidental bumps, or pressure and friction from clothing. Repeated trauma leads to inflammation and *edema* (excess fluid in the tissues that causes swelling), which interferes with local oxygen supply. This reduces your ability to process the wound effectively. Over the long term, friction on your healing piercing will cause complications, including irritation, delayed healing, and ultimately scarring and migration or rejection. To minimize trauma to your healing piercing, follow these guidelines:

- The temptation to play with your new jewelry can be almost overwhelming, but you must resist in order to both avoid trauma and maintain good hygiene.
- Wear jewelry of the proper size and style to minimize friction.
- If your jewelry fits properly and is of high quality, leave it in during the entire healing time. Changing it unnecessarily can damage the fragile tissue.
- Do not handle your piercing roughly during cleaning.
- Avoid cloth towels, terry washcloths, and loofah sponges. The little loops on these materials can catch jewelry and cause damage.
- You may have to modify the position you sleep in to reduce pressure against your piercing. If you are a stomach sleeper, you may have to temporarily sleep on your back or side to protect a navel or nipple piercing. You also may need to adjust the way you rest your head on the pillow if you have a healing ear or facial piercing.
- To avoid accidentally catching or pulling your jewelry, be aware of your actions and the presence of your piercing.

- Take care not to bump or catch your piercing when donning hats, eyeglasses, sunglasses, and so on.
- For below-the-neck piercings, try to wear clothing or underwear that minimizes friction.

Physical Activity and Exercise

Generally, you can exercise during healing if you avoid extremes of motion and prevent impact to the pierced area. Still, your activities often need to be modified—at least for a while—if they cause problems with your piercing.

A direct blow can cause delayed healing, excessive scarring, or traumatic tearing. Especially in exposed areas like the ear and face, jewelry could be snagged or possibly torn out during rough play. Soiled, sweaty equipment such as helmets can expose piercings to bacteria, resulting in infection. Friction from body motion or protective equipment can cause irritation and migration. Before wear, thoroughly clean any sports gear that comes near your piercing. Regular workouts enhance your overall health, which has a positive effect on your healing process. Don't stop all fitness endeavors; just discover what works for you and take extra care during healing.

Protective Patch

Even piercings concealed beneath clothes can be at risk unless you take extra precautions. A hard plastic, vented eye patch secured over the area can shield a nipple or navel from impact. Hold it in place with snug, stretchy workout clothing, or by winding a length of Ace bandage around your torso. Add a sterile gauze square or two between your skin and the plastic guard for a comfortable layer of clean, absorbent padding. These supplies are readily available at any drug store or pharmacy. The patch can be used for a range of circumstances, from shielding a navel piercing against tight pantyhose to protecting a nipple piercing from a bulletproof vest.

Waterproof Protection

Don't expose your piercing to a hot tub, pool, lake, ocean, or any body of water, even if it seems clean. The chemicals in heavily chlorinated pools could be as damaging as the microorganisms and dirt in natural bodies of water. Protect your piercing with a Nexcare Waterproof Bandage, a Tegaderm Transparent Dressing, or similar covering. If you don't use a sealant bandage, then you should avoid submerging (or even splashing) your healing piercing. This type of bandage can also be used to protect piercings from contact with bodily fluids during sexual activities.

Tanning

Tanning during healing can cause the tissue around your piercing to become darker or lighter than your normal skin tone, and the discoloration can be permanent. Some doctors recommend keeping scars out of the sun for a year. If your piercing heals without any visible evidence of scar tissue, this will only be of concern during healing.

Extreme temperatures can disrupt the delicate new cells of a healing piercing. The concentrated heat of a tanning bed could be even worse than the sun. Jewelry that gets burning hot will not feel good on your piercing and could damage fragile cells. Gold is the most heat reactive of the popular jewelry metals, and it can get hot quickly during tanning. Do not get tanning lotion or oil inside your piercing.

Skin Is Sensitive

Avoid exposing your healing piercing to harsh chemicals. Hair spray and dye, deodorant, bug repellent, and other products can irritate or damage your piercing. Stay away from laundry detergents that containing stain-fighting enzymes. These enzymes influence chemical processes, and they include bioengineered products that are designed to break down proteins and other components of fabric stains. They may impede healing by destroying epithelial cells.

Soaps also have the potential to bring on allergic reactions that manifest as *contact dermatitis*, a skin rash from contact with an allergen or irritant (see "Dermatitis," page 212). Depending on the sensitivity of your skin, nearly any product or substance can cause such a reaction. Typically, if you discontinue using an offending product, your problem will resolve. Medical treatment will occasionally be needed. Unless you've used something very strong or caused yourself a secondary infection by scratching an itchy rash, the piercing should not be set back too much by such an incident.

The Soak

One of the best things you can do for all healing or irritated piercings is a saline soak. A warm, mild saltwater solution irrigates, cleanses, and allows the cells to rejuvenate.[9] Saline soaks keep the cells well hydrated while simultaneously flushing out fluid and cellular material that accumulate in the wound. This reduces crusting and helps prevent pockets of trapped matter, which can create unsightly and difficult-to-eliminate bumps. If this debris is not removed, it can impede healing.[10] The warm water also opens capillaries and stimulates blood flow, which transports oxygen to the region, promoting healing.

This is not an invitation to swim in the ocean, where you might encounter numerous microbes, motor oil, and other hazards. The goal is to use a solution with a saline concentration similar to that of the human body. Either make your own by following "The Recipe," opposite page, or use *normal saline* (a 0.9 percent sodium chloride solution).

What to Use and Where to Buy It

Use non-iodized, fine-grain sea salt for your soaks. It is superior to regular table salt, which typically contains additives to prevent it from drying or clumping and other components that could be incompatible with wound healing. Do not use coarse kosher salt or rock salt either, because their large crystals do not dissolve readily. Lastly, do not use Epsom salt; it is magnesium sulfate, which does not share the same properties as sodium chloride.

Sea salt has a long history of use as a curative. It was advocated for wound care by both Imhotep (considered the first doctor known by name, born in Egypt around 2650 B.C.E.) and Hippocrates, the famed Greek physician (born around 460 B.C.E.).[11] Today sea salt is a cooking product, not a medicinal one; it is not sold in pharmacies.

Many piercers sell or supply sea salt, so you might be able to obtain it at the studio when you go in for your piercing. Otherwise, look in the spice section, near the table salt, or in the natural foods aisle of your regular grocery store. It is routinely available in health food stores, or you can order it over the Internet from piercing supply vendors or food and spice websites. Natural sea salt is superior because it usually contains trace elements that are beneficial for health and healing.

An excellent—if more expensive—option is normal saline. It is *isotonic* (it matches the saline concentration of human blood), which is what the sea salt and water recipe is intended to emulate. Normal saline is widely used in the medical field. It is a mild but effective cleaning agent and will not harm normal tissue, unlike many stronger antiseptics.[12] This product is sold in drug stores and can be warmed for soaks.

The saline products sold for contact lenses and ear or nasal irrigation sometimes contain additives that may not be suited to healing piercings. To be safe, a prepared saline solution should be used only if the label confirms that the container holds "isotonic saline," or 0.9 percent sterile saline without additives (meaning that it is, in fact, normal saline).

The Recipe

If you are making your own saline solution, the proper ratio is ¼ teaspoon (*not* tablespoon) of fine-grain, non-iodized sea salt to 1 cup (8 fluid ounces/250 ml) of clean warm water. The correct proportions are critical. If the solution is too strong (*hypertonic*, or containing more salt than your blood), it can irritate your skin. If your soaks cause your skin to become dry, use a mixture of ⅛ teaspoon sea salt per cup of water. Premixing a large batch may be convenient, but it is safest to make a fresh solution every time you soak, as a stored supply can become contaminated.

How to Soak

Pour normal saline into a clean container and warm it in a microwave or mix up the sea salt with warm water. The solution should be the temperature of a drinkable hot beverage. Distilled water is best, and bottled water is a second choice; depending on your local water quality, you may need to avoid tap water unless it is filtered or first brought to a full boil for a minute or longer and then allowed to cool sufficiently before use. Even if you believe your water supply is clean, should you experience difficulty healing, use cleaner water for your saline soaks and final rinses.

Soak your piercing in saline solution for five to ten minutes at least once or twice daily, optimally prior to showering (which will rinse away the salt crystals and piercing secretions). If you're not on your way to the shower, follow your saline treatment with a thorough clear water rinse to remove any residue and debris from the wound, as dried salt crystals and piercing crusties are sharp and can cause damage. Dry with clean paper products. Cotton swabs or sterile gauze squares are helpful for drying ears, navels, and other spots that have nooks and crannies. They can also be used to remove any stubborn matter that remains following a soak. Additional soaks to remove matter can last just a minute or two, but the brief duration won't produce all of the benefits as described in "The Soak," on the previous page.

Depending on the location of your piercing, a mug, glass, or shallow bowl can be an appropriate soaking vessel. A cup or shot glass is perfect for a navel or nipple piercing. Just lean forward and seal the container of solution over the area to create a vacuum. Keep a clean cloth or paper towel handy in case of leaks. For an ear piercing, use a small cup or lay your ear inside a shallow bowl. A mug or small bowl can be used for soaking a genital piercing, depending on its placement. Saturate a sterile gauze pad in saline solution to form a small compress for hard-to-soak spots. Disposable cups are a safe (if not environmentally friendly) option; you can also use clean kitchenware. Before use, clean reusable soaking containers in hot soapy water or in a dishwasher.

Depending on the location of the piercing, the soaking process can be challenging or awkward. Hanging around with your ear in a bowl isn't especially comfy. The process can be time-consuming and seem like more trouble than it's worth. Still, keeping up with soaks for at least the first few weeks will give your piercing maximum support during the early healing stages.

Soaking Etiquette

Do not leave the water you used to soak your Prince Albert (or any other piercing, for that matter) in a mug on the kitchen counter to be sipped by a sleepy spouse or housemate. A former co-worker unhappily fell victim to this situation—but only once.

As your healing progresses, you can try reducing the frequency to once a day or even less. Of course, any time a piercing has a flare-up, you accidentally injure it, or it is aggravated by a stretch, go back to regular saline soaks. Following such a setback, treat your piercing like it is new by following all the guidelines in this chapter.

A good time to do an extra soak is before physical labor, sports, or other movement. This is especially helpful for torso and genital piercings. Crust on your jewelry can get worked into the piercing as you move, causing discomfort and damage. After intense physical activity, you may want to do another saline soak or perform one of your daily cleanings—or at least give your piercing a clear water rinse.

When you aren't able to soak, you may want to use a saline spray that is formulated for use on piercings. Some are normal saline in a clean-delivery can, and others have enzymes or other additives. Barring an inappropriate ingredient or an overly strong stream, these products are safe and convenient. However, spraying does not provide all of the benefits you receive from soaking. See "Specialty Products," page 198.

If you eat a low-sodium diet due to high blood pressure or other medical problem, you may need to limit the use of saline on your piercing as well. Consult your doctor for advice.

Cleansers and Soaps

It is imperative that whatever you use to clean your piercing (see "Cleaning Your Piercing," page 192) helps more than it harms. As healing takes place, new cells grow to form the skin tunnel from the openings on either side. But if more cells are killed each day (through harsh products or trauma) than grow anew, the piercing simply cannot heal. Skin cleansing is a physical process to remove dirt, oils, dead cells, and micro-organisms such as bacteria. Few skin cleansers are designed for long-term use on open wounds. Lots of cleansers and soaps have added dyes, fragrances, and other ingredients that can irritate your piercing and your skin.

To avoid harm to your fragile new cells, use a mild liquid soap suitable for wound care. There can be big differences between this type of product and cleansers meant for use on intact skin, such as most surgical scrubs. Many piercers suggest antimicrobial or germicidal hospital-grade soaps such as Techni-Care Antiseptic Surgical Scrub,

Provon Medicated Lotion Soap, and Satin Therapeutic Skin Cleanser. They are not readily available in stores or pharmacies, so you may need to obtain them from your piercer or a body-jewelry supplier. They contain an active ingredient called *Chloroxylenol* (or *PCMX*), which is not toxic to humans in low doses, but does kill a wide spectrum of microbes. Other piercers advise the use of mild antibacterial soap that is made for sensitive skin, Castile soap, or natural glycerin soap. Any product you elect to use should be fragrance and dye free, as well as low-pH or pH balanced. Products with a pH greater than 8 are alkaline and tend to be very irritating to the skin.[13] Read the label and do not use a product past its expiration date. I typically suggest my clients use Provon Medicated Lotion Soap or Satin Therapeutic Skin Cleanser for cleaning piercings during healing.

Remember, it isn't the soap that heals your piercing: *your body heals itself.* Therefore, depend on a soap product only to help keep the area clean; rely on sound health habits, responsible behavior, and gentle treatment of the wound for the healing to take place.

The Antibacterial Controversy

Triclosan, the common broad-spectrum antibacterial ingredient found in Dial and many other soaps, can cause problems from overuse. Long-term exposure may lead to ultrastrong, antibiotic-resistant strains of bacteria. This chemical has become pervasive: it is in hand sanitizers, household disinfectants, toothpastes, deodorants, plastic trash bags, and numerous other everyday products. Triclosan also demonstrates potential as a risk to the environment and to human health.[14]

Many studies maintain that washing with regular soap kills the same amount of bacteria as washing with antibacterial soap.[15] A particular concern for some piercees is the use of antibacterial soap near the vagina, which can cause a yeast infection by upsetting the balance of normal *flora* (harmless bacteria that inhabit a part of the body). If you choose to use antibacterial or antimicrobial soap during initial healing, it may be best to switch to a milder product later.

What Not to Use on Your Piercings

The products listed below were commonly used on healing piercings in the past, but they are no longer considered suitable. Piercers who do not keep up with industry standards still suggest them, as do friends and even uninformed medical professionals. None of these things, however, is medically advisable for use on fresh puncture wounds, including piercings.

- **Alcohol**: shown to be *cytotoxic* (kills cells),[16] too strong, and drying.
- **Hydrogen peroxide** (in over-the-counter strength): too strong and also cytotoxic.[17]
- **Bactine, "No More Ouchies," pierced ear care solutions, and other products containing benzalkonium chloride (BZK) and benzethonium chloride (BZT)**: these antiseptics and disinfectants are designed to kill germs and inhibit their growth, but they do not necessarily clean the skin. Since the 1970s, both of these active ingredients have been out of use in hospital settings. They have a short shelf life once opened and are not intended for long-term wound care. They can cause dry, flaky skin; but, if you dilute them, their effectiveness is diminished and the solution can become contaminated. Some products in this category contain alcohol,

fragrance, or numbing agents such as lidocaine (xylocaine), which can irritate your piercing. The manufacturer of Bactine specifically states that Bactine is not recommended for use on piercings or other puncture wounds.[18]

- **A+D Original Ointment, Neosporin, bacitracin, and other ointments**: labels advise against use on puncture wounds. Particularly with triple antibiotic products, many people are sensitive to at least one of the three active ingredients. Further, ointments tend to occlude a wound, thereby preventing oxygen from reaching it.[19] Because these petroleum-based products are not water soluble, when cleaning a piercing coated in such salves, you could be washing the ointment rather than your healing tissue beneath the greasy coating.

- **Betadine and other povidone-iodine products**: Studies show iodine is not suited to wound care, as it can damage new cell walls, causing cellular material to leak out.[20] Packaged pads or swabs are excellent for skin prep prior to piercing or other procedures in which skin will be broken, but iodine stored in plastic (PVC) bottles is susceptible to the growth of infectious organisms once opened.[21]

- **Dial liquid soap**: again, too strong and drying. There are plenty of other soaps on the market that clean your piercing effectively without being as harsh to your delicate wound.

- **Colloidal silver**: controversial at best, and its many touted benefits have not been medically proven. The FDA issued a ruling declaring that all over-the-counter drug products containing colloidal silver or silver salts are not recognized as safe or effective.[22]

- **Listerine and other alcohol-containing mouth rinses**: the high alcohol content is damaging to the new cell growth of healing tongue or lip piercings. Overuse can upset your normal oral flora, leading to a yeast infection (see "Oral Piercings and Yeast Infections," page 27).

Cleaning Your Piercing

An obvious step in caring for a healing piercing is washing it. But using the wrong cleanser or too many different products can harm your piercing. Overcleaning causes different problems than not cleaning enough, but either can be damaging.

A once-a-day wash with mild soap is suitable for most piercees; it is usually easiest to do this in the shower. If you live in a hot or humid climate or engage in activities that are sweaty or dirty in nature, then a second daily cleaning—or at least a good clear-water rinse—is wise.

When you take a shower, first wash your hands and your entire body. You may continue to use your regular soap in the shower, but keep it away from your piercing if it is not suitable for wound care. If you have strong water pressure, shield the pierced area from the forceful spray. The steam and warm water will open your pores, soften crusties, and loosen them. This is important to avoid damaging the skin during cleaning, and it is especially helpful if you have not soaked the piercing prior to your shower. Stubborn matter should be removed with moistened cotton swabs or gauze pads, not your fingers or nails.

Soap makes dirt and germs become slippery so they wash away. Lather some soap in your hands and suds up your jewelry and the surrounding area. Friction is a key part of cleaning, but this must be balanced with treating the wound gently. Finally, rinse, then rinse again: you don't want any soap residue to remain on the piercing or jewelry.

To Rotate or Not to Rotate

Most piercers used to advise rotating your jewelry to work soap though the channel. It was believed that this was required to clean the inside, but this has not been proven. In fact, the gentler no-turn approach appears adequate and is less apt to cause trauma. Some piercers argue for the old method, but I am no longer a proponent.

It was also thought that moving the jewelry was needed to prevent it from becoming stuck in the hole, but this reasoning is not valid: sutures are not rotated, and yet they don't become stuck. Jewelry should never be turned just for fun, either. There are, however, a few situations in which it is appropriate to rotate jewelry:

- **During healing**: to clean the interior of the piercing channel if soap, dirt, or other foreign matter has gotten inside it. A small amount of gentle rotation while rinsing is appropriate to ensure that all of the undesirable substance is removed from the interior.
- **After healing**: during daily bathing. See "Regular Maintenance," page 218.

Advice, trends, and products used for aftercare come and go, but rough handling of a healing piercing is never helpful; do not force your jewelry to move.

Aftercare for Oral Piercings

The same principles of avoiding trauma and maintaining sound health habits also apply to healing oral piercings, although lip and tongue piercings are cared for somewhat differently than the rest of the body. For a piercing such as a labret, which intersects the mouth, care of the exterior is the same as for any body piercing; additionally, you should follow the guidelines in this section to care for the interior.

See the tips in "Tongue Piercing: Healing and Troubleshooting," page 109. Below are several additional things you can do to minimize swelling and discomfort during the first few days of healing:

- **Rest**: Don't speak or move your jewelry unless necessary.
- **Ice**: Suck on chipped or shaved ice made from clean water, or small cubes of frozen chamomile tea (big cubes can be uncomfortable and irritating).
- **Elevation**: Sleep with your head propped up on an extra pillow the first few nights; keeping your head above your heart helps to minimize overnight swelling.
- **NSAIDs**: Take over-the-counter, nonsteroidal anti-inflammatory medication according to package instructions.

Cleaning and Hygiene

Your primary aftercare for oral piercings (including tongue, labret, and lip piercings) will consist of rinsing your mouth with an antibacterial or antimicrobial mouthwash for thirty to sixty seconds. Rinse up to five times daily: after meals and before bed. There is no need to actively move your jewelry while rinsing—oral piercings get an abundance of movement, no matter how you try to avoid it. Alternatively, you can rinse with the saline mixture described in "The Recipe," on page 189.

Rinsing too frequently or using harsh mouthwash can cause complications by diminishing your normal protective oral flora. Products that contain alcohol are still recommended by piercers who are not keeping up with industry standards. Your piercing will heal better and you will be more comfortable if you use an alcohol-free germicidal mouthwash or saline rinse. Brush your teeth normally, gently scrub your tongue and jewelry after each meal (before rinsing), and floss daily.

Pay attention to what you put in your mouth while you are healing an oral piercing. Don't chew on pens, sunglasses, fingernails, or other foreign objects; they are likely to harbor germs. Dirty cups, plates, and eating utensils can expose you to bacteria, so keep all kitchenware clean and don't share during healing. Avoid having your teeth cleaned or getting dental work when your piercing is new. It can be irritating to the piercing, and it may increase your risk of infection.

Toothbrush Hygiene

It is prudent to use a new toothbrush when you get an oral piercing. To keep it hygienic, store it in a clean area separate from anyone else's—and well away from your toilet. Studies show bacterial and viral spray from flushing a toilet can land on surfaces (including a toothbrush) up to eight feet away![23]

Your piercing is an open wound so you must avoid others' bodily fluids, including saliva, while healing: this means no unprotected oral sexual contact and no French (wet) kissing. Failing to comply opens you to risks that include STDs, HIV, and hepatitis B and C. Even if you have a long-term partner, you must still abstain due to risk of infection. Performing oral sex is also inadvisable during the first few weeks of healing. This is true even if you use barrier protection for hygiene, as vigorous activity can damage the delicate cells.

Smoking and drinking alcoholic beverages should be minimized or eliminated initially. Chewing tobacco is not safe while you are healing an oral piercing.

The Point

Caring for your piercing can be confusing if you receive different advice from multiple sources. New information and aftercare products are always surfacing, so the current regimen may well be modified again. Ultimately, you must listen to your body and trust your instincts, bolstered by knowledge and common sense.

Emu Oil

For the care of healing and troubled piercings, *emu oil* has proved itself superior to all the other products I've advocated throughout my career. Yes, emu, as in the big flightless bird. Aboriginal people in Australia have used emu oil on wounds for centuries. Today it is used by massage therapists, dermatologists, other medical practitioners, and piercers for its anti-inflammatory, pain-relieving, and wound-healing properties. I believe emu oil is safe and effective enough that it could become the norm for post-piercing care, at least among nonvegetarians. I know I've advised against miracle products, but if there is such a thing, in my opinion, emu oil is it.

Emu oil is safe even for use inside the mouth, and no, it doesn't taste like dead bird or like anything at all. A natural food by-product, high-quality emu oil is odorless and tasteless. It is considered hypoallergenic, and I haven't witnessed any negative responses to it. No adverse reactions or toxicity have been reported in the scientific literature.[24] Laboratory studies show that emu oil has anti-inflammatory properties[25], and in its pure state, emu oil is *bacteriostatic* (restricts the growth and activity of microorganisms).[26]

Emu oil is high in essential fatty acids and keeps your skin moisturized. This establishes favorable conditions: healing is three to five times faster and less painful in a moist environment. Pure emu oil does not clog pores, and it does not prevent air circulation like petroleum-based products. The emollients help keep secretions from drying and adhering to the skin or jewelry, which cuts down on crusting, trauma, and discomfort. Even though it is called "oil," it is more like a lotion. It rubs in well and does not leave a greasy residue. Emu oil feels extremely soothing the instant you put it on. These pleasant attributes help to encourage regular applications.

Emu oil is also economical because you apply only a tiny dab. It is easy to use:

- Shake the bottle

- Two to three times daily, rub a single drop onto the piercing with a clean or gloved finger

- You can use it in conjunction with saline soaks, though many piercees have had excellent results healing with emu oil as the sole care product. Studies have shown that emu oil penetrates the skin, which resolves any debate over rotating the jewelry.

I also suggest applications of emu oil on the tissue of any piercing that is being stretched. Research has shown it can thicken skin, so it may be especially helpful for thinning tissue.[27]

Different manufacturers produce emu oils of varying qualities, and it may not perform equally well in all climates. I once tried an inferior brand that did smell and taste like a big, dead bird. Use only certified fully refined oil on piercings. The idea of suggesting oil for piercings seemed appalling after years of preaching against the use of ointment. All I can say is, "This is different!"

Alternative Aftercare

The standard aftercare guidelines described in the previous chapter follow accepted principles of wound care, and they are safe and effective for most piercees under ordinary circumstances. However, there isn't only one correct method or even a single best way to clean and care for all piercings; each body responds differently.

Some piercers make honest attempts to discover new and better methods to facilitate healing. Others, however, have poor motivations for deviating from the usual care guidelines including:

- A lack of familiarity with the industry-standard suggestions
- The conventional advice doesn't help to heal their bungled piercings—but nothing will
- A desire to do things differently simply to make a name for themselves as innovators

Unless the suggestions are truly horrid, at least some piercees will probably have success with even the most unconventional of treatments. I had a client who managed to heal more than a few piercings by topically applying Bacardi 151 rum. Still, beware of being a human guinea pig. If you don't feel convinced that a proposed departure from the traditional care sounds superior in some way, abide by the commonsense principles of the previous chapter.

This chapter reviews a number of alternative healing methods and products, including those specifically designed for piercing care. It also identifies alternative treatments to avoid and explains why they should not be used. Just because something is *natural* (unprocessed or minimally processed) does not necessarily mean it is safe or effective to use on a healing piercing.

Alternative Healing Methods

Below is an introduction to a few alternative aftercare regimens. Many piercees have successfully used these and other approaches. This is not meant to be an exhaustive investigation of all the possibilities that diverge from the traditional guidelines. If you are interested in pursuing alternatives, there is a great deal of information available in your library and online.

The Better Options

These methods and products are generally accepted as being among the safest and least controversial of the alternatives:

- **Castile soap (such as Dr. Bronner's):** This is a simple soap made from vegetable oil rather than animal fat. Oils used in castile soaps include olive, coconut, almond, hemp, and/or jojoba. Medical professionals have used Castile soap on wounds, and preliminary studies show it may reduce the risk of infection.[1] Simply wash the piercing with Castile soap once or twice daily. Depending on the product, it may need to be diluted with distilled water; follow the package instructions.

- **Lubrication:** Dab a small amount of natural oil such as almond, jojoba, or olive oil around the holes of the piercing several times daily. Apply the lubricant only on the surface without getting it inside your piercing. This keeps the skin moisturized and helps to reduce crust and minimize damage when the jewelry is bumped or moved. Do not use Vaseline or other petroleum-based products on your piercings. Of course, lubrication can also be used in conjunction with the standard care regimen. Emu oil automatically provides lubrication when used for piercing care.

- **Herbal remedies:** Herbs have been used in medicine for thousands of years. There is a large body of well-tested and proven herbal wisdom. When used properly, certain herbs can be beneficial to healing. Herbs can be applied on healing piercings in several ways: you can soak your piercing with an *infusion* (a tea that is steeped longer than usual) or topically apply diluted *essential oils* (concentrated liquid compounds from plants). An infusion of herbs can be used on a compress or as a soaking liquid instead of a saline solution, or in addition to it.

  - Lavender, chamomile, and comfrey are good herbs for healing piercings. Select one at a time unless you are a skilled herbalist or receive advice from one.

  - Add one to two teaspoons of dried herb per cup of boiling water to make an infusion. Let it steep for at least ten minutes before you strain it. Some herbalists recommend infusing for hours. Keep the mixture covered in the refrigerator for two to three days. Heat the tea (a microwave is fine), and use it on your piercing as described with salt soaks. Unlike saline, there is no potentially harmful residue that must be rinsed away, so you can soak with herbs after your shower.

  - Tea tree and lavender in essential oil form are popular for topical use on healing piercings. Essential oils are much too harsh for full-strength application on piercings; they must be diluted first. Since they come in varying concentrations, ask for guidance from a knowledgeable supplier before putting this type of product on a piercing. Tea tree oil is also sometimes used for troubleshooting problem piercings.

  - An *infused herbal oil* (an essential oil that is mixed into an oil base) is milder and can often be used topically on a piercing at full strength.

Interview your piercer about any alternative regimen suggested to you that is not mentioned above. Ask how long he has been using the method, and how many piercees have had success with it. Inquire about potential risks or negative results. Whatever you plan to try should seem sensible for the care of a healing wound.

The Jury Is Out

The jury is still out on the most laissez-faire approach and some other herbal and natural remedies that might work:

- **Leave It the Heck Alone (LITHA):** This so-called "method" is the easiest possible care because it involves doing nothing to your piercing other than providing normal daily bathing or routine oral hygiene, depending on placement. No soaks, soaps, oral rinses, or other special products are used. This lends itself well to oral and certain genital piercings, because the mucosal tissues have faster rates of regeneration than other areas. Key elements to the LITHA method, as with all aftercare, are sound overall health habits and good hygiene. If you work or play in dirty environments, this is probably not a good choice for you.

- **Aloe vera gel:** This plant product has been used medicinally for thousands of years, including for wound healing. The gel—best taken from the living plant—can be applied to the exterior of the piercing several times a day. Some studies on the effectiveness of aloe for wound healing report positive results, but others show no benefit or worsening of the condition.

- **Honey:** This natural substance that not only tastes good, but, according to some evidence, certain types are beneficial for wound healing.[2] No research (or even experimentation) appears to have been done on its use for healing piercings, however, so take this sweetness with a grain of salt. In particular, manuka honey has been studied extensively for reducing inflammation, treating infection, and promoting healing. According to proponents, this honey has been shown to have antibacterial properties.[3]

- **Additional natural remedies:** Other remedies that have been suggested for wound care include elk or deer antler velvet, calendula, marshmallow root, rosemary, gotu kola, echinacea, cocoa or shea butter, oatmeal, plantain, banana peel extract, rose hips, raw garlic, castor oil, sugar, and seaweed, among others. More research is needed for these to be considered advisable for piercing care.

Don't Try This at Home

One alternate approach that I do not advocate is referred to as *dry wound care* or *anti-care*, in which the crust is left undisturbed. There is no wetting or washing of the area for weeks or months, and all care and cleaning products are avoided.

The health-care community is in widespread agreement that regular cleansing with mild soap and water is appropriate in the presence of broken skin.[4] Further, medical research suggests that a moist wound will heal more quickly and easily than one that is kept continuously dry.[5] A wound should also undergo regular *debridement* (removal of dead, contaminated, or adherent tissue or foreign material) to prevent the spreading of infection to surrounding skin.[6] The debridement of body piercings is accomplished by removing the crust, normally through soaking and washing.

Specialty Products

In response to increased consumer demand and sometimes in the name of making a buck, numerous companies are now manufacturing an array of products designed specifically to care for healing piercings. Some of them are safe, convenient options.

Among the choices are liquid-filled swabs, individually packaged pads or towelettes, and sprays. They are often heavily advertised to piercers and piercees.

Consider whether the claims being made by the manufacturer seem reasonable, and when evaluating these products, assess the following:

- **Ingredients:** Does the manufacturer provide enough information about the active ingredients and other components, or does the label seem evasive? Can you determine if the contents include allergens, irritants such as alcohol or peroxide, or other undesirable substances?

- **Application:** Many piercees like the convenience of specialty products. When you can't do a regular wash or soak, such as after the gym, a portable substitute is clearly preferable to nothing. However, when you dab or spray on a product, you miss out on the significant benefits of submerging your piercing in a solution of warm saline: thorough softening of crusty matter, improving blood circulation, and draining excess fluid from the wound. If a spray is too forceful, it can damage healing tissue.[7]

- **Cost:** Some of the specialty goods are quite pricey. Learn all you can about the ingredients and mechanism of action. Weigh the cost and convenience and consider your piercer's opinion; some alternative care products are excellent—but others aren't.

The selection of specialty items is growing as piercing continues to gain popularity. In time, the most effective (and the best marketed) of the new products will endure, and increased competition may drive down prices.

Running Cold and Hot

In addition to the care products you choose to use, ice packs and warm compresses can increase comfort, decrease post-piercing symptoms, and facilitate healing.

- **Ice packs:** Applying ice during the first twenty-four to forty-eight hours can help reduce the swelling, bleeding, and bruising that may accompany a fresh piercing. Use a clean zip-top plastic bag with ice cubes or frozen peas, adding a little bit of water inside to help the contents conform to your body more comfortably. Wrap the baggie in a clean paper towel and replace soggy towels with dry ones as condensation wets them. Too much moisture can disrupt the fresh scab, resulting in prolonged bleeding. Gently place the ice pack on your piercing for ten minutes and remove it for forty-five minutes to an hour before reapplying.

- **Warm compresses:** After the first forty-eight hours, if initial bleeding has stopped, you can begin using warm compresses. They can feel soothing and stimulate circulation and your body's immune response, which is helpful to healing. Using different additives can further aid in healing and serve other functions as described below. Wash your hands and apply a clean washcloth or gauze soaked in water that is warm to hot—not scalding (see "How to Soak," page 189, for information on what type of water to use). Apply the compress directly to the area until it no longer feels warm, then reheat and reapply. Covering the compress with a folded dry towel can help maintain the heat for longer periods. Repeat for fifteen to thirty minutes, a maximum of four to six times daily. Use only clean disposable products for washing and drying, or launder your washcloths and towels with bleach between each use, and store them carefully to avoid contamination.

Additional options that may be helpful include:

- To diminish inflammation, add two tablespoons of apple cider vinegar to one cup of water, and use this mixture to wet your compress. Vinegar is also a natural antiseptic and may help promote healing.

- Add chamomile tea or use a warm, wet chamomile tea bag as your compress to diminish irritation and inflammation.

- Add lavender tea to your compress to facilitate healing. To make lavender tea, boil three tablespoons of flowers in one liter (one quart) of water for ten minutes, then strain.

- Add witch hazel tea (boil two to three grams of witch hazel leaves, twigs, and bark in a cup of water for about fifteen minutes, then strain) to your compress. This will cleanse the wound, soothe it, minimize swelling and bleeding, and promote healing. Avoid commercial witch hazel: it is distilled and contains alcohol, which is drying.

- Add four to five drops of any of the suggested essential oils to a cup of water and use this water to make your compress.

The Point

Regardless of the source for your advice on aftercare, or how many other people have had success with the method or product you use, the ultimate test rests with your own piercing. Unless negative results are obvious, it is reasonable to stick with a routine for a few weeks before deciding it isn't working for you. Should your regimen cause problems or fail to foster healing, there are many other options to try. And, if you run into trouble, read the next chapter.

Trouble and Troubleshooting

Disclaimer: The suggestions in this book are not to be considered a substitute for advice from a medical professional.

Occasionally things go awry with body piercings, even when they are performed by a qualified professional and cared for properly. Depending on what is wrong, the solution might be as simple as a change in your care regimen or jewelry. Sometimes minor complications improve spontaneously, while other times you will need to look after a piercing with an over-the-counter remedy. In more serious cases, doctor visits and medical treatments are called for; on occasion, removal of your jewelry is required. The good news is that grave situations are rare. In the event that you must abandon your piercing, it is uncommon that the site cannot be repierced.

A visit to a knowledgeable piercer is advisable at the first indication something is amiss with your piercing. If you have to see a doctor, your piercer may be able to direct you to a piercing-friendly practitioner. Never let embarrassment or fear of being judged by a medical professional get in the way of treatment you require. Speedy intervention can prevent more serious consequences, so it is crucial to address problems quickly. If you have a history of health problems or you experience any severe symptoms, seek *immediate* medical attention.

Anxiety

If you are concerned about the state of your piercing, take action instead of just worrying. Certain piercings typically become discolored, irritated, and oozy during healing. This can be frightening if you are not familiar with their usual appearance. Clients frequently come to me in a panic over a piercing that looks perfectly normal to my trained eye. Fortunately, all they need is some reassurance. Have a piercer examine you, and she will be able to let you know whether your healing course appears to be progressing normally.

Excess nervousness and anxiety are healing problems—even if they aren't based on the actual condition of your wound. If you are particularly stressed out, your healing is apt to be delayed.[1] Not all medical professionals are familiar with the way healing piercings look. Whether you simply want a little support or urgently need expert troubleshooting, an experienced piercer is an excellent resource.

Serious Problems

Because of the relatively recent growth in the popularity of body piercings, solid scientific data on this topic is somewhat scarce; few research studies include large populations of piercees. Surveys on the incidence of piercing complications often use limited geographic samplings of participants. These appear to reveal more about the quality of piercing in a given region than about industry practices in general. One study adds redness, swelling, drainage, and bleeding to the list of "complications" along with infection and trauma. The first four are normal consequences of piercing and do not generally belong in the category of "problems." This study put "minor complications" at about 20 percent of piercings and major complications at 3 percent, but the piercing techniques included use of the ear stud gun.[2]

Regardless of the "complications" listed, the available literature confirms that the majority of piercing problems are relatively minor and that conditions grave enough to require hospitalization or surgery are rare. However, the frequency of infected piercings reported in the research is as high as 45 percent.[3] This does not reflect my clinical experience, which demonstrates very few infections in piercings that are performed and cared for responsibly. The studies do support my assertion that the quality of both piercing and aftercare affect the rate of infection.[4]

The most serious conditions (including the few deaths that have been attributed to piercing) appear to have been impacted by one or more of the following circumstances of the piercee:

- Did not have the piercing performed in a hygienic, professional setting
- Failed to follow suggested aftercare procedures
- Failed to respond to infection or other complications in a timely manner
- Had a preexisting health problem such as a heart condition or diabetes[5]

What to Do

This chapter contains information intended to help you deal with the most common complications that occur with piercings. The usual signs and complaints are described to help you figure out specifically (possibly with the assistance of your piercer or doctor) what type of problem you are having. Suggestions are provided on the most effective ways to handle them. Try to be patient and understand that everyone is different; frequently, some experimentation is needed to figure out what works best for you.

Leave Jewelry In!

Try to discover precisely what is wrong before taking out your jewelry. Chances are it can be cleared up, and there is no need to take such a drastic measure. In any case, simply removing your jewelry and giving up on your piercing may not resolve your problem. In fact, if you have an infection, this can cause a condition that is much more severe (see "Infection: Abscesses," page 204).[6] Even if you don't have an infection, it is not easier or better to take out your jewelry now and try to get it reinserted or repierced later. Scar tissue, delayed healing, and other issues can occur from repiercing after unnecessarily abandoning a piercing.

When you seek medical care for an ailing piercing, many physicians will immediately ask (or order) you to remove your jewelry. If an infection is suspected or diagnosed, resist this command. If your health-care provider is unfamiliar with piercings, you may need to explain that jewelry or an appropriate substitute must remain in an infected piercing to keep the channel open and enable the wound to drain. Once this is explained, it usually makes sense to a doctor.

If metal jewelry will be left in a troubled piercing, it must be made of high-quality material and be in good condition. Wearing an appropriate style is crucial, as is a good fit. Problem piercings frequently swell and thus require a larger size. If you aren't sure what is causing your complication, a jewelry swap is often a good idea. It is best to have a piercer help you with this when your piercing is distressed.

An inert plastic retainer is a good substitute for metal jewelry; you can obtain one from a piercer. Their flexibility makes them more comfortable to wear in a tender piercing, and a negative reaction to metal will obviously be ruled out or resolved. If a retainer is not readily available, the catheter tubing found in medical settings can suffice in an urgent situation. Details can be found in "Medical and Dental Emergencies and Appointments," page 247, and "Retainers," page 248. If you have recently abandoned an infected piercing, your piercer may still be able to insert an appropriate retainer or piece of jewelry. Even if it is thinner than your original gauge, this can help the wound to drain and prevent more serious problems.

Localized Infection

When a piercing acts up, it is commonly assumed that it is infected. However, not everything that is wrong with a piercing is an infection. When piercings are performed and cared for according to accepted practice, an *infection* (invasion and multiplication of disease-causing microorganisms that have a detrimental effect) is not as prevalent as you might think. Other complications, such as irritation, are far more common; however, when a piercing is infected, it requires prompt care. Left untreated, an infection can worsen to become extremely dangerous and, in rare cases, life threatening.

Many *minor* (or *self-limiting*) *infections* are successfully self-treated. If your condition is recent, mild, and you do not take steroids or have a chronic illness or other health condition, you can try the suggestions listed below for a few days. Numerous products for this purpose are readily available in drugstores. If your piercing is visible to the public, show it to a pharmacist and ask for his suggestion on the best over-the-counter product[7] or whether he thinks you need to see a doctor right away.

Identifying Minor Localized Infection

- Skin is pinkish or reddish, swollen, and warm to the touch
- Localized tenderness
- A small amount of pus
- Swollen lymph nodes

You can have an infection even if you don't have all of the symptoms above. Conversely, having several of them doesn't guarantee that your piercing is infected. Some redness, swelling, and tenderness are normal in fresh piercings, especially during the first two weeks.

What to Do for a Minor Localized Infection

The following suggestions are for *minor* infections only:

- Take ibuprofen or acetaminophen to diminish swelling and tenderness.
- Keep the area clean and wash it twice daily with a fragrance-free soap, rinse well, and dry with clean, disposable paper products.
- Perform mild saline soaks and/or apply warm, moist compresses to encourage drainage and relieve discomfort (see the information on warm compresses under "Running Cold and Hot," page 199).
- Apply topical over-the-counter antibiotic cream or gel (not ointment) according to package instructions. While this type of product is not suggested for routine aftercare, this is the time to put it to use. The topical antibiotic products usually contain bacitracin, neomycin, or polymyxin B, alone or in combination, to fight different types of microorganisms. Combinations of the three ingredients work against a broader spectrum of bacteria, but allergic reactions to neomycin are common.[8] Stop using the antibiotic if you notice redness, itching, or skin eruptions surrounding the area, and consult your physician.

See a doctor right away if you experience the following:

- Your symptoms last for a week or markedly worsen.
- You experience a fever, chills, nausea, vomiting, dizziness, or disorientation.
- The piercing is very painful, swollen, has red streaks emanating from it, or there is a loss of function in the region.
- You have copious pus discharge that is greenish, yellowish, or grayish.

For topical treatment of localized piercing infections, a cream or gel called *Bactroban* (mupirocin antibiotic, available only by prescription) is recognized as an effective medication.[9] A doctor who is unfamiliar with piercings may be unsure what to recommend, so you can inform him this product is commonly prescribed for bacterial infections in piercings. Never try to self-treat an infection with leftover antibiotic medication or someone else's prescription.

Infection: Abscesses

An *abscess* is a pocket of infection containing pus, trapped under the skin, surrounded by inflamed tissue. Medical research shows that abscesses usually occur long after the initial piercing—on average from four to twelve months later.[10]

An abscess can be created when jewelry is removed from an infected piercing, thus eliminating the pathway for pus and matter to leave the body, trapping the infection inside. Occasionally an infection will occur and an abscess will form adjacent to a piercing when jewelry is in place. This is more apt to happen if your jewelry constricts the tissue because the initial size was too small, or because of an unexpected amount of post-piercing swelling.

Identifying an Abscess

- Tenderness, pain, inflammation, heat, and swelling at the site of a hard localized mass (feels like a marble under the skin). In the case of nipples, the duct system can result in an abscess forming inches away from your piercing.
- Redness or darkening of skin (if the abscess is closer to the surface, rather than very deep underneath).
- Worsens over time and may cause nausea, fever, and chills if severe.
- Infections caused by the bacterium *Mycobacterium abscessus* have been described as *cold abscesses* because of the absence of tenderness and inflammation. This means you could have an abscess when a hard mass is present, even if you don't have any of the other symptoms.

What to Do for an Abscess

- For milder cases (a localized abscess without systemic symptoms such as fever or nausea), saline soaks or application of warm-to-hot moist compresses might cause spontaneous drainage.
- Switching to jewelry of a thinner gauge may also help to encourage drainage if the mass is close to an opening of the piercing.
- Elevating the area and taking over-the-counter analgesics according to package instructions may help to make you more comfortable.

If the abscess does not drain within forty-eight hours as a result of these steps, or if symptoms worsen, a visit to the doctor is urgent. Infection can spread to deeper tissue or the bloodstream if untreated. This is serious!

- If red streaks emanate from the site, the lump is larger than ½ inch across, or a fever is present, you *must* visit the emergency room right away, as the infection may have spread and become cellulitis (discussed next).
- An incision and drainage procedure to empty the pus-filled cavity is commonly needed. If the abscess is in close proximity to the piercing, the channel may be lost (cut) in the process.
- Antibiotics alone will not necessarily resolve an abscess. It usually must be cleared out as well. In fact, doctors sometimes drain an abscess without prescribing antibiotics.[11]

Cellulitis

Cellulitis refers to an inflammation of the cells. When it spreads beyond a localized area throughout the deeper layers of the skin and surrounding tissue, immediate medical attention is required. **Without proper care, this can enter the bloodstream and lymph nodes and become septicemia (a severe total body infection), which is potentially deadly.**

Identifying Cellulitis

- Inflammation and redness of the skin further than ½ inch from the wound, possibly including broad areas of redness, or red streaking
- Tight, glossy, stretched appearance of the skin, or dimpling like an orange peel
- Warmth, tenderness, and swelling
- Drainage of clear yellow fluid or pus from the skin

Emergency medical care is required immediately if:

- The rash is changing rapidly, or a large area is already involved.
- Fever, pain, chills, weakness, vomiting, joint or body aches, swollen lymph nodes, or mental confusion accompany the other symptoms.
- The infection is on your face, especially in the area of the eye.
- You are immunocompromised (have AIDS, diabetes, or lupus) or have other medical history of concern, including a heart condition.

What to Do for Cellulitis

You must visit a doctor for treatment; do not delay. Cellulitis is not a condition that can be handled with home care. If the infection is deemed severe, you may need to be hospitalized for intravenous antibiotics or surgical intervention.

Hypergranulation Tissue

The terms *hypergranulation tissue*, *granuloma*, and *pyogenic granuloma* are all fancy words for *benign* (noncancerous) types of growths that form on wounds, including piercings. These can simply be a consequence of injuring the body, or they can be caused by excessive trauma, moisture, or infection. If you are taking Accutane or certain other medications, you are at increased risk for this complication, though you may see improvement if you lower the dosage or discontinue taking the medicine.[12] Always take prescription medications according to your doctor's instructions.

These bumps are comprised of cells that are normally formed during wound healing but that have overgrown, often quite rapidly. These unsightly lumps are most common on piercings of the navel, outer labium, nostril, and the inside of the lip, though they may also occur elsewhere. In some cases, they can successfully be treated and the piercing may be maintained, though healing of the piercing is suspended while excess granulation tissue is present.[13] You may need to be patient and to try different treatments or combinations of remedies to achieve a satisfactory resolution.

Identifying Hypergranulation Tissue

- Bump of tissue protrudes above the surface of your skin
- Looks like raw hamburger, or like the inside of the piercing is on the outside of your body
- Oozing clear or yellow sticky drainage
- Bleeds easily
- Usually looks worse than it feels, though it can be tender

What to Do for Hypergranulation Tissue

Keep the area as dry and free from friction and irritation as possible. Do not try all the listed products at once, and keep careful watch on the area to gauge your response to treatments.

- Frequent saline soaks, or more aggressive sodium chloride treatment: use a *hypertonic* product (one that contains more salt than the body's fluids do) such as Curasalt (20 percent sodium chloride–impregnated gauze), or Hypergel Hypertonic Gel (20 percent hypertonic saline gel). Use according to the package directions, but be careful to cover only the hypergranulation tissue, or you will cause drying and irritation to the healthy skin surrounding the problem.[14]
- Topical application of over-the-counter cortisone cream according to package instructions.
- Use a styptic pencil to stop bleeding and dry out the tissue.
- Topical application of rubbing alcohol, 3 percent hydrogen peroxide, iodine, Campho-Phenique, *or* undiluted tea tree oil, twice daily for one to two weeks. Seek medical care if you don't see improvement or your symptoms worsen.
- Topical application of a paste made from bottled or distilled water and aspirin tablets or powder. Apply only to the hypergranulation tissue for ten minutes and then rinse well, two to three times a day for two to three weeks. This can burn your skin. Discontinue if irritation results.

If none of these help your condition, visit a doctor for treatment. These often recur, especially when a problem with moisture, jewelry fit, or friction is not resolved.[15] If the condition proves intractable, the piercing will need to be abandoned. Frequently the bumps diminish significantly or disappear completely when you remove your jewelry.

"Localized Piercing Pimple"

This complication is somewhat common, but, unfortunately, the piercing-friendly medical professionals I polled failed to come to a consensus on a diagnosis or suggested treatment. Therefore, I've named this complication based on its appearance and address it below using my professional piercing experience in conjunction with accepted health-care principles. Overall, the symptoms are similar to those of folliculitis, which is an inflammation and infection in or near a hair follicle.[16] This type of complication routinely occurs near nipple piercings, where hair follicles are not plentiful. Piercers sometimes mislabel this as a "follicular cyst," but that is a condition of the ovary.[17]

Sometimes a *pustule* (a small round area of inflamed skin filled with pus) will appear under the skin near the opening of a piercing. It may be caused by trauma or a mild infection that remains contained locally. A small pocket forms close to the surface and repeatedly fills, and drains. Sometimes it seems to be gone for good, and then the cycle begins again weeks or months later. The best way to resolve the problem appears to be by helping your body to break down and absorb the sack or pocket that has formed. You may be tempted to pop this pimple-like eruption yourself, but never lance your skin with nonsterile implements; use soaks and compresses to encourage drainage. If you have a localized pustule that won't open or drain and needs to be lanced, seek medical assistance.

Identifying a Piercing Pimple

- Small, slightly elevated pus-filled bump or pimple adjacent to the piercing
- Red and inflamed, but contained locally
- May be tender, itch, or burn, though some are painless
- Usually secretes pus and/or blood when drained (or popped)

What to Do for a Piercing Pimple

- Follow the suggestions under "What to Do for a Minor Localized Infection," page 204.
- Over-the-counter antihistamines taken according to package instructions can diminish itching and inflammation.
- Do plenty of warm saline soaks or hot compresses. Continue them for two weeks after the problem seems to have been resolved.
- Light massage of the area may help break up the pocket and prevent it from refilling.
- If you do not respond to treatment, lab analysis for an invading microorganism may be needed to determine if the cause is fungal or bacterial so your doctor can prescribe appropriate medication to target the problem.[18]
- You must see a doctor if you have increased pain, a fever over 100°F (37.8°C), or the infection obviously worsens or spreads.
- If you have a verified diagnosis of folliculitis, laser hair removal can destroy the hair follicle, prevent future episodes, and reduce the scarring of repeated eruptions.

Discoloration

Some discoloration extending from your piercing in an area the size of a pea is a standard part of the healing process. It can remain for many months. Shades described as purplish, pinkish, reddish, or brownish are normal, depending on individual complexion. This discoloration is apt to diminish over time; still, a mark beyond the borders of your piercing could be permanent, depending on your skin type, healing course, and piercing placement.

Certain piercings, including the ever-popular navel, have a tendency toward discoloration around the openings, especially if you experience problems or trauma during healing. After your piercing is no longer an open wound, try one of the options described in "Scar-Reduction Products," page 211, to minimize any residual discoloration. Sometimes the best resolution is to wear jewelry that has a ball, gemstone, or other ornament that obscures the discolored area.

Scarring

A *scar* is simply defined as "a mark left on the skin after the healing of a cut, burn, or other area of wounded tissue,"[19] so scar formation is a normal process following any type of breach in the tissue, including piercing. Unfortunately, however, the body sometimes fails to perform this job properly and complications occur. Below are some of the most common scarring problems with suggestions on how to handle them.

Atrophic Scarring

Atrophic scarring, a depression or pitting below the normal skin level, sometimes occurs when a piercing migrates. Unfortunately, this type of scarring is usually permanent. Navel and facial piercings are the most common sites to find this type of pockmark. There are no easy fixes, but a dermatologist can explain treatments such as dermabrasion or laser resurfacing that might be effective. If the piercing can be maintained, generally the best way to deal with this problem is to leave jewelry in place. This will usually mask the scar or at least part of it.

Excessive Scarring

The presence of jewelry causes prolonged healing and predisposes the wound to chronic inflammation. Both of these conditions increase the likelihood of excessive scar formation. Keloids and hypertrophic scars are the types of bumps and lumps commonly found on ear cartilage piercings, though other pierced sites also fall victim to these conditions.

A *keloid* is a very large, dense mound of scar tissue that becomes significantly bigger than your original wound. They can be extremely unsightly, and some grow to shocking dimensions. Unfortunately, once you have formed a keloid, you can seldom fully recover from it and will always have some amount of scar tissue.

A *hypertrophic scar* is a lumpy scar that sits above the surface of the skin. This is the smaller and far more common growth that forms around a piercing. They are not as big or severe as keloids, respond better to treatment, and are more easily resolved. Hypertrophic scarring sometimes goes away spontaneously, or it may recur and recede in cycles for an extended period of time before improving substantially or disappearing.

Hypertrophic scars are frequently mislabeled as keloids—even by doctors—possibly because both are types of excessive scarring. These problems tend to run in families and occur in about 5 to 15 percent of wounds.

Identifying Hypertrophic Scarring

- Raised fleshy bump surrounding a piercing that stays within the bounds of the injury
- Usually somewhat pink or red in color, at least initially
- Not tender; may itch
- Tends to form during the healing period
- No pus or other drainage

What to Do for Hypertrophic Scarring

Try one of the following methods at a time:

- A simple and inexpensive form of *compression therapy* (continuous mechanical pressure on a scar to flatten it) using Micropore breathable paper tape. It comes in "flesh tone," which will not be visible on certain shades of skin. I personally found this to be effective in diminishing a hypertrophic scar that had formed on the back of one of my ear cartilage piercings. This is best used on healed piercings.

- Use scissors to cut a piece of paper tape that will fully cover the entire bump plus a millimeter or so of unaffected tissue. Use a clean hole punch to create a tiny dressing for the smallest of bumps.

- Cut a slit to the center of the bandage so you can place it around your ring or bar; you should be able to completely seal the piercing without covering the jewelry, as a Band-Aid would.

- Wear the tape continuously and change it when necessary. It can be left on during normal bathing.

- Discontinue if you do not see improvement in two to three months.

- Frequent mild saline soaks plus topical application of alcohol, 3 percent hydrogen peroxide, tea tree oil, or Campho-Phenique twice daily for two to three weeks. If you don't see any improvement, try one of the other options. (The phenol in Campho-Phenique is a caustic substance that destroys tissue, so use it carefully.)[20]

- Over-the-counter alpha hydroxy acid (AHA) cream used according to package instructions. This exfoliates skin and may diminish scar tissue over time. Use only over-the-counter strength (containing less than 10 percent AHAs). This concentration promotes exfoliation but is not potent enough to generate collagen production, which can increase the size of your hypertrophic scar. This product can cause sun sensitivity.

- Daily massage with emu oil or other nonirritating oil or lotion to soften the tissue can be added to the following methods:

  - Topical treatment with an over-the-counter corticosteroid cream according to the package instructions.

  - Topical application of a chamomile tea bag compress for fifteen minutes, three times a day, for two weeks.

- Some piercees find laser or other medical treatments are effective for hypertrophic scars. See a dermatologist for other treatment options.

Identifying Keloids

- Bulbous and large, extending well beyond the boundaries of the original wound
- Sometimes tender, painful, or itchy
- Usually red or hyperpigmented and vascular, containing broad bundles of collagen, which are absent in hypertrophic scars
- Can develop over many months, or even up to a year following the piercing

What to Do for Keloids

Prevention is best: avoid piercings if you or a member of your immediate family has had keloids. Treatments are often ineffective and there is a high rate of recurrence, especially for those with a family history of keloid formation. There is a greater incidence of keloids in black and Asian populations, though anyone can get them. Combination approaches are common using multiple modalities as suggested by a doctor.

Scar-Reduction Products

There are many scar-reduction products on the market. You may try to use them for any type of scarring, but they are less likely to be effective on atrophic or keloid scars. Unfortunately, even when you consistently comply with instructions, these treatments are effective for only some piercees. Certain products do have guarantees, however, so check before buying them. Listed below are some of the scar-reduction products available. Silicone strips may be the most economical treatment because they are washable and reusable.

- Scargo, Scar Freee, and other oils and lotions with natural ingredients such as cocoa butter, shea butter, aloe, arnica, calendula, or camphor (available at health food stores).

- ScarEase, ReJuveness, and other silicone sheets, and Biodermis, Kelo-cote, and other silicone gel systems. It isn't understood exactly how silicone helps scars heal. Some researchers believe that static electricity from the silicone helps align collagen fibers in the scar, while others believe it might help to trap moisture, which can help scars to fade.

- Mederma, Derma E Scar Gel, and other products containing *allicin* (onion or garlic extract). This is intended to act as an anti-inflammatory and may inhibit the overproduction of collagen in a scar. These need to be rubbed in several times daily over an extended period of time.

Dry Skin

If the area surrounding your piercing is excessively dry, chapped, or cracked, this can cause discomfort, delay your healing, and increase your risk of infection. To keep your skin moisturized and in good condition, follow the instructions under "Lubrication," page 197; or apply a low-fragrance, water-based, nonirritating moisturizing cream (with clean hands, of course) on the exterior of the piercing, two to three times daily.

Here are some ways to troubleshoot dryness:

- Don't overclean; washing once a day could be sufficient, depending on your environment and activities.

- Bathe in a shower rather than a tub and use cooler water.

- Avoid harsh products; switch to a milder soap and thoroughly rinse at the end of your shower.

- Use no more than ⅛ teaspoon of salt per cup of water for saline soaks, and carefully rinse off saline residue. Limit soaks to once or twice daily.

- Use fragrance-free, dye-free laundry detergent.

"Tarnish Tattoo"

No, this isn't a new type of body art that's gaining popularity; it's a complication caused by wearing inappropriate jewelry. When sterling silver, low-karat or poorly alloyed gold, or other unsuitable metal is worn in a piercing, especially during healing, a residue can turn the interior of the hole dark blue, gray, or black. The technical term is *localized argyria*, and it is caused by skin exposure to silver or silver salts. This dark bluish blotch is largely a cosmetic issue, but once the discoloration sets in, it is permanent unless you have it surgically excised. Avoid wearing silver jewelry in nostril and facial piercings, where a tarnish tattoo can be particularly unbecoming.

Dermatitis

Contact dermatitis is a skin rash caused by an allergen or irritant. When it appears near your healing piercing, it is usually from a care product or poor-quality jewelry containing unsuitable materials. Harsh soaps and cleansers are apt to cause irritation, inflammation, and sometimes dermatitis in the adjacent tissue (in addition to killing off some of the delicate new skin cells that are formed during healing). When you have sensitive skin, problems can develop even if you use a mild soap.

A red rash that surrounds your piercing or one that covers a large area (without pain and swelling) usually indicates contact dermatitis from your cleaning product or jewelry. Skin eruptions below your piercing (where soap suds run during bathing) obviously demonstrate contact dermatitis caused by the product you are using to clean your piercing.

Many people are sensitive to nickel (it is one of the ten most common causes of allergic contact dermatitis).[21] Unfortunately, it is used in cheap jewelry of all sorts, including body jewelry. A nickel allergy may develop after your initial exposure to an item containing nickel or after repeated or prolonged exposure to it. So even a piece that seems fine initially can cause trouble over time if the nickel content is too high. A lasting allergy can form that has ramifications on many aspects of daily life. If you become highly sensitized to nickel, you should not eat foods that contain traces of nickel, including nuts, chocolate, beer, tea, coffee, and apricots. Skin contact with metal, including watches and other jewelry and clothing with metal snaps, buttons, rivets, or zippers can all cause localized itchy rashes that can spread to other areas of your body.[22] Treatments, whether prescribed by a doctor or over-the-counter, are temporary solutions to deal with an outbreak, but they cannot desensitize you or cure an allergy.[23] It is not advisable to use clear nail polish to coat offending jewelry because it contains chemicals including toluene, formaldehyde, or dibutyl phthalate, which can actually cause dermatitis in nickel-sensitive individuals.[24]

Identifying Dermatitis

- Redness, rash (blisters, multiple pimple-like eruptions, or hives), and inflammation; sometimes cracking, flaking, or peeling skin follow the initial outbreak
- Localized swelling, tenderness, and possible warmth
- Oozing clear fluid
- Itching and possibly burning (not present in local infection or cellulitis, which share some of the same symptoms)
- The hole of your healing piercing becomes visibly larger than the jewelry in it (the skin appears to be receding from the ornament)

What to Do for Dermatitis

- Replace your jewelry with a more inert material or stop using an offending care product. This usually results in rapid improvement; no other action may be required.

- Ease symptoms with over-the-counter topical hydrocortisone, allergy-relief medications such as Benadryl (diphenhydramine), and/or topical anti-itch products.

- If your allergy is severe, visit a doctor for prescription medication.

- Do not scratch an itchy rash with dirty fingers, as you can cause yourself a secondary infection.

Embedded Jewelry

When you fail to change out jewelry that is too short, it can become embedded. It is much easier to prevent this from happening than to treat it after it does. If your jewelry is starting to sink into your tissue, see your piercer for a longer piece right away.

Tongue and lip jewelry normally *nest* (sink a millimeter or two) into the soft oral tissues, but if more than half of the ball has disappeared into your piercing or the skin appears to be growing over your jewelry, visit your piercer as soon as possible. Oral tissue regenerates extremely quickly, and jewelry can end up embedded overnight. If you cannot immediately get to your piercer for help, use elevation, rest, ice, and over-the-counter anti-inflammatory medication to minimize the symptoms until you are able to get your jewelry changed.

In the unfortunate event that the tissue completely grows over the jewelry and you or your piercer cannot push it back through the surface, you must seek medical care. A small incision will be made (generally under local anesthesia) to allow for removal of your unintentional implant. If you want to preserve the hole, obtain jewelry of the proper size beforehand, as it might be possible to insert it after the embedded piece has been liberated.

Traumatic Tear

Skin is pretty tough, so a serious snag is needed to cause real damage. When you wear jewelry of the suggested minimum thickness and exercise some awareness of your piercing, this type of unfortunate event seldom occurs, but accidents do happen. Piercings occasionally catch and tear. If your jewelry is ripped through your piercing, control the bleeding and clean the gash. Visit a medical facility if you cannot join the edges of the split tissue together properly or if direct pressure does not stop the bleeding, which is rare.

If the jewelry is not completely torn out, it might be possible to preserve your piercing using a plastic retainer, depending on the original placement and the amount of damage. Place the plastic piece in the original location as close to the body as possible and use medical tape such as Micropore to secure it. Resume the care regimen as if you had a new piercing and replace the tape as needed. If the tissue heals satisfactorily, you may be able to reinsert regular jewelry in a few months. Your piercing may permanently require gentle handling following a tear because scar tissue is only about 80 percent as strong as normal skin.[25]

Catching the Tube

This isn't about surfing; it's a type of trauma that can happen when you force your jewelry to turn and there is a tube of skin on it that used to be the lining of your piercing. Removing the interior of a piercing may cause tenderness or bleeding. It also sets back your healing as your body repeats the process of generating new cells to line the channel. Your cleaning and care must start all over again. Multiple episodes can result excess scar tissue. Be gentle!

Dealing with Rejection and Migration

When your jewelry moves closer to the surface or your tissue gets narrower between the openings of a piercing, you are experiencing migration. The piercing may move only a little and then settle and stay in a different position. For safety and longevity, a piercing should have at least 5/16 inch (almost 8 mm) of tissue between the entrance and exit holes. If your piercing is narrower than that, there is a strong possibility you will lose it.

Don't allow jewelry to come all the way through to the surface or an unsightly split scar will often remain (unless you undergo plastic surgery). Also, future repiercing could be more difficult if you permit the jewelry to be completely expelled from your body.

A body piercing should be abandoned if the tissue between the entry and exit progressively gets smaller or thinner over time and any of the following happen:

- The skin between the openings is flaking and peeling, red and inflamed, or hard and calloused-looking.
- You have less than 1/4 inch of tissue between the openings.
- Just a thin filament of nearly transparent tissue is left, and you can virtually see the jewelry right through your skin.

These issues can arise long after you are healed. I know of piercings that were stable for ten to twenty years, and then migration or rejection occurred without any indication as to why. This is especially distressing when it happens to a piercing you've had for a long time because it feels like you are losing a part of yourself. Whether your piercing is old or new, if you catch the problem before the point of no return, there are some measures that might help.

Check the fit, quality, and condition of your jewelry. Wearing inferior metal or a piece with a scratched finish can cause serious trouble. Even if the jewelry seems okay, swapping it out is sometimes all you need to stop the movement of your piercing. Wearing inert plastic may calm a piercing that has started to migrate, whether jewelry was the apparent cause or not.

If ring-style jewelry won't rest flat against your body (after the first few weeks of healing), or barbell ends sink into your tissue, these are signs that your jewelry is too small. Inserting a piece that fits properly often stops migration that has been caused by constriction, if the change is made while sufficient tissue remains.

Repiercing after Loss

When trauma, migration, or rejection results in the loss of a piercing, you can often be repierced—unless you were left with an excessive amount of scarring or lack of tissue pliability. After losing or abandoning your piercing under difficult circumstances, it is prudent to wait a year or more before repiercing.

Consider what caused your problem and what you can do differently so that it doesn't happen again. When you do repierce, it is best to try a different size or style of jewelry, or alternate material or care regimen if you are not sure what went wrong previously. In cases of migration or rejection, ask yourself relevant questions: Did I sleep on the piercing? Did I experience an unusual amount of physical or emotional stress? Did I care for the piercing properly? Was my jewelry suitable?

Your piercer will usually position the new piercing behind any scar tissue, though this does not assure success, because scar tissue is weaker than regular skin, contrary to what many piercers believe.

Sometimes a migrated piercing that has been abandoned will remain an open channel, but it is too shallow to safely support jewelry. You can ignore an empty hole because it does not represent a health risk. But, when it comes to repiercing, sometimes an old channel becomes inflamed or infected after a new piercing is placed nearby. Due to continuous secretion or irritation from the previous piercing, occasionally these situations cannot be resolved satisfactorily and you will not be able to wear jewelry in the site.

Choking

Although it is not a common occurrence, it is possible to accidentally choke on body jewelry, which could be very serious. Most oral body jewelry, however, is too small to become lodged or cause an obstruction in the throat if it becomes unfastened.

What to do for jewelry caught in the throat:

- *Immediate* emergency medical care is required if you cannot breathe. Dial 911, or have someone do it for you, if possible.

- If you cannot speak or cough, the *Heimlich maneuver* (upward abdominal thrusts) may be used to force air from your lungs in an attempt to dislodge the obstruction. If you are alone, you may be able to perform the procedure on yourself using the back of a chair or other object.

- If you can breathe but feel jewelry lodged in your throat, cough vigorously to attempt to bring up the jewelry. If this is ineffective, seek emergency medical attention.

Swallowed Jewelry

Much more frequently, jewelry is swallowed and then passed through to the stomach and intestines. This seldom causes any negative consequences in the digestive tract. The aftermath may include some anxiety, the loss of your adornment, and the expense of buying a replacement.

If you swallow jewelry, do not attempt to induce vomiting. A lost ball will simply pass on through; a ring or barbell post usually will, too. If you were wearing a treasured piece of jewelry, whether precious in price or sentiment, you may wish to hunt for it over the next few days by checking your stool. A strainer can be helpful for this process. An advantage of finding your jewelry is that you can be assured it is not stuck inside. It is doubtful that a ball smooth enough to be worn safely in your mouth will cause internal damage on the way through. Barbell posts are less apt to be ingested but could be more dangerous.

Identifying Intestinal Damage from Swallowed Jewelry:

- Abdominal pain or vomiting
- Abnormal bowel sounds emanating from your abdomen
- Dark stools containing blood

Jewelry can pass though the digestive tract, all the way to the end, where you might encounter a rare (perhaps hypothetical) complication: it gets lodged on the way out.

Identifying Jewelry Stuck in the Rectum:

- Sudden, sharp pain when eliminating
- Fresh red blood in the stool

Should you experience any of the above symptoms after swallowing jewelry, *seek immediate medical attention*. Diagnostic tools such as X-rays can determine the position of lodged jewelry, and a variety of methods are available to remove it, depending on its location.

Prevention is best: check threaded ends daily to ensure that they are securely fastened.

Aspirated Jewelry

If you *aspirate* your jewelry (inhale into your lungs rather than swallow it), this is extremely serious. This grave consequence is frequently cited in warnings about piercing risks, yet no verified cases can be found in the available literature on piercing complications.[26]

If you manage to inhale jewelry without choking, you must *seek medical attention right away*. A foreign object that remains in the lungs usually causes inflammation and infection, including pneumonia.

The Point

When complications occur, the best chance you have to resolve them is to correctly identify what is wrong and follow the suggestions accordingly. Prompt attention and optimal treatment of problems can prevent more serious conditions. Never hesitate to seek assistance from a qualified piercer or health-care provider when you need it. On those occasions when a piercing truly is lost or must be removed, you won't win by fighting. The good news is that with proper handling, you can achieve a positive outcome most of the time.

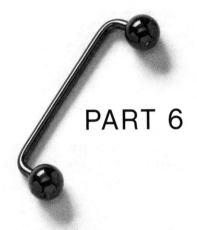

PART 6

Living with Your Piercings

Upkeep and Stretching
Advanced Jewelry and Practices
Special Situations
Sex!

17

Upkeep and Stretching

After your piercing has healed it still requires routine maintenance, however minimal, for life. This chapter covers the necessary upkeep as well as activities such as changing your jewelry, stretching to larger gauges, and retiring.

Regular Maintenance

Your piercings and jewelry should be included in your daily personal hygiene routine. When you bathe, simply wash your jewelry and piercing with soap and water, rotate, and rinse well. This keeps the area clean and free of matter and removes the normal (and smelly) secretions that can coat jewelry and lodge in a healed piercing.

Check regularly to make sure hair does not become tangled around earrings or body jewelry. Just a single coiled strand that remains next to your tissue can cause an accumulation of secretions and lead to irritation and even infection.

Body jewelry does not necessarily need to be removed for regular upkeep. It can often be left in place for maintenance and worn for years on end. However, once you are healed, if your jewelry looks or feels dirty and you've done everything you can while wearing it, your adornment will need to be taken out for more scrupulous attention. Bar posts, nostril screws, and other snug-fitting styles will require at least brief removal for thorough cleaning.

Steel and other body jewelry metals lose their luster when coated with personal care products or natural body oils and secretions. Gold jewelry may tarnish (it is actually the other metals in the alloy that discolor) when worn in a piercing. This can happen even to high-karat, quality pieces; it is not necessarily a sign of cheap jewelry.

Commercial jewelry-polishing cloths help return a shine to the metal. Different types are available, so use a cloth intended for the jewelry metal you're wearing; a gold-polishing cloth, for example, will not be very effective on steel. Keep harsh jewelry cleaning products away from your skin. Many chemicals that are appropriate for use on rings and necklaces could be dangerous to put on jewelry that will be returned to your body or mouth. Toothpaste on a firm toothbrush is effective for polishing body jewelry whether your ornament is in an oral piercing or not. Jewelry that contains durable gemstones (like diamonds, rubies, and sapphires) can get the toothbrush treatment, too; it will keep settings clean and stones sparkly.

Small home-use jewelry cleaning machines that use steam or ultrasonic technology are not expensive and they do a more thorough job than polishing cloths, but all require temporary removal of your jewelry. The steam units use distilled water, and an ultrasound will still clean when filled with a mild soap solution or even plain water instead of a strong chemical cleanser. Check with your jeweler/piercer before using such equipment if your jewelry is set with genuine or synthetic gemstones. Certain setting styles and stones, such as opals and emeralds, are too fragile for this treatment.

If you don't have a spare ring or bar to wear during cleanings, buy a retainer to keep the channel open or a taper to facilitate the reinsertion. Some piercings shrink so quickly that it can be difficult to put your jewelry back after it has been out for cleaning only briefly.

Regular Maintenance: Oral Piercings

Any jewelry worn continuously in your mouth is subject to plaque formation, just like your teeth. Most people don't take their teeth out to clean them, and if you are extremely conscientious, you may be able to perform sufficient upkeep without taking out your oral jewelry either. However, it is challenging.

Regular use of an antiplaque oral rinse can help keep jewelry clean. Still, there is no substitute for a vigorous scrub. Meticulously scour each end of the jewelry with a firm toothbrush as you hold the other side between your fingers. The hard-bristle toothbrush suggested for use on body jewelry may be firmer than your dentist recommends for brushing your teeth. The junctures where your barbell balls or discs connect to the post should be cleaned with a loop of dental floss. Daily brushing of the in-the-mouth part of lip and labret jewelry is as much a necessity as brushing your teeth. The ball on the underside of your tongue is particularly susceptible to collecting plaque.

> **Brush Up**
>
> I'll never forget changing a client's tongue jewelry and grasping a white acrylic ball on the underside between my gloved fingers. On closer inspection, I saw that it was, in fact, a metal ball that had become completely encased in plaque from inadequate maintenance. Yuck!

If brushing, flossing, and rinsing don't do a thorough enough job, jewelry can be removed and submerged in hydrogen peroxide or a denture-cleaning soak, according to the manufacturer's directions.

Changing Jewelry

Quality body jewelry can be worn indefinitely. If you like what you're wearing, there is no need to change it. Most piercees don't have the requisite know-how, dexterity, or sanitation to safely insert new jewelry into a healing piercing at home. A clumsy attempt to swap out the jewelry on a healing piercing can cause irritation, delayed healing, and infection. See a piercer if you experience problems; otherwise, your initial piece of jewelry should remain in your piercing until you are fully healed.

Once you're healed, however, it should be safe to replace your jewelry when all of the following conditions are met:

- Your piercing is no longer secreting and getting crusty.
- It is not tender.
- The minimum healing time has passed (see "Minimum Healing Times Chart," page 276).

Many piercees prefer to have a professional change their jewelry, especially the first time. Depending on placement and whether you can see and access your piercing, you may be able to perform the job yourself. Studios ordinarily offer free jewelry insertion or charge a nominal fee when you purchase something new. Ask for a lesson on how to deal with your own jewelry; good piercers are amenable to educating their clients.

Insertion Tapers for Jewelry Changes

If you are a novice and you wish to swap out your own jewelry, an insertion taper is invaluable to keep the channel open and avoid excess trauma. Its tapered shape helps to slide the existing ornament out and ease the new one into place.

A taper that does not correspond to the gauge and style of the jewelry you are putting in can be worse than not having one at all. Internally threaded jewelry uses a *pin-coupling* taper (the back end is formed into pin that fits into the hole tapped in the jewelry) or a *threaded-pin* taper (the back end screws into the jewelry). Fixed-bead rings, captive bead rings, and most externally threaded jewelry use a *concave taper* (the concave back end of the taper connects with the convex end of the jewelry). See "Insertion Tapers," page 63. To avoid an unpleasant surprise, check the fit of your taper with your new jewelry before removing what you're wearing.

If you feel confident that you can follow the old jewelry with the new (and you are not stretching up), then the taper is not required. But, if your old jewelry comes out before the new piece passes through, finding the hole can be harder than you think. Trying to shove jewelry through a channel that has shrunk is not only painful, but it is also traumatic to the tissue, especially for a recently healed piercing.

Jewelry Change Procedure

I've had many a piercee show me an inflamed or empty piercing and recount a painful tale of trying to change jewelry at home for "over an hour." When properly handled, the procedure should take only a few moments. Learning what to do and using the correct tools will ensure your comfort and safety.

- **Prepare yourself:** Swap out your jewelry after a shower when your skin is clean and the tissue is looser. Your hands must be clean and dry. You may find it easier to get a grip on the jewelry while wearing latex medical gloves, but a tight fit is key if they are to help rather than hinder.

- **Prepare your work area:** If you are near a sink, plug it carefully. Many pieces of small body jewelry have been lost down a drain.

- **Assemble everything you will need for the process from beginning to end:**
    - ☐ Jewelry: Clean or sterile and open, ready for insertion
    - ☐ Lubricant: A water-based product such as K-Y Jelly
    - ☐ Tissues or paper towels: To keep your fingers dry and wipe off the jewelry after insertion
    - ☐ Clean zip-top bags: To store your jewelry after removal
    - ☐ Snug-fitting medical gloves (optional)
    - ☐ An insertion taper that connects with your new jewelry (optional)
    - ☐ Jewelry tools (RXPs, RCPs, hemostats, and/or brass-jaw pliers) (optional)

- **Choose the right jewelry:** Buy body jewelry only from a reputable dealer. New jewelry is often sold in individual packages, but you can't tell if it is sterile by looking—you have to ask (and you must trust your source). If you are unsure, have a piercer sterilize the jewelry in an autoclave before you wear it.

- **Prepare the jewelry, if it has been worn before:** If it you were the only wearer and you stored your own previously worn jewelry in a clean environment, wash it with soap and water. If another person wore the jewelry in their piercing or it was your own but not kept in a hygienic location, it must be autoclaved before you wear it. Your piercer may charge a small fee or provide free jewelry sterilization.

- **Open the jewelry:** Unscrew a threaded end, remove a ball from a captive, twist open a fixed-bead ring, and so on. Rings must be spread wide enough to clear your tissue without pinching your skin.

- **Assemble the right tools:** If your hands aren't strong enough for the job, you will require the help of tools. They must be appropriate or they can harm you or your jewelry (see "Jewelry Tools," below). Regular workbench pliers are not recommended. If you scratch the metal (which is easy to do with improper tools), your jewelry will be unwearable. If you have to use regular tools in an emergency, clean them thoroughly and wrap each tip with a strip of cloth tape or adhesive bandages to form a protective cushion. Be certain you have a very firm grasp before attempting to bend a ring that is in your body.

- **Lubricate:** Apply a small amount of lubricant to the jewelry you are wearing and work it into the piercing channel. Apply some to the end of your new jewelry or the tip of your taper, too, but try to keep it off your fingers.

- **Make the swap:** Try to keep something in the piercing at all times. Support the tissue on the exit side to facilitate the transfer. Push out the old jewelry using your new jewelry (or a taper). If you're using a taper, chase your old jewelry out with the thin tip; or, if the taper matches the size and style of jewelry you're wearing, you can use the thicker end of the taper to back your jewelry out. Next, connect your new jewelry to the back end of the taper and push the tool out of the piercing with your new jewelry.

- **Close the jewelry:** Wipe off the lubricant with a clean tissue and fasten your new jewelry.

- **Wash up:** Clean your worn jewelry and insertion tapers with soap and water and dry well with clean paper towels. Store the items in clean zip-top bags or another hygienic location, keeping jewelry made of different metals in separate containers to avoid scratches.

Jewelry Tools

Your piercer may use these during a piercing procedure or jewelry change, and you can purchase them for home use if you need them to change your own jewelry. If you have personal tools that you do not share, washing them with soap and water between uses should be sufficient if you keep them stored in clean zip-top bags.

Large-gauge, small-diameter, or unannealed captive rings usually require tools for removal and insertion.

Ring Expanding Pliers (RXPs)

RXPs are reverse pliers, with tips that spread apart when you squeeze the handles. RXPs help widen the gap on a captive ring so you can insert or remove the bead. Make sure that there is no tissue between the tool and the jewelry, or you will suffer a mighty pinch. It is equally important to be careful when releasing the handles to avoid nipping the skin as the pliers close.

You generally need RXPs only when the metal is too hard or thick to bend by hand or when you are inserting a bead that is larger than usual. Squeeze the handles slowly so you do not spread the gap any more than you absolutely have to for the bead to be inserted or removed. If you do open the ring too wide, then you'll need the next jewelry tool, ring closing pliers.

Tip: When removing a bead, grasp it in your fingers to pull it from the ring as you use the tool to spread the ring just enough to engage its spring tension (rather than enlarging the gap of the ring so far that the bead simply falls out).

Ring Closing Pliers (RCPs)

These pliers have a grooved rounded head that is used to close the gap on captive rings. If a ring has been opened too far by RXPs or you are inserting a smaller bead than the one that was previously in the ring, this tool is indispensable. Some small RCPs also have a grooved end that can be used to unscrew barbell balls that have been affixed too tightly to open by hand.

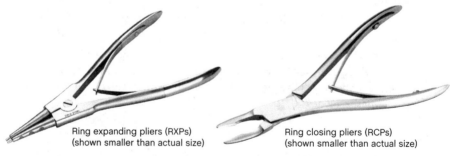

Ring expanding pliers (RXPs)
(shown smaller than actual size)

Ring closing pliers (RCPs)
(shown smaller than actual size)

Tip: Whenever possible, use RCPs to make adjustments to your ring when it is not in your piercing. If you are wearing the ring when you use the tool, exercise extreme caution to ensure that the pliers do not slip and pinch your skin.

Hemostats (Hemos)

This multipurpose tool can be used to bend small rings open and closed, adjust nostril screws, and hold jewelry or a bead during insertion and closure. Hemostats used on metal body jewelry must have smooth jaws, never serrations. Brass-jaw hemostats, RXPs, RCPs, and pliers diminish the risk of damaging jewelry because brass is softer than the body jewelry metals.

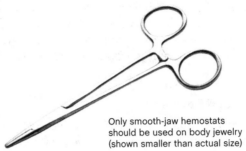

Only smooth-jaw hemostats should be used on body jewelry (shown smaller than actual size)

Jewelry Emergencies

Mishaps occur on occasion, even with quality pieces. To minimize the likelihood of losing your jewelry (and avoid the problems described at the end of the previous chapter), check threaded ends regularly for tightness, and see to it that captive beads are inserted properly. Purchase an extra bead or ball at the time of your piercing so you will always have all the parts needed to keep your jewelry where it belongs. If you lose a ball and have no spare on hand, there are temporary measures you can take to prevent your jewelry from falling out. Try one of the following until you can obtain a replacement:

- **Eraser:** Use a small piece of clean pencil eraser and cut it to the desired size and shape. Press it onto the end of a barbell post or between the ends of your empty captive ring to keep jewelry in place.
- **Band-Aid or surgical tape:** Apply it to your jewelry and/or body in a way that keeps the piece from falling out.

Here are some tips:

- Never assume that a piece of jewelry will fit simply because it looks like what you have at home. Jewelry made by different manufacturers, especially threaded items, is frequently not interchangeable. Variables include the size and depth of the threads and thread counts per inch. Captive rings have different size gaps, and so on. Bring your jewelry with you when shopping for replacement parts.
- Other than your take-along spare, don't carry body jewelry around with you unless you are transporting it to your piercer for assistance with an insertion or for some other purpose. Keep your spare jewelry in a secure place at home.
- Don't underestimate the ability of a piercing to shrink quickly. Plenty of piercees have learned the hard way that it was a bad idea to leave a hole empty for "just one night."
- Thick carpeting and home jewelry changes don't mix. Pick an area where jewelry will be easy to find and retrieve if you drop it.

New Jewelry

To be assured of a good fit when you shop for new jewelry—especially for your first change—buy from a studio where a piercer can do the insertion for you. Jewelry for some piercings comes in increments as small as ⅛ inch or even fractions of a millimeter. A piece that looks right might not fit properly once it is in your piercing.

Use the "My Piercings and Jewelry Chart" on page 274 to keep accurate records. Write down the style and gauge with length or diameter and other details. When you go to buy new jewelry, you will know exactly what size you're wearing. This is useful whether you would like to purchase a duplicate of a ring you already have, obtain a different style in your current size, or if you intend to stretch. Record all changes and you will always have an up-to-date list.

Post-Healing Ups and Downs

After putting in new jewelry you might experience some irritation. This can occur from the process of swapping out the jewelry, even if your piercing is well healed and the process was handled smoothly. Or, your body may be adjusting (or objecting) to the new ornament. If you do not improve within a week, you may need to return to your old jewelry. Visit your piercer for advice if your condition worsens.

On occasion, tenderness, secretion, or other symptoms of a fresh piercing occur long after your healing period. These flare-ups can result from emotional stress or hormonal changes, but sometimes no cause is apparent. Some follow-up with your piercer or a medical professional could become needed long after successful healing. Whenever your piercing flares up, it is always best to treat it like a healing piercing. If you believe something is wrong beyond the normal ups and downs, seek assistance from your piercer or doctor.

Stretching

If you've seen photographs of African women with huge plates in their lips, you have witnessed the astounding elasticity of the human body. The practice of stretching piercings (sometimes referred to as *gauging up* or simply *gauging*) for the purpose of wearing larger jewelry has gained popularity and acceptability, much like body piercing itself. Some of today's stretching harkens back to the appearance of primitive tribesmen with enlarged ear, septum, or lip piercings. Other stretching is done on nipple or genital piercings for increased sensation. You may want to go up only one size from your initial jewelry, or you might yearn for a gigantic perforation in your body. Regardless of your motives or goals, the method is the same: stretch piercings slowly and gradually.

Typically even old piercings can't usually go up more than one size at a time, barring heavy play, wearing weights, or tearing from trauma. You must allow a sufficient interval of time between each enlargement for your tissue to fully regain its suppleness and integrity; only then is it safe to go further. Skin is remarkably resilient if not abused, but if you become impatient and try to force your piercing, the consequences can be severe. Overstretching tends to result in a buildup of scar tissue and reduction of flexibility, which can limit your capacity to stretch in the future—or shrink back to normal, if desired. Failure to adhere to appropriate procedures can cause the total destruction and loss of your piercing from tissue *necrosis* (death).

I am often asked, "How large can I go and still have the hole return to 'normal' when I take the jewelry out?" Many factors, including your age, piercing placement, sun exposure, and the speed and extent of your stretches, affect the outcome. The slower you go, the better you will preserve your tissue elasticity, which increases the chances that the hole will shrink back down if jewelry is removed. A quick, brutal expansion to a modest 8 gauge could leave a void that daylight can be seen through, and an unhurried stretch to a much larger size might shrink and close to just a dimple. There are no guarantees, so think before you stretch.

Ancient Practice
The oldest mummified body in the world, found in an Austrian glacier in 1991, had earlobe piercings that were enlarged to a hefty 7 to 11 millimeters in diameter.

When most people see an enlarged piercing for the first time, their initial thought is, "Ouch! That had to hurt." But the process of gauging up should be close to painless, if not completely without some sensations. Safe stretching involves paying careful attention to the responses of your body, and heeding warning signals.

When to Stretch

Human tissue varies considerably, so there is no set timetable that is correct for stretching each type of piercing. In fact, it is possible to have a pair of matching piercings with one side that stretches easily and the other that just won't give.

Before attempting any expansion, it is safest to wait a minimum of two to three times the duration your piercing took to heal. For quick-mending areas, doubling the initial healing period is sometimes sufficient, but the longer your healing period, the more extended your delay should be before gauging up.

After stretching to a thicker gauge, you generally need to let the tissue recuperate and stabilize for a minimum of several months before attempting to fit in the next one. The gauge measurements become progressively bigger, so the stretch from 14 to 12 gauge isn't sizable (.43 mm), but going from 4 up to 2 gauge is a significant jump (1.36 mm). The larger you go, the longer you usually need to wait between stretches. This is due to the escalating size differences between gauges, and also because the tissue often becomes more difficult to expand as you strain its capacity.

The type of jewelry you wear is another factor to consider. A metal ring or other style with added weight helps you by passively enlarging your piercing. Plugs, eyelets, and other lightweight jewelry styles do not cause any stretching over time, so you may need to wait longer before you are ready to gauge up.

How to Stretch

Many people go to a piercer for help with stretching, and this is advisable if you are not acquainted with the process. If you have the right equipment and you can see and access the area, you should be able to stretch your own piercing at home. When your piercing is ready to go up, use the technique explained in "Jewelry Change Procedure," page 220, but with a taper of the next larger size (smaller gauge number).

When you change jewelry with a lubricated insertion taper, the tool glides right through your piercing because it is the same size as the channel. However, when actively stretching tissue with a larger taper, you will feel resistance, so you must push the taper through. You have to know how much pressure you can exert before causing damage to your tissue. If a taper the next size up slides right in with a minimal push and results in only slight warmth or pressure, you may be able to safely stretch to the next gauge. Only Prince Albert, inner labia, fourchette, and ear lobe piercings routinely stretch that quickly and easily. You are clearly not ready for the bigger gauge any time you push quite hard but the taper won't progress further, or if only the tip of a taper fits in comfortably. Agony is not a part of safe stretching; if it hurts that much, you are applying too much force and causing damage.

Gauging up should never cause obvious tearing or bleeding, but it is routine for stretching to weaken the skin and cause micro-tears. This invisible damage makes you susceptible to infection, so always handle fresh stretches gently and hygienically.

Stretching Tips

- Do not attempt to stretch shallow piercings without consulting a piercer.

- Do not stretch piercings that are irritated, inflamed, or infected.

- Do take a shower or perform a warm soak to loosen the tissue before stretching.

- Use plenty of lubricant, working some throughout the piercing channel using the existing jewelry or the tip of a taper before attempting to stretch.

- Keep the lubricant off the surfaces you need to hold for the jewelry transfer.

- An oil-based lubricant such as bacitracin ointment is acceptable for stretching, even though it is not suggested for use on fresh piercings. Some piercees use liquid soap (like Techni-Care) as a lubricant, and this should be rinsed out afterward.

- Don't use cheap tapers that aren't properly graduated. Some are too bullet-shaped and can cause damage as they pass through your tissue, especially if your skin is tight. A smoothly sloping taper is imperative for your safety and comfort. Some of the plugs and eyelets that are popular for enlarged ear piercings require specific styles of tapers for smooth jewelry transfers.

- Support the tissue at the exit (where the taper comes out) with a two- or three-finger grasp. This helps to increase the comfort and evenness of the stretch.

- Don't rush! Stretching should be done in a slow, controlled manner. Never jam the taper through.

- Don't screw the taper in, though a slight bit of rotation or twisting is sometimes helpful.

- As the tissue expands, you may feel discomfort in the form of tightness, warmth or burning, or a pinching sensation. It should not be excruciating, nor should you experience sensations of tearing or splitting.

- Don't force it! It should not require much muscle to work the tool through. If it does, stop pushing and go back to your previous size. See the next two sections for techniques to help you enlarge your piercing more gradually.

- Insert jewelry of an appropriate material and style. Many large ornaments are not suited to a fresh stretch. It is best to choose one of the materials approved for new piercings, and to use an alternative only after the area has settled.

Weights

Stretching with a taper is a common method, but there are other approaches. One alternative is to add weights or wear heavy jewelry so that the piercing enlarges itself over time. Some people affix additional weight for a certain duration each day. Others attempt to wear something heavier full time. It is crucial to pay attention to your body's responses. Soreness, redness, or inflammation of your tissue indicates a problem. Lighten the load for a while and try again later with less weight, wear the weight for shorter intervals, or wait longer between additions.

To supplement the weight, you can add multiple rings onto a hoop worn through a piercing (rather than adding rings through your tissue). This affords good control of the added load, is a creative way to use surplus jewelry, and can look attractive, too. Another option is to wear an eyelet through the hole (once it is large enough to accommodate one) and add weight through the eyelet. This helps to distribute the burden over a somewhat larger area.

Note that using weights or simply wearing heavy jewelry sometimes causes thinning or irritation of the tissue at the bottom of the piercing due to excessive pressure. And, of course, wearing a heavy adornment is apt to enlarge your piercing whether you want it or not.

Tape Wrap and Heat-Shrink Tubing

Another stretching technique involves wrapping your jewelry in *plumber's tape*, which is extremely thin. It is made of Teflon, so it is inert and can be used safely by most piercees. It is inexpensive and available in the plumbing section of any hardware store. Each time you wind the jewelry with a little more tape and reinsert it, you enlarge your piercing minutely.

Follow these tips to stretch using plumber's tape:

- A good time to add tape is after a shower.
- Wrap a few layers of the tape around the portion of the jewelry that goes through your body. The tape is not adhesive, so use a tiny dab of oil to help it to adhere to your jewelry.
- Put the tape on smoothly to avoid an uneven surface that could irritate your skin.
- Reinsert your taped jewelry using lubricant to make the transition easy.
- Affix a few new layers several times a week, or even daily if it feels comfortable and your body responds well.
- Don't put on too much new tape at once, and observe whether your body is accepting the material and the larger sizes.
- Remove all the tape and start over at least once a week to preserve hygiene.

This method will enlarge your hole very gradually and help you to avoid making a large jump from one gauge to the next via insertion taper. The various enlarging techniques can be combined; first use tape wraps to stretch your piercing part of the way, and then use a taper to achieve the rest of your expansion to the next jewelry size.

Heat-shrink tubing made of Teflon is stocked in the electrical supply department of the hardware store. This tubing can enlarge jewelry in the same way, but it isn't as thin as plumber's tape. Heat-shrink tubing provides smooth, even coverage for a piercing channel that is wider than the plumber's tape, so it is excellent for long barbells. Cut the tubing with some extra length to allow for the usual contraction. For barbells, leave enough excess so that the end of the bar post is sheathed in the tubing when it shrinks. This forms the tip into a tapered shape that eases reinsertion. After the jewelry is in place, carefully trim off the surplus tubing with clean scissors to expose the bar post and screw the end in place.

To use heat-shrink tubing, apply the same principles as above but use a heat gun or lighter to make the tubing shrink. Be careful not to burn yourself or scorch the tubing. Allow it to cool before reinserting your jewelry.

Dead Stretching

Dead stretching is the term used for simply pushing a larger object into a piercing. This is safe only when the tissue is ready and the object is no bigger than your piercing can handle; otherwise, damage will occur. Adding multiple thin rings into a piercing over time is one relatively safe way to accomplish dead stretching, but this sometimes results in a piercing that isn't smooth and round.

Pierce and Stretch

This technique is fairly common, but it is even less advisable than dead stretching. A piercing is made with a piercing needle and then immediately stretched with a taper to a larger gauge. This takes a wound that was neatly formed by a sharp needle and distorts it, which can make it more challenging for your body to form the base layer of cells, the literal basis of tissue healing. Doing immediate damage in this way can also predispose the piercing to trouble, including delayed healing or excess scar tissue formation.

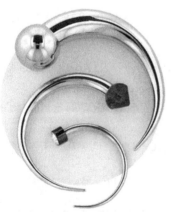

A selection of tapered ear talons

Tapered Jewelry: Caution

Many graduated jewelry styles come in metal, glass, acrylic, and an array of natural materials. A popular type is called a stretching crescent or stretching ring, and these are basically curved or circular insertion tapers. Variations include talons that are hooked or bent, spirals, and straight pieces that look just like insertion tapers. These can be dangerous because piercees have a tendency to cause tissue damage by stretching too quickly with them. Also, when tapered jewelry is used for stretching, the O-rings that are required to keep the ornament in place can cause irritation from excessive pressure against the skin. Tapered jewelry is safest in holes that have already been stretched.

Maintenance of Stretched Piercings

Because a stretched piercing has an increased surface area, the amount of sebum is also amplified. You need to be especially vigilant with your hygiene routine to get rid of these deposits. After your stretch has settled, if your jewelry is easy to remove, slip it out daily to wash it and the inside of the channel. Many piercees with enlarged holes find that wearing jewelry made of natural materials helps to diminish sebum formation.

Some piercees can easily swap back and forth between two jewelry gauges; others can fit only one size because the piercing shrinks too quickly.

Resting

A technique called *resting* or *relaxing* is the practice of removing large-gauge jewelry (approximately 2 gauge and thicker) for a time each day or night. This is to relieve the tissue of the jewelry's weight and pressure. It may help to promote healthier skin by increasing circulation, especially at the bottom of the piercing, which supports most of the burden.

Experiment to determine the amount of time your jewelry can be removed without the hole shrinking too much. Generally, the longer you have worn a particular size, the easier this becomes. Some individuals leave jewelry out overnight and slide it right back in the next morning. Others go without their jewelry for only an hour or so before the hole starts to feel uncomfortably tight during reinsertion. Try removing your jewelry for successively longer periods until you find your comfortable interval. Ideally, you want to leave it out for as long as possible but reinsert it before the hole shrinks enough to cause you discomfort during reinsertion. If you run into trouble getting your jewelry back in, do a warm saline soak and use some lubricant and possibly a taper, too. Wait until the tissue has recovered for at least a week or two before making another attempt at resting your piercing.

Tissue Massage

Daily massage of stretched tissue can be a tremendous help in maintaining elasticity and vascularity, keeping your piercing in top condition, and facilitating future stretching. Use a biocompatible moisturizing lubricant such as jojoba or emu oil. Wash your hands, apply a small amount of oil, and for a few minutes during your rest period massage the tissue firmly, especially on the bottom of the piercing. Roll and rub the skin between your fingers to work in the oil. If the piercing is large enough to fit a cotton swab or fingertip inside, massage the interior of the hole especially well. This treatment moisturizes the skin, which is essential; dryness can result in brittleness, weakness, and tears. The manipulation also helps to break down scar tissue and stimulate circulation to promote healthy, vital skin.

Trouble and Troubleshooting

If you experience pain or bleeding, a lot of secretion, or excessive redness (some is normal for a few days after a stretch), you have enlarged too fast. You will need to regress to your previous jewelry size, or possibly even smaller, depending on the extent of the damage. Don't wear heavy jewelry in an irritated stretch, and stick to the materials suited to new piercings.

If you end up with a painful weeping wound from impatient stretching, you may decide to give up and abandon the piercing completely. Be aware, however, that tissue inflamed by overstretching sometimes responds even more poorly to being left empty than it does to simply having smaller jewelry in place.

Treat an overstretched piercing like a brand-new one and follow appropriate care and cleaning. Failure to do so can result in serious consequences, including infection and tissue loss. If you make the mistake of stretching until your skin thins and splits in two, the piercing is lost; reconstructive surgery will be needed to repair the deformity to your bifurcated tissue.

Another nasty consequence of stretching too quickly is a *blowout*, in which a section of skin pushes out from the interior of the channel. In essence, the piercing twists itself inside out due to excessive pressure. The most common location for a blowout is the back of the earlobe. It may not be as painful as it looks, but it clearly indicates a problem. You must immediately remove the offending ornament, try to realign the tissue, back down at least one gauge, and resume aftercare procedures. If the skin is allowed to remain distorted, it will generally stay that way. A blowout might be improved by doing your next stretch from the opposite direction to force the tissue back inside the channel, or by treatment with a compression technique. Wear tube- or plug-style jewelry with an inert plastic (PTFE) washer (available at hardware stores) against the tissue on each side to compact the blowout back into place. Use O-rings to hold everything firmly together. Remove the jewelry to massage the tissue daily with emu or other oil. Also take it out at night to rest the tissue, if this seems to help.

If you overstretch, wait at least a few additional months before attempting further expansion. Slow down! Whatever method you choose, being patient and heeding the signals from your body are key elements for success.

Retiring a Piercing

Retiring a piercing is permanently removing your jewelry and abandoning the hole. Though body piercing has the potential to be a lifelong adornment, there is no doubt that a piercing—especially one that hasn't been stretched too fast or large—is easier to be rid of than most other body modifications.

It is best to retire your piercing when it is in good health. A notable exception is when you have a rejecting piercing in which the jewelry has migrated too close to the surface. The main risk of removing jewelry is the potential to trap an infection inside. If there is any purulent drainage (pus), pain, inflammation, or suspected infection, do not abandon your piercing. See "Leave Jewelry In!" page 202, and subsequent sections for more information.

If your piercing is fine but you have decided the time has come to get rid of it, simply wash your hands and the area, open your jewelry, and remove it. A little bit of water-based lubricant such as K-Y Jelly can help to make the transition smooth. Wash the area daily when you bathe. Abandoning a piercing is that simple.

Will It Close?

Depending on the size, age, and location of a healed piercing, along with the course of stretching, if any, it may not seal up completely. Most holes contract fairly rapidly and can continue to shrink over time. Over the ensuing weeks, the area will stabilize and the channel is apt to remain in whatever state it has achieved within a month or two—smaller, or fully closed.

It is nearly impossible for a foreign body to accidentally enter an average abandoned piercing channel after the jewelry is out and the tissue has shrunk. You will not have an opening into your body if the piercing was fully healed before removal. A healed piercing has formed a tube (fistula); it is sealed off from the rest of your body. If you abandon a piercing before healing concludes, the cells of your body continue to grow together and seal the wound up completely. Neither is harmful or dangerous.

A fully healed piercing that is abandoned but does not seal up may excrete sebum. A simple test can be used to see if a channel could still be open: squeeze the tissue as if trying to push something out of it. If a thick white secretion of sebum comes from one or both holes, there is a strong possibility the channel is intact. This is not harmful and does not indicate a problem. The area will stabilize and can be ignored if you have no itching, swelling, or inflammation. Should your empty piercing discharge sebum spontaneously, you may wish to periodically assist with expressing it. One method is to squeeze the tissue in an attempt to release the matter from each side. Another is to use a small, clean insertion taper (usually 18 or 16 gauge, depending on how tight the channel shrinks) and run it through periodically to clear out the interior of the hole. The taper should fit snugly but pass through without irritating the tissue. Beyond this annoyance, there is seldom any problem from retired piercings.

The only way to be entirely rid of all traces of a previous piercing is by having the residual fistula removed by surgical excision. There is almost never the need to go to that extreme, and, of course, such surgery will leave some scarring of its own.

Many regretful piercees who have abandoned their piercings return to me to have their jewelry reinserted or to be repierced. Carefully consider whether you are truly done with a piercing before removing your jewelry. Reinserting jewelry in a piercing that has shrunk can be much more painful than the original piercing—but if a hole is still present and can be stretched, then repiercing is not usually appropriate. If the initial placement was correct, relocating the piercing is undesirable. However, if your piercing closes and leaves you with diminished tissue pliability or excess scar tissue, repiercing the original location might not be possible. Additionally there is potential for complications when piercing near an open channel. See "Repiercing after Loss," page 215, for details. If you think you might want to put your jewelry back in later, don't take it out in the first place.

The Point

For many body art enthusiasts, part of the attraction to piercings is their versatility. Not only does a piercing change your body, but you can also change your piercing, both by swapping out the jewelry and by stretching. Whether you have a collection of ornaments that you change daily with your mood, or you replace your jewelry infrequently, the choice is yours.

Advanced Jewelry and Practices

This chapter delves into advanced jewelry, including natural and man-made materials, for healed and stretched piercings. It also describes certain advanced piercings, more extreme modifications, and alternative practices.

Jewelry for Healed and Stretched Piercings

The form and function of initial body jewelry are all about safety, so relatively few materials and styles are suitable; however, after your piercing has healed, a whole bounty of beautiful ornaments is yours for a price. They come in countless materials, sizes, and styles. These factors, along with the weight and finish, contribute to whether the jewelry is suited for daily wear in the body.

Some pieces are safe and comfortable for continuous wear, but others are acceptable for only a few hours of dress-up fun. And, unfortunately, still others are best left in a display case for viewing enjoyment only. Adornments that are extremely heavy will seldom be appropriate for everyday wear. Anything with an uneven, etched, twisted, or matte finish has the potential to cause irritation. Quickly replace jewelry that does not agree with your piercing, no matter how much you like the way it looks.

Natural Materials[1]

In addition to the metals commonly used for fresh body piercings, healed piercings may tolerate (or even thrive with) jewelry crafted of alternative materials, including horn, bone, wood, amber, stone, and others created by Mother Nature. Often referred to as *organics*, these materials have been worn in piercings throughout the ages and all around the globe. Many modern piercees favor natural alternatives, especially for enlarged piercings in the ear, septum, or lip, though you should avoid wearing them in fresh stretches—and, of course, new piercings.

Some body jewelry is produced with consideration to avoid harming the earth and its creatures. Socially and environmentally conscious piercees can obtain natural jewelry made from sustainable or renewable resources including woods that are reforested, horn harvested from animals that die of natural causes, and antler that is shed seasonally.

Like all body jewelry, these products vary in quality and wearability. Natural materials are very fragile compared to metal. This jewelry with pointy or narrow areas or in thin gauges can easily be broken. Many alternative materials and styles are not safe to wear during sports or sleep, and organic pieces should be removed for bathing and swimming. Choose your jewelry to suit your lifestyle as well as your budget and aesthetic preferences.

Natural materials are too delicate to be autoclaved, so you must disinfect (rather than sterilize) them before insertion. Do not soak organic jewelry in anything, including water. Wash new jewelry with soap, then rinse, and dry it thoroughly without delay. To be safe, a chemical-free product such as Dr. Bronner's liquid soap is recommended. If you prefer a stronger cleaner, use tea tree oil, though this can sometimes cause drying or cracking. Be vigilant to avoid exposing your jewelry to chemicals such as bleach (no swimming pools), strong soaps or cleansers, and harsh personal care products. Contact with chemicals can be harmful to the jewelry and to you; in some cases they may be absorbed and then deposited into your body. Extremes of temperature can negatively affect organics, as can overexposure to light and humidity; drying, splitting, or warping may occur.

Cracks, pits, and uneven surfaces are not uncommon in organic jewelry, and they may encourage the growth of microbes. You must pay ongoing attention to the condition of the jewelry and your piercing. Depending on the material, you will need to rub natural jewelry with oil or wax to preserve and maintain it properly. Some people use jojoba, vitamin E, or mineral oil, and others favor food-grade oils such as olive, coconut, or peanut, though these can become rancid over time.

Handle natural body jewelry only with washed or gloved hands, and clean and oil it before wear, and also periodically, even if it is not being worn. If your jewelry appears to be dry, oil it more frequently. Body jewelry made of natural materials needs to be removed and washed regularly with mild soap and water.

Countless styles and variations of spirals, claws, tusks, pincers, and even captive rings are fashioned of natural materials, though plugs and eyelets are among the more common designs. Ears are unquestionably the most popular location for this type of jewelry. Nonstandard sizes are sometimes available, and these are useful when you cannot make the stretch to the next full gauge in one jump and want to wear something in-between.

A Sample of Natural Materials

- **Wood:** There are numerous varieties of wood, and some are safe for body jewelry styles such as plugs, eyelets, spikes, spirals, and elaborately carved pieces for ears. Wood's lightness makes it functional for large jewelry, and its properties allow handcrafted items to be affordable. All types of woods are not equally biocompatible. Many are inert, but some cause irritation or worse, and others are toxic; patronize a knowledgeable distributor. Porous woods can harbor bacteria and other germs. Do not expose wood jewelry to excessive heat or moisture, and dry it very thoroughly after washing it. Wood is not well suited for wear in moist areas of the body. Some jewelry may need to be sanded periodically as the grain expands in response to moisture. Do not wear wood if you have irritated or sensitive skin.

- **Bamboo:** This is actually a type of grass rather than a species of wood. There are many different kinds of this lightweight material, and it comes in colors ranging from yellow to green and even close to black. It may be mottled or even in coloration. Because the bulk of it is hollow, bamboo is an ideal material for a natural eyelet design. Nonstandard sizes are common because the natural plant dimensions form the jewelry diameters. When the *skin* (smooth coating) is left on the surface, only the ends of the jewelry need finishing.

- **Bone and horn:** Even though these are different materials, they largely share the same properties: both are porous, semihard, and lightweight. Bone is white, while horn ranges from tan to black. They both absorb moisture and skin oils, so a natural sealant such as beeswax is recommended. Horn is *thermoplastic* (it can be heated and then shaped, to some extent, and will retain its new form once cooled). Avoid exposing horn jewelry to hot water, as it can cause the material to revert to its original shape.[2] Most horn body jewelry is fashioned from water buffalo horn.

- **Amber:** Amber is a fossilized tree resin. Although it's best known for its yellow and orange shades, it can range from nearly colorless to brown or black. It can be clear or cloudy and may contain visible inclusions of fossilized insect or plant life. Amber is among the most delicate of natural body jewelry materials. Heat and chemicals can cause damage, including softening, cracking, and breaking. Be certain the amber is genuine, as faux products may not be sufficiently inert to wear safely in your body. Real amber is buoyant in salt water, feels warm to the touch (compared to gemstones), and, when rubbed briskly with a cloth, emits a piney odor. Most low-priced pieces containing a whole, clearly visible insect are imitations.

- **Gemstone, semiprecious stone, and rock:** These natural materials are dense and heavy, so they are seldom fashioned into big pieces or large plugs, which are liable to fall out. This category includes hematite, fluorite, agate, onyx, jasper, lapis, tigereye, amethyst, turquoise, and many others in a full range of colors. Some stones are durable, while others are more fragile and apt to crack, though any piece that is dropped on a hard surface can be expected to chip or break. Some stones may fade from exposure to sunlight.

- **Porcupine quills:** These are sometimes worn in septum piercings without alteration save cleaning, and possibly waxing or oiling the surface.

- **Fresh ivory:** *Ivory* can be defined as the dentine portion of a mammal's tooth,[3] though a purist may say that it comes only from elephants. Body jewelry can be crafted from the tusks of walrus, boar, warthog, and hippopotamus. These are acceptable sources of *fresh ivory*, since trade in new elephant ivory is illegal. Worldwide restrictions are in place to protect the elephant population, which is dwindling because of the demand for their tusks. Sunlight may bleach ivory or cause yellowing or brittleness, and it is also susceptible to damage from sudden changes in temperature.

- **Fossilized ivory:** This material from animals that lived during the Ice Age—the walrus, mastodon, or mammoth—is found in the tundra or permafrost of Alaska and other frigid places. It is at least 10,000 years old. Colors vary from creamy white to brown. This sensitive material can crack from rapid changes in temperature or humidity.

- **Antler:** White antler from moose, deer, or elk is a great substitute for ivory since it is similar in appearance yet more affordable and readily available. It is durable and not as liable to crack from exposure to moisture and skin oils. It also comes in shades of brown and gray. Antlers are comprised of bone and they are shed annually.

Man-Made Materials

A variety of nonmetal materials are frequently fashioned into body jewelry, including acrylic and glass. PTFE (Teflon) and Tygon are autoclavable plastics commonly used in fresh piercings, so they are discussed with the other materials used for initial jewelry in "Nontoxic Plastics," page 77.

- **Acrylic/plastic:** *Acrylic* is a general term for many varieties of plastic, including those sold under the brand names Plexiglass and Lucite. Certain plastics are better suited for wear in the body than others. Some are described as "FDA approved," though none are suggested for fresh piercings or new stretches. Acrylic threaded balls, acrylic-topped metal nostril screws, and other styles in which the acrylic does not pass through the tissue may be fine as initial jewelry. They may not be safe for everyone or suited to long-term wear, even in healed piercings. Most acrylic cannot withstand the pressure and high temperatures of an autoclave so it must be disinfected rather than sterilized.

  - Because acrylic is lightweight—about half the weight of glass—and inexpensive, it is commonly worn in enlarged piercings. It comes in a tremendous range of colors and also in clear and flesh tones, so concealment and retainer styles are frequently fashioned from acrylic. Watch out for glow-in-the-dark plastic jewelry: it is considered unsafe for wear in the body, and possibly carcinogenic. However, UV varieties that fluoresce under black light can be safe.

  - Most types of acrylic are quite fragile, especially when exposed to cold. Extended exposure to direct sunlight or heat can cause warping. Alcohol and other chemicals can crack, degrade, or even destroy this material. Use your hands or warm water to heat an acrylic captive ring before attempting to change its bead or it could snap due to brittleness. Acrylic can be scratched easily, so check the condition of your jewelry regularly, avoid the use of tools, and store it carefully. If you screw on an acrylic threaded end too tight, you can crack it or cause the threads to come out of it.

  - *PMMA* (polymethylmethacrylate) is a type of acrylic that has superior impact strength and is better suited for wear in the body than some other varieties; it is used for many medical and dental applications. Some body jewelry is referred to as *dental acrylic*, a hard, biocompatible form of the plastic. I've seen some of these products melt or warp at high temperatures even though they are supposed to be able to withstand autoclave sterilization.

  - *Silicone* is another type of plastic that is soft and flexible. It is used for ornaments that add onto, or take the place of, balls or beads, and is also worn in piercings, usually as eyelets. The softer the silicone, the stickier it will be, and this can be a source of irritation if it adheres to your tissue. Clean silicone jewelry regularly and carefully and keep it as dry as possible. A tight fit can trap secretions and cause irritation and infection. Your skin cannot breathe well with snug-fitting silicone occluding the tissue. Not everyone can tolerate this material in piercings.

- **Glass:** Though there are many varieties of glass, the two most popular types for wear in piercings are *borosilicate* and *soda-lime*. You know them as the materials used in laboratory glassware and kitchen cookware. These types of glass are safe, inert, and biocompatible when they are lead free. They are nonporous, stable, resistant to chemicals, and strong—but still potentially breakable. Glass doesn't get as cold as metal jewelry, and, unlike most of the alternative materials, it isn't harmed by the range of temperatures to which body jewelry is ordinarily exposed, including autoclaving. Glass is lighter than metal, transparent, and colorful. Countless color and design variations are possible. Some glass jewelry has harmful metals or objects such as insects inside; however, these are still safe to wear when a layer of glass encloses and protects you from the interior.

- Glass should be stored separately because it can be scratched by steel and certain other metals and materials. It is suitable for wear in ear and septum piercings but generally should not be worn in oral, genital, or nipple piercings, where there is a higher risk of breakage. With the exception of plug or eyelet styles, it is safest to avoid glass body jewelry in 8 gauge or smaller. It is advisable to remove glass jewelry when playing sports, sleeping, swimming, or showering.

- *Quartz glass* (or *fused quartz*) is a form of glass made from almost pure silica, which is quite biocompatible. On a molecular level, it is similar to natural quartz. Quartz glass is made only in clear, and it comes in thinner gauges than other types of glass. This variety is even stronger and more resistant to cracking than the types described above, though it still can break; be careful with small sizes. It is used for clear retainers, including those made for eyebrow and nostril piercings. Because glass nostril screws cannot be custom-fit like metal jewelry, finding a comfortable piece in this material can be difficult.

• **PVD (physical vapor deposition):** These high-tech films represent a modern version of electroplating. They are applied at an atomic level to coat the surface of other materials, including metals. PVD coatings are used in everything from firearms to the medical and dental fields. Jewelry with a PVD coating has a shiny, metallic-looking surface. It comes in colors that were previously unavailable in piercing jewelry, such as deep black, and shades corresponding to materials that are potentially harmful to wear in the body, like brass and copper. Gold-colored PVD jewelry can be a good alternative to unsafe colored gold, potentially dangerous gold-plated pieces, or pricey high-quality, high-karat jewelry. Some PVD coatings have been certified biocompatible by a lab that tests medical devices that contact bone, skin tissue, or blood.[4] Body jewelry featuring a black coating, called DLC (diamond-like carbon), goes by various trade names, including Blackline and BlackOut. Not all piercings respond equally well to these finishes, and product quality varies.

Advanced Piercings

To the uninitiated, all piercings may seem alike. However, certain piercings, including surface piercings, industrial projects, and orbitals, call for a piercer with a higher level of skill.

Surface Piercings

In recent years, the chest, back, wrist, and other nontraditional piercing sites have become more common areas for wearing body jewelry. As the name implies, *surface piercings* are situated on areas of the body where there is no fold or protrusion of tissue in which to place them. Stable areas subject to minimal movement and trauma are best. Most surface piercings are fraught with more healing problems than other piercing placements. Some last for months or longer before they migrate and reject; others stay in place for only a few weeks before being ousted by the body.

Seek a piercer who is skilled in surface piercings and check her qualifications carefully. If she can't show you photos of healed surface piercings she has done, don't stay. There is a huge difference between performing these piercings and placing them so they heal well and remain in the body long-term. Never have just a little pinch of your skin pierced or wear ordinary metal body jewelry in a surface placement. A piercer who does these things lacks the knowledge to perform these piercings correctly or doesn't care that your piercing won't heal.

Some people are predisposed to healing surface piercings. If you are not among the lucky few, then migration, rejection, and significant scarring are all probable consequences. If you can't live without attempting a surface piercing, be prepared for a lengthy healing period (usually six to nine months or longer) and the possibility you will be wearing a scar instead of jewelry by the end of it all.

When I perform surface piercings, I use Tygon, and I have had excellent results with it. However, when someone asks me to pierce an area of the body or a type of tissue that in my experience seldom heals successfully, I simply decline. I've seen only one surface placement that routinely heals easily and remains in place for a decade or longer: the *nape* (back of the neck).

Some piercers are having success with a broader range of placements by using *surface bars* (see "Surface Bars," page 73). Another method combines Tygon tubing with the staple shape of a surface bar by inserting a thin wire inside the lumen of the tube to shape it. Some of the work with surface bars seems promising, but there is no data available on long-term success rates.

You may have an ambitious vision of being covered in rows of multiple surface piercings, but it is wise to first try just one to determine your body's willingness to accept foreign objects in unorthodox locations. Also, if you are overloaded with too many piercings at once, it is probable that none of them will heal properly. If a qualified piercer counsels you against a piercing because she believes it would not be successful, heed her advice.

Industrial Piercings

The *industrial, industrial project,* or *scaffold piercing* is a single barbell that connects two or more piercings in the ear. The most popular configuration threads a long barbell through two piercings of the upper ear cartilage from close to the head to the outer edge of the ear. A variation passes from the tragus through the conch. Another style pierces vertically behind the ear through the upper and lower edges of the conch so that a long span of barbell post is visible from the front. Possibilities are limited only by your imagination, and more importantly, your anatomy.

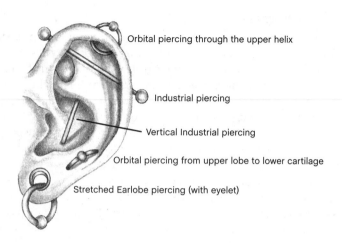

Orbital piercing through the upper helix

Industrial piercing

Vertical Industrial piercing

Orbital piercing from upper lobe to lower cartilage

Stretched Earlobe piercing (with eyelet)

Many people are not good candidates; they simply lack sufficient tissue where the piercings should be placed. You must have the ideal anatomy so the piercings can be angled without distorting or causing stress on the tissue. Alternatively, your piercer must have the proper equipment and know-how to custom-bend your barbell. Attempting to cheat tissue into the piercing is common but injurious. Along with the grief of troubled healing, an ear cartilage piercing that is under constant pressure will feel downright agonizing.

It is normal for any piercing to swell during initial healing. Even minor inflammation in one or both wounds, however, can be disastrous for an industrial because the piercings are connected. Excess scar tissue formation, migration, and rejection are common in poorly placed industrials.

I use a needle receiving tube or freehand support on the exit side of the piercings. I create the second hole while the back end of the needle is still in the initial piercing, directing me to the perfect, natural angle.

In the event you experience swelling or scarring during healing, you can attempt to preserve your piercings by replacing the single long bar with two individual pieces of jewelry such as short barbells. But, once released from their conjoined status, the piercings may heal at slightly different angles. Similarly, making two new cartilage piercings with separate jewelry and the plan to unite them later won't always work.

The subtle jewelry curves usually suited to industrial piercings are easier to create than the sharper bends of a surface bar. Some piercers are capable of safely modifying barbells in the studio, but they must use appropriate equipment. Bending jewelry, even just a little bit, must not produce any burrs or scratches in the metal. If nonsterile tools are used to customize a bar post, the jewelry must be sterilized before being inserted into your new piercings.

A *nasallang* is the only industrial piercing that is ordinarily performed on an area other than the ear. A single barbell is worn horizontally across the nose through piercings of both nostrils and the stiff cartilage of the septum. The nasallang can be difficult to access inside, especially when the placement is high on the nose, so extra diligence is needed for cleaning and maintenance.

Orbitals

Similar to the industrial, the orbital joins two piercings together, but it uses a ring instead of a barbell (see illustration, previous page). This style can connect two holes in the lobe, the upper cartilage, or other regions such as the cartilage of the tragus and antitragus. It is rarely used in other areas of the body. Unlike the industrial, it is often best to start the piercings with separate pieces of jewelry and insert one ring through them after healing; or, connect one piercing that is healed with one that is new. Depending on placement and ring size, it is sometimes possible to link two healed piercings.

One problem is the tendency for a ring to rest unevenly between the holes and constrict one or both piercings, which causes the same healing problems as any ill-fitting jewelry. To wear a captive ring, orbitals must be placed the correct distance apart to fit one of the standard diameters. Otherwise, a widened circular barbell or custom jewelry is needed. Earlobe tissue is forgiving, and an imperfect fit may be tolerated, but the same is not true for the cartilage.

Surface Anchor/Dermal Anchor/Microdermal

This relatively new technique with multiple names is becoming explosively popular. During the procedure, a tiny ornament is inserted into a single L-shaped opening that is formed in the tissue. The surface anchor is similar to surface piercing because it is done on flat areas, but placement options are greatly expanded all over the face, torso, and other locations of the body. Unlike the pairs always present in piercings, these have a single adornment per perforation. The embedded jewelry remains under the skin, while the visible threaded end can be changed. Multiple surface anchors are sometimes arranged in patterns.

The procedure is performed with a piercing needle or a small dermal punch (see page 240) to make an opening. The jewelry is placed into a small pocket that is formed with the needle, a taper or similar tool, or the jewelry itself. Though surface anchors may bleed more than the average surface piercing, they appear to be easier to heal and not as subject to complications.

The mini jewelry used in this procedure has a flat plate (only about ¼ inch long) that is inserted under the skin to affix it. The longer toe is placed in first, followed by the nublike heel that helps to hold the piece in the tissue. A short upright threaded post passes through the skin and extends to the surface where a gem, disc, or other threaded ornament screws onto the end of it. When inserted correctly, the jewelry appears to be glued onto the skin. Some of the plates are drilled with holes so the tissue grows into the base as it heals to secure the jewelry in place. Variations on the jewelry design are under investigation in the body art community. Healing time is reported to be one to three months.

Migration, rejection, scarring, and catching accidents, including traumatic removal, are risks, but the extent of scarring is apt to be limited due to the diminutive size of the wound. To remove it, the jewelry is firmly grasped, the tissue is held steady, and the ornament is forcibly taken from its pocket. If tissue has grown to the plate, a needle may be needed to free the piece. It appears they may be more likely to fall out than surface piercings, but they are less likely to grow out.

Single-point piercing (yet another name used for the process) is a relatively new and experimental modification, so there is no data on long-term successes or complications.

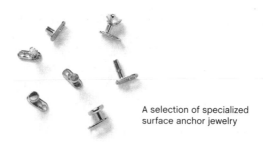

A selection of specialized
surface anchor jewelry

However, this apparently promising alternative may be superior to surface piercings. Surface anchors are more like ordinary piercings, much less invasive to insert, and certainly not as risky as most of the advanced body art forms described next.

Extreme Modifications

Within a body art studio you expect to find piercing or tattooing, but a number of techniques go further in modifying the body. Some of these processes are much more severe than ordinary body piercing. Modifications such as branding or cutting are more akin to tattooing than piercing and are not covered here; those that involve some type of ornament are discussed below.

The Dermal Punch

A *dermal punch* or *biopsy punch* (a medical tool designed for use in tissue biopsies) is sometimes used to create a piercing. The tool has a razor-sharp circular blade on a handle. Unlike a piercing needle, the punch does remove tissue during a procedure. When small punches (1.5 mm and 2 mm) are used by a pro, the risks of the punch are similar to those of an ordinary piercing. Larger holes are commonly created with them, however, and with increased sizes come greater risks.

Before you decide to have a piercer/puncher remove a substantial chunk of your tissue, you must feel confident that she is qualified. If she makes a mistake with the angle of a big punch, or if you abandon a large punch (over 6 or 4 gauge, or 4 or 5 mm), you may be left with a void people can see through, unless you get reconstructive surgery.

If the jewelry is removed during healing, there is some chance that your skin could grow over and seal the hole, depending on its size. The cartilage that is removed, however, is gone forever.

The process and the equipment may seem frightening, but most "punchees" report that a skillful procedure causes only a brief, intense sensation of pressure. I have not heard clients describe it as more painful than regular cartilage piercings. Perhaps the most disturbing element of being dermal punched is the sound. Since the action usually takes place on your ear, the c-r-r-runch of cartilage can be quite loud. The nostril and nasal septum are also sometimes punched with this tool.

I perform the punch using a firm surface on the exit side to support the tissue and receive the instrument. Even though the tool is razor sharp, it can take a fair amount of force to push through cartilage. Unlike a piercing needle, this instrument might be rotated as well as pushed to make the perforation. Even when your piercer uses

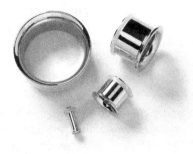

A selection of single-flare eyelets with clear silicone O-rings

illumination to map the position of visible vessels nearby and avoids them, heavy bleeding is to be expected from a large dermal punch. It could last for several days, so prepare by purchasing sterile gauze in advance.

If you are a dedicated body art enthusiast and you desire a cartilage piercing that is bigger than normal, you may find the dermal punch is a viable option. I do not use this tool for ear lobe piercings or other soft areas that are amenable to stretching. Piercings of the cartilage, however, are notoriously difficult to enlarge, and making a hole with a needle 10 gauge or larger can result in excessive damage to the dense tissue. From stretching my own conch piercing, I have painful personal knowledge (and professional experience) to support those assertions.

According to one school of thought, dermal punches are superior to needles for all ear cartilage piercings, and some piercers routinely use them instead of a needle. In certain regions of the United States, however, nonmedical personnel are forbidden to use a dermal punch.

For comfort and safety, initial jewelry must be lightweight and minimal (no large rings). A plug or single-flare eyelet that secures with one O-ring, and a tube that uses two O-rings, are popular jewelry styles. Dermal punches are sized by millimeter, but American body jewelry is generally measured by gauge or fractions of an inch, so there may not be an exact size match. When the jewelry is even slightly smaller than the punch, the hole is inadequately plugged, so extra bleeding is to be expected. There is also a higher risk of jewelry falling out if the flares or O-rings aren't large enough. But, unlike a piercing made with a needle, the dermal punch removes the hard cartilage, so the opening is looser. This makes it easy to slide in jewelry that is marginally larger than the punch without damaging the wound.

Before you leave the studio, your piercer should give you sufficient time to recover and be certain bleeding is under control. Both can take a little longer when you get a dermal punch rather than a regular piercing.

Punch-and-Taper Surface Piercing

The dermal punch is sometimes used in an alternative technique to create surface piercings. A surface bar is inserted into a prepared channel: each hole for the legs of the bar is made using a dermal punch, and the tissue in between is lifted with an insertion taper or an instrument called a *dermal elevator* (or *separator*) at the correct depth for the jewelry post. The theory is that there will be less pressure against the tissue because the piercing is made with angles that match the shape of the jewelry and suit the anatomy. Because a small punch is used, this technique is not as severe as other extreme modifications, including the next one.

Scalpelling

Scalpelling is the technique of using the familiar razor-sharp instrument for creating or enlarging a body piercing. As with the punch, nonmedical personnel are prohibited from using this tool in some regions of the United States and abroad. Piercings of the ear, body, and genitals are sometimes performed with a scalpel. The opening is generally stretched (or at least shaped) with a taper to make the incision round and facilitate jewelry insertion.

This procedure can be more extreme and make larger openings than dermal punching. The relative safety of this method is undocumented, but excessive bleeding is an obvious risk of scalpelled incisions, even in the hands of an expert. **This act should not be undertaken lightly; mishaps may require medical attention and could conceivably result in the loss of a body part such as a nipple or earlobe.**

When a needle or dermal punch is used, the size of the instrument automatically limits the dimensions of the aperture. However, during a scalpel procedure, your cutter/piercer must have the skill to use the blade to create an opening of the desired size in the correct spot. Enclosing the area being modified in forceps provides the protection of a solid perimeter to limit the extent of a cut.

Proponents explain that the scalpel method for enlarging existing piercings offers greater control than traditional stretching techniques. For example, a low original placement or a thinning spot at the bottom of an earlobe can be "fixed" by cutting upward, effecting a minor repositioning of the piercing. Another possibility includes merging adjacent ear piercings into a single larger hole by cutting the tissue that divides them.

Implants

Implants are similar to piercings because foreign objects are placed within the body, and because piercers and body modification artists perform them. There are, however, notable differences. In *subdermal implants* (as opposed to *transdermal implants*, described next) no portion of the object remains outside the body, as jewelry does in a piercing. The procedure is also different from body piercing: a hole or incision is made, usually with a scalpel, the tissue is lifted to form a pocket, and an object is placed in this cavity. The skin is then closed with sutures or medical tape. Sometimes several implants are inserted through a single incision. Generally they are made of silicone or Teflon, though metal is also implanted. Balls, hearts, stars, and other shapes are used. This is intended to create a textured, 3-D effect of the object(s) under the skin.

This procedure is surprisingly common, but beware: there are serious risks involved. After insertion, the implant is usually taped or bandaged to encourage it to heal in the desired position. But, similar to a piercing, an implant may migrate under the skin and heal crooked, after which it cannot be adjusted. To fix it, the implant must be removed and then, if desired, reinserted in another location or at another time. Rejection and loss sometimes occur with implants, much like they do with piercings. These complications are minor when compared to some of the other dangers.

One critical hazard is the potential for tissue damage in the area beneath the implant due to stress, friction, and diminished blood supply. Over time, the continuous pressure of an implant rubbing on bone or cartilage can cause *resorption* (erosion). This can ultimately result in total bone loss beneath an implant. Soft tissues may also be affected, as an implant can press into muscles, tendons, or nerves, resulting in pain and impairment or dysfunction of the affected structures. Implants made of softer materials such as cast silicone may help to slow this process, but damage is likely, and perhaps inevitable, over an extended period.[5] **In an area such as the skull, where horn implants are sometimes embedded, bone resorption can result in an implant wearing through the cranium.** This disturbing danger is not much publicized.

Infection is a serious risk because the wound is closed following the implantation. An infection cannot easily drain to the surface as it does with a piercing, so it could spread to deeper tissues more quickly. This has the potential to be very severe. **In the event infection is suspected, medical attention is required.**

Reversing an implant is also much more difficult than taking out a piercing because removal requires another incision. This often takes place at the site of the original cut, or a new opening will be made. If tissues encapsulate or adhere to the implant during healing, removing it can be considerably more challenging than inserting it. Even if a body artist puts in an implant, you may need to visit a doctor or surgeon to remove it.

Genital Beading and Genital Ribs

Genital beading is a form of implant in which round beads are placed within the genital tissue to add sensation. It is more popular with men, but it can be performed on women as well. This is done using the same procedure as a regular implant, or with the pierce-and-taper method. A large piercing is made with a needle, and then a taper is used to expand the hole. A bead is left in the channel, and sutures or surgical tape is used to close the wound. *Genital ribs* are a variation in which rod-shaped pieces are used for a different sensation and appearance. The pierce-and-taper method is the most common technique used for inserting genital ribs.

Transdermal Implants

Transdermal implants use a procedure similar to the one described for subdermal implants. However, an opening (apart from the incision, which is closed after insertion of the implant) is made to allow an ornament to screw together with the implant so it shows above the surface. Larger pieces are sometimes implanted, and multiple holes made to attach rows of spikes or other ornaments. These are subject to the dangers of resorption, like the subdermal implants, and are reported to have a long-term success rate as low as 20 percent.[6] Rejection is a possible complication; alternatively, the whole implant can become unintentionally embedded.

Pocketing

In pocketing, two adjacent cavities, or pockets, are formed in the tissue and a single ornament (often a simple rod) is placed with one end in each side. This is akin to a pair of externally connected half-piercings. These, too, have had poor long-term success rates.

Unproven Territory

Some experimental practitioners are testing the limits of the human body in an active effort to invent new techniques and modifications. Risks and failures are common consequences when you enter unproven territory or when radical procedures are performed by anyone other than a licensed medical professional. If you are considering a modification that is beyond the scope of ordinary body piercing, exercise extreme caution and use common sense. If the technician does not astonish you with her skill and experience and cannot demonstrate successful, fully healed examples of extreme forms, it is safest to walk away.

Alternative Practices

Some practices are related to piercing but are not traditionally performed within a piercing studio. They include play piercing, which is commonly done by laypersons rather than professional piercers, and different types of pulls and suspensions, for which a piercer with more knowledge is required.

Play Piercing

Play piercing is the insertion of a needle or needles temporarily for a ritual, performance, or BDSM or erotic scene; it frequently takes place between intimate partners. The piercing or piercings are made in the skin (usually surface-to-surface), but jewelry is not often inserted. When the session or event is over, nothing will remain in the skin, as it does in permanent body piercing. Play piercing routinely involves multiple needles (sometimes many of them), which may be as thin as acupuncture needles or as thick as those used in body piercing. The needles can be placed nearly anywhere on the body, including the face, arms, legs, torso, and genitals. Sterility and hygiene are imperative, as always, because the skin is broken. All types of people engage in play piercing, and they seldom have the sterilization equipment required in piercing studios. Therefore, disposable packaged products such as sterile hypodermic tips should be used and then discarded carefully. Of course, needles must *never* be reused or shared.

If you find yourself getting pierced because you enjoy the experience of it but don't care to heal piercings and wear jewelry, then play piercing may be a good alternative for you. It is possible to do this safely in the privacy of your home, but you must seek input and guidance from an experienced mentor before attempting it. A book on the subject, simply titled *Play Piercing*, can provide you with additional information.[7]

The Pull

Other types of temporary piercings require more knowledge and expertise. The *pull* (or *energy pull*) involves temporary piercings in which needles or hooks are inserted, usually in the chest or back, and two or more people tethered together by these piercings literally pull in opposite directions. This is not an all-out tug-of-war, but a cooperative, mutual experience. A solo pull is possible if the rope or cord is attached to an immovable object. Multiple people can engage in a pull when joined to a central point. Pulls are enacted using a wide variety of materials, from thin 18-gauge hypodermic needles lassoed with dental floss or suture material to large hooks. The individual(s) involved control the intensity and extent of the pull, and motivations can include seeking a physical rush or trance state, facing fears, or connecting people in body and/or spirit.

Suspension

Suspension is another form of temporary piercing that is practiced privately for ritual purposes or performed publicly, usually for entertainment. During a suspension, large, sterile hooks are temporarily inserted through the flesh of the back or other areas of the body, and special rigging is used to lift the individual so that he is fully or partially suspended from these hooks for a (usually brief) period of time. Specialized knowledge about the size, number, and placement of the hooks required, as well as about the mechanics of the rigging, is imperative for safety.

Do not attempt a pull or suspension on your own. If you want to undertake such experiences, you must seek qualified assistance. Clearly these activities are not for everyone, but those who have pulled or been suspended usually describe achieving profound effects: enhanced self-confidence, altered states of consciousness, and spiritual awakening among them.

The Point

From common ear piercings to advanced modification techniques and alternative activities, the world of body art is vast and varied. An amazing wealth of jewelry styles and materials is available to wear in body piercings. Depending on your desires and level of involvement, changing your jewelry for the first time can be as exciting as a getting a new dermal punch or trying out suspension. Each person is unique, so follow your own path, do it safely, and enjoy yourself along the way. Respect others who make choices different from yours, including the decision to be heavily pierced, or not to be pierced at all.

Special Situations

Various facets of your life are noticeably affected when you coexist with a piercing. I've worn a number of mine for over a quarter century, and we have endured some piercing-related ups and downs together. Dealing with daily activities can sometimes be a challenge for a pierced person. For instance, women have a unique set of considerations when it comes to piercings as they relate to pregnancy, childbirth, and breast-feeding. Whether you are wearing body jewelry while traveling or dealing with planned or emergency medical care, life is just a little more interesting with a few extra holes. This chapter addresses some common situations and concerns.

Fitness and Sports

If you are involved in athletics or physical fitness activities, evaluate the effect of your activity on your piercing. Participation in rough sports can be dangerous to a piercing, regardless of how long you have had it. Wear close-fitting jewelry that extends from your body as little as possible, or consider a flexible plastic retainer, which can be more forgiving if bumped or struck.

Make use of protective gear such as athletic cups or chest protectors to shield genital and nipple piercings during heavy contact sports. Note, however, that the gear itself can sometimes cause problems. Wearing a helmet for football, bicycling, or other activities can exert pressure on above-the-neck piercings. This mechanical stress increases the chances of irritation and migration, even when your piercing is well healed.

Certain physical activities and piercings just don't mix. Try all the different jewelry options and protection possibilities you can find. Ultimately, you still might decide that your piercing gets in the way of your game, or your sport gets in the way of your piercing. Regardless of deep dedication to both, you may need to make a decision about which to sacrifice.

Weight Loss or Gain

Most piercings are not at all affected by a modest weight gain or loss. Even a profound change will have a negligible impact, if any, on above-the-neck piercings. Piercings in or near areas that contain a lot of adipose tissue, such as the abdomen, breasts, and thighs, are more apt to experience effects from a substantial weight gain. A change in the size or shape of your chest or breasts can have cosmetic affects such as a shift in the angle of your nipple piercing, but this will not be harmful.

Adding inches to your waistline might cause a navel piercing to become irritated, even if it is well established. Genital piercings can be subject to additional pressure or friction from weight gain due to proximity to the inner thighs. Swapping out your jewelry for a different size or style often helps to alleviate these setbacks.

Medical and Dental Emergencies and Appointments

If you are in an accident or need to be rushed to the hospital in an emergency, it is possible that your body jewelry will be cut off along with your clothes. Ongoing efforts are being made to educate health-care professionals about the proper way to open common body jewelry designs, but paramedics and emergency room personnel will be more focused on handling your urgent situation than preserving your personal property, and rightly so. When your life is on the line, the loss of jewelry or a piercing is a minor consideration.

Circumstances are quite different, however, when you undergo scheduled medical or dental procedures or get treated for a non-life-threatening health problem. If you think it may be difficult to put jewelry back in once it is removed, take precautions to preserve your piercing. You might need to educate your care provider, but your time and effort will be well spent to avoid leaving a hole empty, risking shrinkage or closure.

Many health-care workers insist that you remove body jewelry for all procedures or tests, especially when the area in question is adjacent to a piercing. This is sometimes a reflection of ignorance or thoughtless adherence to policy rather than genuine medical necessity. Locating a piercing-friendly medical or dental care professional can sometimes prove challenging, but if you do find one, consider him a treasure. Your piercer may be able to supply recommendations for practitioners who are knowledgeable about piercing, or help you to educate your own.

Discuss your piercing with your doctor or dentist, preferably prior to scheduling an appointment in which the presence of your jewelry may be an issue. Inquire about the feasibility of wearing a nonmetallic replacement when you are asked to remove metal from your body. Obtain one before your appointment and arrange for an insertion if you will require help. If you cannot get a retainer in advance, a sterile floss threader (available in a dental office) or sterile tubing from a catheter needle (available in a hospital) can function as a retainer.

Studies have shown that removing piercing jewelry is generally not necessary for magnetic resonance imaging (MRI), X-rays, and many other procedures, unless the piercing is directly in the area of examination or treatment.[1] High-quality metal body jewelry is *non-ferromagnetic* (nonmagnetic), so it will not react to the MRI equipment. Beware, however, that cheap body jewelry may indeed be a dangerous problem when getting an MRI.

If you wear metal jewelry, it will be visible on the test results, of course, but this is only a problem when the ornament obscures the area of concern. Computed tomography (CAT or CT) scan images, however, do become blurred if metal is present, so all metal jewelry in the region of the examination does need to be removed for this type of analysis.

Dentists, orthodontists, periodontists, and hygienists are often particularly disapproving of tongue and other oral piercings. Sometimes they are downright hostile, and this can make dental procedures even more challenging for piercees than they usually are for most people. You may be subjected to poor treatment, lectures on the dangers of tongue piercings, or even the refusal of urgent procedures unless you remove your jewelry. There is justification for dentists to have a negative attitude: poorly fitted jewelry and excessive play do cause substantial damage to the teeth and oral structures. But there is never an excuse for a health-care professional to mistreat you.

Many dentists don't know about the important and effective measures that can be followed to diminish the risks of oral piercings. Explain to yours that you wear jewelry of the proper size and avoid playing with it to preserve your oral health. Once he knows that you care about your teeth and that you are educated about piercing safety, you may earn his respect. Show your dentist chapter 11 of this book or bring him a copy of the APP brochure "Oral Piercing Risks and Safety Measures."[2] Sharing the information will educate him, and he can pass along this newfound knowledge to his colleagues and other pierced patients who have not been provided with essential facts. Your health is the priority, always. Do your best at proactive planning, but never sacrifice medical or dental treatment to avoid a reprimand or the risk of losing a piercing.

Retainers

Most piercers offer a selection of retainers. Some are specific to a particular type of piercing, while others can be used in a variety of placements. These retainers can be worn to conceal piercings or keep them open when ordinary jewelry must be removed, such as for sports or medical care. The possibilities for safe and effective concealment of most piercings increase considerably after you have healed. You might merely want to downplay the visibility of a facial piercing for a friend's wedding, or you may require total invisibility for your job or a court date. Most above-the-neck piercings can be concealed using jewelry so tiny that it can barely be seen, or using clear or flesh-colored retainers or ends for barbells and labrets that blend in with the surrounding tissue. Replacing a threaded end may prove easier than changing out an entire piece of jewelry. For example, if you wear a labret stud, you can swap your ornamental end for a small concealment disc as needed.

Acrylic retainers are common. They may have a ball, dome, or disc on one end and an O-ring closure on the other. Unfortunately, the O-ring is fairly easy to dislodge, especially in oral piercings. The best of these retainers has a groove in the post to help hold the small O-ring in place, but it can still fall out or worse: the O-ring can become embedded in your tissue. This jewelry is made as thin as 16 gauge, but acrylic is fragile in small sizes. Bioplast in the same gauges is not breakable, but the lack of a secure closure is still a drawback.

Compared to such retainers, nonmetallic barbells of PTFE and Bioplast are superior because they stay in much more securely.

Another style of retainer is made of clear flexible monofilament nylon of the sort that is used for sutures. In one design, the ends are slightly bigger than the piercing and the piece must be forced through your tissue. This may be difficult to get in and out of a snug piercing, or it might easily fall out of one that is looser. The monofilament nostril screws and septum retainers provide excellent camouflage for these facial piercings.

The hook-shaped eyebrow retainer and any other design that is held in by gravity are apt to come out during sleep or physical activity.

DIY Retainers

You can create your own retainers for concealment or to avoid wearing metal jewelry. One camouflage method is to select the smallest or flattest body jewelry available for your piercing and coat the visible portion of it with nail polish that matches your skin tone. To minimize the smooth, shiny appearance, tap it with your finger while the lacquer is still a little tacky. Once dry, the piece can safely be worn. Examine your concealment coating regularly and maintain it by repeating the process as needed.

Another type is a custom-fit retainer that you can make yourself from Tygon or other clear, inert plastic. Some piercers sell suitable materials that are generally quite inexpensive. For thinner gauges, small, clear pieces of monofilament (like thick fishing line) may work. Use scissors to trim a piece to fit the length of your piercing and burn one end into a small knob with a lighter so the retainer doesn't slip through. Remove your jewelry and insert the plastic into the hole. These are very discreet, but they aren't useful for daily wear because this type of unsecured retainer is held in place almost solely by gravity and the tightness of your tissue; it can easily fall out when moved or bumped. Most nipple, navel, and ear cartilage piercings have snug channels and may keep in the retainer reasonably well, but earlobes are quite loose, so the piece may fall out.

Body Jewelry and CAT Scans
I once had a radiology tech who was as curious as I was to find out what would happen if we attempted to do my cranial CAT scan without removing the jewelry from my twenty-five above-the-neck piercings. The results resembled a modern art piece with lots of small geometric lines extending from every ring and bar in my head. It looked interesting, but it was not at all useful for an analysis or diagnosis of anything. I was convinced: I had to remove all of my oral and facial ornaments for this test, which was no quick or easy task—even for a trained professional.

Piercees in the military and others who are under close inspection can use this type of retainer trimmed just shy of the full length of a piercing. Once inserted, the plastic keeps the interior of the hole open, and the ends shrink down. This is as invisible as a retainer can get, but it should be worn only if your piercing is healed and you are familiar enough with it to be certain you can retrieve the plastic at will. To prevent embedding, this type of internal retainer should be used only for short periods of time on fully healed piercings.

A plastic piece that is a little longer than the piercing can be fastened with small, clear silicone O-rings. This will be somewhat more stable, but also more apparent.

It may take some experimentation to find the retainer that works best for you. Healed piercings can be disguised for many situations; but, if you must endure harsh scrutiny and piercing is absolutely not permitted, you will have to go without jewelry or a retainer.

Traveling with Piercings

Travel is taxing under any circumstances, but being away from home with piercings can present additional challenges. Eating exotic foods, riding in crowded buses, changing time zones, and having jet lag all add to the strain on your body. Even old piercings can flare up from differences in temperature, humidity, water quality, and the stress of being on the road. They may become red, irritated, or secrete fluid, even after a long dry spell. Don't panic; simply resume saline soaks and your cleaning routine. Your piercing will usually settle down when your body accommodates to a new location or you return to your familiar environment.

Anyone who has suffered from Montezuma's revenge knows that foreign fauna and flora can make traveling quite disagreeable, with or without piercings. Exposing your system to unfamiliar microorganisms can lead to illness or infection. It is a good idea to boost your immune system prior to and during a trip with extra vitamin C. Take precautions against infection and wash your hands frequently. If you are planning to visit a part of the world that might prove risky, bring along waterproof bandages to cover your piercing. Going on a desert safari, trekking across everglades, and surfing untried waters are perilous journeys when you have a new piercing. These and other travels can also aggravate a healed one.

Especially if you are still healing, be prepared to keep up your aftercare regimen during your trip by bringing supplies with you. Ready-to-use products such as saline spray or emu oil are especially convenient when you're camping or staying in environments that make it hard to bathe as usual. You might need to use bottled water for rinsing, depending on the quality of the local supply on tap. If you're advised not to drink the water or brush your teeth with it, that's a sure sign that you should also avoid getting it on an open wound, including a healing piercing.

Metal Detectors and Security

Many piercees are concerned that their piercing(s) will set off a metal detector in an airport or other venue. Precautions have intensified markedly since the events of September 11, especially in airports. Security personnel will react differently to the presence of piercings, and so will the metal detectors.

Many heavily pierced people will tell you in all honesty that they have traveled extensively without so much as a single beep. Other stories circulate regarding piercees enduring strip searches or being required to remove body jewelry before boarding a plane.

When your travel companions are unaware of your penchant for piercing, you may be concerned about an unplanned disclosure during the security screening. If revealing your piercings during travel is unacceptable, wear nonmetallic jewelry. Quality metal body jewelry is non-ferromagnetic and will not set off the large walk-through metal detectors. However, the hand-held wands are often more sensitive and frequently do sound an alarm when scanning directly over metal body jewelry.

This is precisely what happened to a woman who was required to remove a nipple ring with pliers in order to be permitted by Transportation Security Administration (TSA) agents to board her plane. This sparked a lawsuit and a change in policy by the TSA. As of March 2008, a passenger has the option to request a visual inspection in lieu of removing body jewelry.[3]

Depending on the location of your piercing, you may be examined in a private room by a security officer of your own gender. If you wish to take your trip, it is best to be calm and cooperative. Don't wear or carry long spike-style jewelry during travel, as these are sometimes construed as weapons and confiscated. Spikes aside, you should not be compelled to remove body jewelry, since it isn't a security threat.

Shaving

Shaving when you have piercings can be tricky. Here are some things to keep in mind:

- Hygiene is of paramount concern when shaving around a healing piercing. Rinse your razor well and change the blade frequently. Finish by washing the shaved area with soap and water to guard against infection. Store your razor carefully.

- Even if your piercing is fully healed, always rinse the area well after shaving. Hair particles can cause irritation and infection if they get into the channel.
- Although somewhat painful, plucking can get the last stubborn hairs that are closest to the jewelry and cannot be shaved off. Use clean tweezers.
- Waxing is an option only if you have a skilled technician to assist. To avoid pulling the jewelry or injuring the delicate tissue, a small margin should be left around a fresh piercing.
- Don't use cream depilatories near a healing piercing. These contain strong chemicals that can cause irritation.
- Depending on placement, it might be easier to remove jewelry during shaving once a piercing is healed.

Infant and Child Ear Piercing

The debate about piercing the ears of infants and children has two principal elements: the philosophical considerations, which include ideas about cultural identity and ownership of the body, and the practical aspects. As examples of different philosophies about body modification, Western parents readily subject their own children to bands of metal that painfully force their teeth into new positions, but they shudder to see youth of the Matsés tribe of the Amazon sporting sticks through their pierced lips. Similarly, many people think nothing of circumcising a male baby but condemn practices like *female genital cutting,* or *female circumcision,* in which the external genitalia of an underage girl is altered, or partially or entirely removed, for cultural or religious reasons.

Every society has its own customs, standards of beauty, and marks of identity; they are part of the glue that holds groups together. Parents naturally want to adhere to established norms and create their children in their own image. Piercing the ears of young girls is a fairly established practice in the Western world, and some piercers are amenable—but no ethical piercer would consider piercing any other part of a youngster.

I will perform piercings only on individuals who specifically consent to the act and agree to comply with maintenance procedures during healing. Obviously, this includes declining to pierce babies or toddlers who are too young to grasp the situation—and all animals, of course. I will pierce the earlobes of a child who is old enough to knowingly make the request for it. He or she must also comprehend the need to keep dirty fingers away during healing and promise to abide by my instructions, usually with a parent's help. Many of my colleagues share my standards, though some are more accommodating, and others even stricter.

If you decide to proceed with piercing the ears of your child who does not meet those common minimum requirements, one practical consideration is that you might find it difficult to locate a qualified piercer who is willing to do the job. You may be tempted to visit a jewelry kiosk or accessory store that uses an ear-piercing gun. Don't. Your best option may be to seek a sympathetic pediatrician or dermatologist who is trained in ear piercing.

If you are interested in having your child's ears pierced, consider the following practical matters.

- The risk of infection is high if your child is not old enough to refrain from touching the piercings, either because she is too young to understand the instructions or she does not yet have the self-discipline.

- A piercing positioned in the center of your baby's earlobes sometimes ends up being too low or close to her face when she's grown.

- Established earlobe piercings seldom close completely, and they do leave a permanent mark (however small) if abandoned later.

- Doctors blame the rise in nickel allergies on the popularity of ear piercings done with inferior-quality jewelry. Once they have developed, these allergies may be severe and lifelong. For more information, see "Dermatitis," page 212.

Menstruation

The menstrual cycle causes a complex set of physical changes in a woman's body that can affect piercings. During menstruation and just prior to its onset, breasts and genitals may swell and become tender. Even established piercings in these areas may have a flare-up during this time of the month. Therefore, if you are planning to get a nipple or genital piercing, it is generally best to schedule it shortly after your period ends so you will have some time to heal before your cycle starts again.

Your menstrual fluid will not adversely affect a healing genital piercing, but it is vital that your hands are clean before you touch the area to change sanitary products. Make sure that the string of a tampon is not looped around genital jewelry before you pull it. If you wear pads, change them often and soak your piercing in warm saline or rinse the area with clear water several times daily.

Piercing and Pregnancy

It is not appropriate to get a new piercing while you are pregnant.[4] Beyond the fact that no reputable piercer will perform a piercing if he knows you are expecting, your body is already occupied with a momentous and complex task: creating and nurturing your baby. Getting pierced during pregnancy also exposes your unborn child to unnecessary risks of infection (particularly because of changes to your immune system when you are pregnant), allergic reaction, bloodborne disease, and medication used to treat complications.

If you anticipate becoming pregnant in the next year or so, postpone getting a piercing with an extended healing time, especially the navel. Even if your navel piercing is almost healed, as your abdomen grows and the area changes, further healing of this area cannot take place. If you have a fresh or unhealed piercing, remove your jewelry once it is confirmed that you are expecting. Bolster your system to contend with your pregnancy instead of depleting it by trying to heal a piercing.

Established Piercings

Other than those of the navel, nipples, or genitals, most healed piercings do not experience particular problems as a result of pregnancy. However, any piercing can be affected by the powerful changes that take place in your body. Even old ear piercings can have flare-ups due to the normal hormone fluctuations that occur during pregnancy.

Genital Jewelry

Some women deliver babies with genital jewelry in place without experiencing adverse consequences. However, it is prudent to remove all metal jewelry from genital piercings prior to childbirth to avoid the possibility of tearing the piercing or causing trauma to the baby during birth. It is improbable that piercings of the hood (HCH, VCH, or triangle) could cause problems; labia piercings are more apt to get in the way. Talk to your doctor or midwife about their policy on piercings so that you can be prepared when delivery day arrives. If you intend to wear a genital piercing during childbirth, it should be small enough to avoid catching or interference, but large enough to accommodate engorgement and local swelling. Depending on hospital policy, you may be able to leave genital jewelry in place if a caesarean section is planned.

Navel Piercings and Pregnancy

If your navel piercing is healed and does not cause any problems, simply leave the jewelry in place. However, dramatic alterations to the size and shape of your navel are normal; your innie can become an outie. Once the tissue begins to stretch, many women experience discomfort, inflammation, and sometimes migration. Switching to flexible plastic jewelry usually resolves these problems. If the piercing still doesn't feel comfortable, you should abandon it until after delivery.

Nipple Piercing and Breastfeeding

Many pierced women express concerns about breastfeeding, but there does not appear to be any evidence that nipple piercings negatively affect the ability to breastfeed.[5] A normal female nipple has a multiplicity of up to twenty porelike milk ducts, rather than a single spout. Therefore, a nipple piercing of ordinary size and uneventful healing won't block them all. The ability to nurse could be impaired if a troubled nipple piercing causes excess scarring. When jewelry is removed from a well-healed nipple piercing, some colostrum or milk might seep or flow from the empty channel.

Leaving out your nipple jewelry during breastfeeding is safest for your infant, although some women do successfully nurse with it in place. Jewelry removal eliminates the most serious risk of your baby choking on a ball, ring, or bar that becomes unfastened. You also diminish the potential for other nursing problems such as difficulty latching on or damage to the soft tissue of your infant's mouth. Another concern is that body jewelry might be a source of bacteria that could enter a baby's system. Some women have had success nursing with flexible jewelry like PTFE barbells instead of metal. Do not wear a retainer that has an O-ring closure because it is not sufficiently secure to stay on during nursing.

If you decide to take out your jewelry and leave it out until you are done nursing, the piercing may shrink or close up by the time your baby is weaned. If your piercing is fully healed, there is some chance the hole could remain open. It may be possible to encourage a well-established channel to stay viable by passing a small, clean insertion taper through it on a regular basis. If the piercing has sealed shut and you wish to be repierced, it is best to wait at least three months after you stop nursing to allow the tissue to normalize.

The Point

Even if you don't plan to keep your piercing "through sickness and in health, for as long as you both shall live," coexisting with it can take some effort and patience. Body piercings are likely to have some good times, and bad ones—just like a marriage. It can be difficult to anticipate all the ways in which a piercing can impact you throughout the years. For better or worse, you are likely to be faced with the need to make decisions and perhaps even compromises due to the ongoing relationship between your piercing and your daily life.

Sex!

The act of piercing is exotic and primal, perhaps because penetrating the body with a needle is a metaphor for intercourse itself. While sexual enhancement is a primary impetus for certain piercings, it is not a universal motivation. The assumption that all piercees wear tongue, nipple, and genital piercings for erotic reasons is erroneous. On the other hand, piercings can be experienced as erotically charged even when they are located in areas that are not inherently erogenous. Piercees have described experiencing sensual pleasure from ear, navel, and neck surface piercings, and from improbable spots including the nasal septum and eyebrow. Virtually any piercing has the potential to arouse.

Can Piercings Enhance Your Sex Life?

> "My genital piercings have made my orgasms different, better, and more frequent. . . . I am more self-confident, I know more about my body now . . . and I like having the little surprises down there." J.

Piercings can improve your love life; however, they are not a panacea for problems, including unskilled or incompatible partners. Intimate piercings can also help—or hurt—the genital size match of a couple. If you and your spouse have a snug fit already, adding a genital piercing such as an ampallang may be not be helpful because it increases width at the head of the penis. However, if you have more ease between you, the added jewelry could be just the thing to make you more compatible, resulting in greater satisfaction for both parties.

Safer Sex

There is no set period for abstinence from sexual activities while genital piercings are healing. There are, however, two nonnegotiable rules:

1. **Be gentle.** Pay attention to your body. If your piercing feels sore, you must stop what you're doing, or at least ease up. As you begin to heal and the piercing feels less tender, you must still be vigilant to avoid injuring the fragile new cells.

2. **Be clean and hygienic.** Protective barriers *must* be used to prevent the sharing of bodily fluids. For oral sexual contact, use a *dental dam* (sheet of latex) to shield female genitalia and a flavored or unlubricated condom during fellatio. Thoroughly wash hands and sex toys before contact near a healing piercing, and use condoms for all intercourse and on insertables like dildos and bullet-type

vibrators. If other barriers aren't suitable, apply a waterproof dressing such as a Nexcare or Tegaderm before sexual activities to keep your partner's body fluids from getting on your piercing. All of these precautions are mandatory to prevent infection during the *entire initial healing period*, even if you and your partner are monogamous and healthy.

Appropriate body jewelry is smooth, so high-quality condoms that fit properly should perform well. Water-based lubricant helps reduce excess friction to protect the integrity of the latex. The sensitivity of your healing piercing can make up for the addition of an unfamiliar barrier. Pleasure Plus condoms are made with extra room that is suited to frenum and Prince Albert jewelry. Avoid condoms and lubricants with the spermicide nonoxynol-9 (N-9), as this harsh chemical may burn or sting and can harm the delicate cells of a fresh piercing (as well as vaginal or rectal tissue).[1]

Preventing Catching Accidents

There are some potential drawbacks to genital piercings: they can physically get in the way or cause damage from accidents or rough sex. During the healing period, this risk is virtually eliminated because you and your partner must always be gentle and use barrier protection. If you will not be using barriers after healing, wear body jewelry that is compatible with your significant other's to avoid catching during sexual activities. When one partner wears a circular barbell and the other a closed ring, there is a likelihood of mishaps. Consider adding a captive bead to close off the center gap of the circular barbell.

An accidental entanglement can result in disaster:

"My circular barbell got caught in my wife's captive bead ring that was in her VCH. . . . She pushed me back. I screamed, 'No!' but it was too late. In pushing me back, my PA ripped away her ring and took her entire clitoral hood, or at least a good 80 percent of it, with it. If you get caught, don't try to rip apart, and don't panic. Stop and work the problem [out]. Move easily and gently, and unhook yourself." B.

Piercings and Partners

If intimacy with a new sweetheart is imminent, it is probably a good idea to talk about your genital piercings or at least provide a hint before your clothes come off. In a way, being pierced can both attract and limit possible mates:

"I've been approached by women because of them. At the same time, I've been shunned by others. To me, it's balanced out . . . but at least I have a sense of contentment." R.

Piercings can be a source of conflict when you are involved with somebody who does not appreciate your taste in body modification. You may have to decide whether your piercings are a bigger priority than your relationship and who controls your body. Marriages have ended over such matters.

"My girlfriend left me when I got my first eyebrow piercings. . . . Now I have a girlfriend that loves my piercings and wants to get some with me!" F.

Overstimulation, Sensation, and Desensitization

There is often a period of localized hypersensitivity during the first few days or so following piercing. The overstimulated nerve endings calm as healing begins and the body grows accustomed to the constant stimulus of the jewelry, usually within the first week. For better or worse, genital piercings are not permanently stimulating. Regardless of piercing placement, there is no concern—nor hope—of becoming a continuous human orgasm machine. That said, increased pleasurable sensations are a common consequence when nipple or genital piercings are touched or fondled, whether new or healed. Some piercees experience spectacular enhancements, and a number of piercees also report having an improved libido, at least for a while.

When piercings are properly placed and handled according to accepted practice, there is no physiological basis for permanent damage to sensation from any of the common piercing placements. Piercings (including those of the nipples and genitals) are often rumored to result in eventual desensitization of the area. I've even been asked by an anxious, uninformed piercee, "Two years after my piercing is done, will I lose all feeling in my nipple like my friend told me I would?" Urban myths abound, but there is no empirical evidence that the continued presence of jewelry will diminish any of the sensation with which a person is naturally blessed.[2]

Women occasionally report diminished sensation in the localized area after genital piercing. This can usually be attributed to the typical spike in sensitivity following the piercing, and normalizing of sensation once it has settled and the wearer has become accustomed to it. Rather than a decrease in original sensation, this is usually a matter of getting used to a piercing that felt highly responsive when it was new. These are seldom concerns with male genital piercings because the nerve endings are distributed over a much larger area.

Just Once

I've performed thousands of genital piercings since the 1980s. In that time, I can recall only one case in which a woman complained of decreased sensitivity, about a year after getting a vertical hood piercing. She removed her jewelry, and everything soon returned to normal.

Which Piercings Are Best?

Innumerable variables in anatomy and motivation make that a question without a standard answer. Whether to appeal to your aesthetic sense, increase your own sensitivity, or stimulate your partner, there is a piercing to suit your preferences, and hopefully your build, too.

Specific placement and jewelry selection can affect function. For example, some women enjoy the added stimulation of a VCH, but you might be too hypersensitive. If you like the look of a clitoral hood piercing but don't want the jewelry to have direct clitoral contact, there might be a way to accomplish this. If your hood is long enough, a VCH can be more ornamental than stimulating when you have it placed a little lower and wear smaller jewelry. See chapter 13 for further details on a wide range of genital piercing options for both men and women.

Which Female Genital Piercing Is Best?

First you have to pose the important question: best for what?

- Fastest healing: VCH or inner labia
- Jewelry a partner feels during penetration: Outer labia or fourchette
- Highest visibility: Christina, high outer labia, or a high HCH
- Most clitoral stimulation: VCH, HCH, triangle, or clitoris, depending on anatomy

Which Male Genital Piercing Is Best?

- Fastest healing: Prince Albert
- Jewelry a partner feels during penetration, and potential G-spot stimulation: Ampallang, apadravya, or reverse Prince Albert
- Most clitoral stimulation: Pubic piercing (with a ring that has a large or textured bead)
- Highest visibility: Upper frenum, pubic, or scrotum piercing (side placement)
- Jewelry that is not inserted during penetration: Pubic, lorum, scrotum, or guiche
- For your own sensation and delight: Personal preferences vary, so try the piercing(s) to which you are attracted

Even sound can contribute to the effects:

"The jingling of the scrotals and frenums as I walk around turn her on as well, and the jingling that occurs during sex I think heightens her pleasure . . . kind of like 'copulation music.'" S.

Kissing and Oral Sex

In general, enjoyment of kissing relates to compatibility. If your lover is fond of wet, sloppy kisses but you favor a drier variety, it won't matter whether jewelry is present; your pleasure will fall short. Oral piercings can add an obvious focus to the act of kissing, but they aren't as intrusive as you might imagine.

Similarly, there are differences of opinion about receiving oral sex from someone wearing tongue or lip jewelry. Some men say nothing is better, yet others don't feel anything different. Multiple factors affect the experience including technique and enthusiasm of the giver; jewelry size, type, and placement; and the sensitivity of the receiver. When a woman is the receiver, jewelry seems to make more of an impact, but there is no unanimous accord as to whether it feels good or is "too much."

Male genital jewelry can cause challenges for performing fellatio. Be careful with large jewelry, as it can chip or crack teeth.

Infibulation

In prior eras, infibulation was used to enforce abstinence (see page 12); today, however, it is usually part of a BDSM relationship with a trusted partner. If you have a desire for infibulation, certain piercings and body jewelry can be used to prohibit physical stimulation, erections, or penetration. It may be hard for the uninitiated to understand that infibulation itself can be a form of erotic interaction through the consensual exchange of power and control.

Piercings must be well healed before attempting anything of this nature. The fine, malleable nature of genital tissue makes it difficult to achieve long-term chastity using piercings. Continuous pressure and heavy weight nearly always cause soreness or migration eventually. An ordinary padlock is sometimes used to connect the rings worn in multiple piercings but should never be worn through a piercing. Special body jewelry padlocks are made that can be placed through the tissue. Other devices and closures can be used to control the genitals via piercings.

For women: The inner labia are generally too stretchy for the job of preventing sexual access unless your piercings are placed at the base of the tissue, near the body, and tightly fastened. If you have elongated inner labia that are pierced near the edge, penetration may still be possible, even if you wear a single ring through both sides. Affixing multiple piercings on the upper portion of the outer labia may prevent clitoral stimulation (or, depending on jewelry, could augment it). Connecting outer labia piercings adjacent to the vaginal opening is effective for infibulation. Jewelry may need to be changed if tampons will be worn for monthly periods; otherwise, pads will need to be used.

For men: The most common infibulation techniques for men are to connect a pair of foreskin piercings, or to fasten a Prince Albert (or frenum) to guiche or scrotum jewelry. Piercings are sometimes used to affix cages or other chastity devices.

The Point

"Physically I pretty much look the same, but I definitely smile more when I look in the mirror. My confidence makes everything better, including the bedroom." C.

A piercing is sometimes what you make of it; if you want yours to be an aphrodisiac, then it can function as one. If you just like the way it looks, that's valid, too. Piercings can boost your self-esteem, inflame passions, and bring your sensuality into focus. Joining your lover for a visit to a studio to get intimate piercings may deepen your connection and even inspire new forms of love play. If you feel attracted to a genital piercing, go for it!

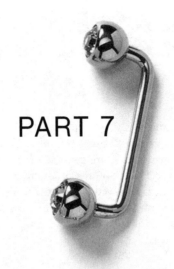

PART 7

Piercing in Modern Culture

Piercees and the Establishment

Most people who get piercings derive great personal enjoyment from them, but, unfortunately, body modification can cause problems when dealing with society at large. The authority figures in Western culture are generally not sympathetic to the practice of piercing. The devout cite sacred scriptures prohibiting body art; medical professionals see only the threat of disease; psychologists decry piercing as self-mutilation; and lawmakers view it as a problem to be regulated. Since the powers that be tend to regard piercing as deviant or disgusting, people with visible piercings sometimes experience discrimination and prejudice.

Doctor/Patient Hostility

At the most fundamental level, body piercings can seem *wrong* to doctors. They are trained to close wounds, not keep them open. Furthermore, many physicians still have no specific training in dealing with piercings. They often incorrectly assume that whatever is wrong with you is because of your piercing—even if you are confident that the healed nostril piercing you've had for eight years has nothing to do with your current headache.

Though body piercing has become pervasive in recent years, psychologists and mental health professionals still often associate it with pathologies like depression. Further, piercing uses instruments familiar to doctors, such as needles and forceps, so many in the health-care field find the procedure uncomfortably close to practicing medicine.

Medical professionals may have negative opinions about piercings because body modification generally comes to their attention only when complications arise. By reading this book, you almost certainly have more education about the subject than most medical personnel are afforded in their curricula.

Your Piercing or Your Job

People with visible piercings frequently run into problems with employers who have negative attitudes about pierced and tattooed individuals. Even those in jobs outside the white-collar realm, such as bartenders and exotic dancers, often find they are prohibited from wearing body jewelry at work. So, unless you are a body artist or among the self-employed, you will likely be limited in the piercings you can display at work.

A 2001 survey indicated that 58 percent of managers would be less inclined to offer a job to a pierced applicant, and not much seems to have changed since then: in a 2008 study, researchers found that even managers who had piercings and tattoos themselves were critical of applicants with body art.[1] This is not discrimination in the legal sense, because appearance is always a key component of getting and keeping a job.

Try to downplay visible piercings by wearing small jewelry or concealment pieces whenever possible. The basic rules always apply: punctuality, preparedness, and good grooming are vital.

Some mainstream businesses hire people with visible piercings. Ask modified friends for job leads and watch for pierced employees in action. Modified Mind (www.modifiedmind.com) and Tribalectic (www.tribalectic.com) post lists of piercing-friendly employers.

Health and safety issues sometimes impact piercings in the workplace. Those who wear earphones or other headsets can end up with irritated ear piercings. Cooks, landscapers, and those who work in dirty environments may find that their piercings simply do not fare well.

Dirty Business

I had a client who experienced endless problems trying to heal ear and facial piercings, though she assured me that she followed all aftercare instructions without fail. It finally came to light that she worked in a waste treatment plant and the environment was simply prohibitive to healing.

Dress Codes

Whether you attend school or go to work, you may have to contend with a dress code that prohibits piercings. Trying to combat this type of imposed conformity can be frustrating. One problem is that dress codes often contain ambiguous standards: jewelry must be "in good taste" or "not distracting."

If you run into trouble, determine whether there is a written policy, and if so, read it. If the guidelines are vague or do not specifically refer to piercing, or if there is no printed policy at all, you may be in a better position to negotiate. Some dress codes are changing in response to current trends. To her delight, a registered nurse discovered that her employer had loosened restrictions against body piercings:

"This means that I can finally get my nose repierced after all these years. . . . I'm glad to see that employers in health care are realizing that people with piercings are capable of being professional and hard workers. I've had many elderly patients and their families notice my tongue, and all they said is, 'I don't understand why you kids do that.' When asked if their opinion of me as a nurse changed, all have quickly replied no, they still think I am professional." E.

Pierced Professional

Joe Rohde, one of Disney's leading "Imagineers," wears a large conglomeration of earrings in his stretched earlobe, in defiance of the more restrictive dress code that is enforced for other employees at the company.

The Halls of Learning

Private and parochial educational institutions have almost unlimited power to formulate rules about the conduct of their students, including dress codes. Dealing with school authorities can be a challenge at the best of times, but if you are brazen enough to make an attempt at defying your school bureaucracy, it helps if you are well behaved and earning good grades. Arguably, wearing body piercings in school is not nearly as distracting to students as puberty, and no one can ban that—although parents have tried.

The Military

Despite a long history of tattooing among military personnel, the armed forces rigidly require conformity of appearance. In recent years all branches of the United States military service have banned body piercing, issuing edicts like U.S. Army Regulation 670-1, which asserts that personnel may not "attach, affix, or display jewelry through the skin while in uniform, in civilian clothes on duty, or in civilian clothes off duty."[2] Trying to fight against their strict standards is a losing proposition; if you can't obey the rules, don't join.

Piercing and the Law

Tattooing has a long history of regulation, but since piercing has more recently come into the public consciousness, legal systems have scrambled to catch up. Everyone agrees that laws establishing minimum standards for preventing the spread of disease are beneficial, but there are disagreements about the content and reach of proposed legislation. Consumers often assume that piercers have laws that they must follow, but this isn't always the case. Even states that heavily regulate tattooing do not always have legislation covering body piercing. To find out about laws that have been enacted in your area, ask a reputable piercer, use the Internet, or contact your local health authorities.[3]

Lawmakers often have very little knowledge about piercing. An extreme example of this lack of understanding was illustrated by the Georgia state legislature in March 2004. When someone mentioned the existence of female genital piercings to Republican state representative Bill Heath, his response was, "What? I've never seen such a thing. . . . I, uh, wouldn't approve of anyone doing it. I don't think that's an appropriate thing to be doing."[4] Rep. Heath immediately added a provision to an existing bill under consideration to ban all female genital piercing. The bill proposed a maximum punishment of twenty years in prison for performing a clitoral hood piercing. The bill passed in the state senate, but fortunately it later died in committee. If enacted, the law would have prohibited women—though not men—from getting genital piercings.

Some legal issues are matters of intense debate even among the body modification community. For instance, if sixteen-year-olds are treated as adults in mature tasks such as driving motor vehicles and consenting to sex (in many states), why can't they make independent decisions about getting a body piercing?

One of the Lucky Ones

"I often get questions, especially when I travel, as people try to find context for who I am, because in their professional lives they are not accustomed to seeing an adult male with a septum piercing, in addition to my eyebrow, earlobes, and other piercings. . . . In fact, I am a tenured full professor in health education and had my first piercing (ear lobe) twenty-five years ago. I'm in my eighteenth year in my current faculty position. My septum piercing—no, I do not remove it when I work—has been a part of who I am for more than a decade. Am I treated differently because I have piercings? Yes. Do I have colleagues who think my piercings are unprofessional? Yes. Why do I have piercings? Why not? . . . I am who I am and I have no desire to be like anyone else. I desire only to be the best and most unique me that I can be. That's what should be truly important in life. I am past president of a national professional association. I have published in scholarly journals in my field and fortunately continue to excel in my profession. I am sure that there are times when I am overlooked because of my appearance, my race, and/or my sexual orientation. Therefore, everyone, particularly a new professional or a student in secondary school or in college, should think very carefully before getting body art. There will be those who will treat us differently because of the decisions we have made to tattoo or pierce our bodies. However, if I were to do it over again, would I obtain body art? Yes!" —Reginald Fennell, PhD

Freedom's Just Another Word

Ultimately, as a pierced person, you must consider your priorities when interacting with society. You may have to sacrifice some of your piercings in order to feed yourself or your family; there is no disgrace in that. On the other hand, a young man who once dreamed of being a firefighter told me, "I wanted to be a firefighter for a while, but to be honest . . . I loved my mods more. Sometimes you've got to make a choice."

As Shannon Larratt of BME fame says:

"Looking like yourself will force you to work much, much harder than people who all look the same. Being free requires a lot more work than being a slave. Running your own business is more effort than working for someone else . . . but there are still people left in this world who believe that sometimes the difficult—but free—path is the more rewarding. . . . The fundamental question in becoming publicly modified is a question of finding a balance between how free you want to be and how hard you want to work."

22

A Career in Professional Piercing

Most piercers are regularly confronted with enthusiastic inquiries, such as "Piercing is awesome; how can I become a piercer?" and "Hey, will you teach me to pierce?"

Piercing seems like a totally cool career: you don't have to go to college for a degree, you can have your own personal style, including all the body modifications you want, and you get to be in a hip studio where it's probably more like a party than drudgery.

Unfortunately, if that's what you think, you have a rude awakening coming. Professional piercing *is* a real job—and it isn't about you; it's about your clients. A long period of training is followed by years of demanding work and the certainty that you won't become a millionaire. Unless a piercer is extremely talented, businesslike, and skilled in self-promotion, her line of work is likely to be close to a subsistence-level job.

To be a good piercer you need certain talents and abilities. It also takes extensive education, even though there are no courses in body piercing offered at your local university, community college, or vocational school. Obtaining training is difficult because there are limited opportunities for instruction.

Attributes

Perhaps surprisingly, a piercer's main concern isn't with jewelry and needles—it's with people. If you are considering becoming a piercer, first ask yourself if you have the personal qualities required in this service-oriented profession. Are you tolerant and able to interact closely with all types of people? Can you summon the patience and empathy necessary to deal with nervous clients? Do you have strong verbal skills to communicate effectively with them?

Piercing is a profession that also demands specific physical and practical attributes. A quality piercer must have natural artistic aptitude (to place piercings aesthetically), good vision, excellent eye-hand coordination, and manual dexterity. You must have the stamina to perform your last piercing of the day with the same energy and concentration as your first. If you get sick easily or have allergy-prone skin, think twice about choosing piercing as a profession. While few piercings are gory, if you faint at the sight of blood, this is obviously not a job for you.

Risks

When you pierce, you assume a real risk: a disease could be transmitted to you via a needlestick accident. To avoid the health hazards of working with needles, extensive training and consistent focus are indispensable, because hepatitis and other bloodborne pathogens are widespread. You also run the risk of developing illnesses or allergies from contact with harsh chemical disinfectants or latex gloves.

Formal Education

At a minimum, all piercers should undergo training in CPR and first aid and study bloodborne pathogens. Some regulations require a piercer to pass courses on all these subjects to receive a license. If you are seriously interested in pursuing a future in professional piercing, classes in biology, chemistry, anatomy, medical terminology and ethics, phlebotomy, and patient relations are recommended. These are available in nursing, emergency medical technician (EMT), and medical assistant programs at most community colleges, and some can be taken online.

Even if you never intend to manage or own your own studio, general business classes in accounting, computers, customer relations, marketing, and entrepreneurship can only be of benefit. If you are unable to locate a piercer willing to take you on, you will have some familiarity with alternate fields you may want to pursue instead.

Piercer Training

There is no recognized program for obtaining a certificate or diploma in body piercing, so don't be fooled into thinking you could get one, hang out your shingle, and start poking holes in people for a profit. There are a number of ways piercers learn.

Some receive all of their so-called "training" by watching how-to videos. This method provides a bare minimum of information and is not recommended. Videos are a poor substitute for hands-on training, and some of them contain techniques that are harmful or even criminally negligent. A beginner does not have the ability to distinguish piercing facts from fabrications. The best videos offer valid tips, but they should never be used as a sole form of piercing instruction. Some of these videos provide excellent training—for what *not* to do. I've actually used them for this purpose in the course of teaching my staff to pierce.

Other piercers learn using the "trial-and-error" method: they practice on friends and/or the paying public. Obviously, this is not recommended either.

Still other piercers attend a workshop or seminar to learn to pierce. These courses usually last a few days to a week, and the participants may do several piercings on friends, volunteers, or each other under the supervision of an instructor. The top programs provide an abundance of vital information about hygiene, sterilization, and cross-contamination control, as well as piercing techniques, appropriate jewelry, aftercare, and more. Depending on the quality of the program, this is preferable to no instruction at all, but even the best short course is not a substitute for comprehensive hands-on instruction under the guidance of a mentor. There is simply no way to impart thorough instruction in such a brief period. Even the most apt of pupils will still require additional one-on-one training to pierce skillfully, or her clients will suffer through considerable trials and errors.

So remember that a piercer who posts a handsome "Certificate of Training" on her wall may have received it in the mail with a video and "piercing kit," she may have had a week or so of solid instruction—or she may have taken a substandard class from someone who was out to make a fast buck.

Apprenticeships

An apprenticeship is an extended training period in a studio under a qualified mentor. In an ideal situation, an apprentice spends several months learning about body jewelry and acquiring counter-help skills. This interval allows the piercer to assess the apprentice's capabilities, trustworthiness, and work ethic. Later, the apprentice observes piercings, and eventually performs them under close supervision. In the best case the instructor will be a truly accomplished expert, and she will teach the apprentice everything she knows. One year of full-time training under a mentor is a reasonable minimum for most apprentices. Apprentices are frequently paid as employees, although they commonly receive a rather low hourly rate or salary. Most ethical piercers will not take you on as an apprentice unless they intend to keep you on staff. There is little point in devoting intensive time and energy to training you if you will leave to set up a competing studio or have to seek a job in a glutted market.

Some piercers take on trainees as cheap labor or to make extra income by requiring that apprentices pay for their training. These apprenticeships are seldom fruitful. Be very suspicious of any instructor who claims you can be taught body piercing in a brief period—especially if you must pay a substantial fee. You could find yourself in the same position as the piercers who pay thousands of dollars for a three-month program only to find that it was dangerously incomplete and unprofessional.

Openings for legitimate apprenticeships are rarely advertised because piercers can pick from a flock of hopefuls they already know. Networking and persistence are needed to land a position. Talk to piercers and develop a rapport with any you trust and admire. Have piercings done on yourself and make it clear to your piercer how interested and serious you are about piercing as a career. Consider volunteering your time to help out around the studio so you can get to know one another better; be persistent but not pesky.

Evaluating an Apprenticeship

There are no standardized criteria for specific apprenticeship terms or curricula, or for the credentials of a piercer who is eligible to teach. Unqualified mentors can only turn out inferior piercers, bringing down the overall level of competency. A top-notch instructor is crucial. Even a respected and experienced piercer is not necessarily blessed with the ability to impart her knowledge to others. Find out how long she has been piercing, how she learned, and if she has previous experience teaching others to pierce. Did she train any of the staff at the studio? Ask to speak with them or other former students, and check around to determine her reputation in the body art field and the community at large.

The terms of an apprenticeship can range from a casual agreement—"Yeah, come on over. I'll teach you"—to a formal contract. You may be asked to sign a confidentiality agreement, a noncompete clause, or other legal forms. Even if you are walking on air over landing an apprenticeship, don't sign anything you don't feel comfortable with or don't understand. If it is not written in plain language, consider having an attorney look it over. Even if you don't have a pact on paper, it's a good idea to work out specific terms before starting. Will you be paid, and, if so, how much? Does the instructor have a formal program in mind? What exactly will your duties include? How long is the anticipated duration of your training? When will you actually start to pierce? A comprehensive apprenticeship should provide instruction in anatomy, hygiene, sterilization, bloodborne pathogens, jewelry quality and selection, aftercare, troubleshooting, and customer service, as well as plenty of supervised hands-on instruction in piercing procedures.

Ethics in Apprenticeships

"A Piercee's Bill of Rights" (see page 273) addresses ethical considerations between piercers and clients, but what about those between a piercer and his apprentice?

A piercer should:

- Be honest with an apprentice about her own training and skill.
- Take on an apprentice only if she has sufficient knowledge, competency, and time—not for financial gain.
- Fully and clearly disclose the details of the apprenticeship.
- Instill a love of the craft and professionalism in the trainee.
- Instruct competently on all aspects of body piercing for a sufficient length of time.
- Encourage the apprentice to explore further education, especially health courses.
- Supervise all piercings until the apprentice is well qualified to perform solo.
- Welcome all questions and be patient with the trainee.

An apprentice should:

- Show respect to the piercer.
- Commit to the course and show good work habits; be responsible and on time.
- Keep the piercer informed of progress, questions, and problems.
- Disclose trainee status to prospective piercees.
- Perform all piercings under supervision according to the piercer's instructions.
- Be enthusiastic and committed to the profession of body piercing.

Continuing Education

Experienced industry leaders sometimes offer workshops or seminars. These can be a worthwhile way to supplement knowledge, particularly in technical or advanced topics. The Association of Professional Piercers offers a wide range of continuing education classes to piercers during an annual conference. It is a unique and inspiring educational event for beginning and experienced piercers. You need not be a member of the organization to attend classes.

The Point

Some of this industry's veterans learned by piercing themselves and their friends, but there were no other options when they began. Better opportunities should be available now. If you are serious about becoming a piercer, spend a few years getting pierced and studying related subjects. Make an honest evaluation of your own character and capabilities to decide if a career in professional piercing is right for you.

23

The Future of Body Piercing

Body piercing has undergone a truly explosive revolution in recent decades. After a long history among tribal peoples followed by years of obscurity at the fringes of Western society, body piercing has now achieved massive worldwide popularity in contemporary culture. Whether done as a reaction to the high-tech world, a display of peer bonding, or a statement of rebellion, modern body piercing has touched the lives of countless people. If you don't wear a piercing of your own, surely you know someone who does (even if you are unaware of it). Whatever the reason for getting a piercing, there is something special about body piercing and other forms of modification that stirs the human desire to adorn the body. This deep-seated drive is an important element that will help to sustain the popularity that body piercing has achieved.

While body art still is not considered entirely mainstream, virtually everyone is now aware of the concept. As recently as the 1980s, this was not the case. Time and repeated exposure have helped to lift piercing from the dark realm of subversive activities, and it continues to develop into a more "normal" activity. Ongoing familiarity leads to ever greater acceptance.

Growth of the Industry

In addition to the original groups who engaged in piercing, a number of other subcultures embrace the practice. Belly dancers, bikers, goths, Wiccans, skateboarders, and naturists/nudists often share piercing as a common interest. Piercing is not mandated by any of these groups, but it can strengthen connections between people who meet to share other mutual interests. In some cases, piercing functions as a formal or informal ritual or rite of passage. This can have great meaning for those who participate, and it may serve to deepen their bonds.

The Internet has also contributed enormously to the escalation of piercing. Millions of people around the world every day share information and photos and participate in blogs, forums, and chats on the Web. These virtual communities help to connect fervent piercing fans to each another and form an important backbone for piercing in today's world.

Openly pierced celebrities continue to inspire fads and fashions in piercing when they are shown in print and on TV flaunting their latest adornments. They continuously generate trends as fans emulate their favorite stars' piercings and styles of jewelry.

Stereotypes and Negative Perspectives

Even though piercing is widespread, negative stereotypes about visibly pierced people still persist. Unfortunately, we sometimes perpetuate disapproving perceptions ourselves. If we are to gain respect, all piercers and piercees must demonstrate to the people around us—families, neighbors, and strangers alike—that we are human like everybody else (though a bit more fancy and full of holes).

When you show off your body art, you become a liaison for the modified whether you want to or not. Try to be tolerant with strangers. It does require patience when you are asked, "Didn't that hurt?" for the thousandth time, but through your behavior, you can foster acceptance wherever you go.

When you are visibly adorned, it is unreasonable to expect that people will not look—or even gawk—at you, depending on the extent of your modifications. Handle the attention with tact and maturity; don't react with the "What are you looking at?" sneer. You know what inspires their stares. Instead of fulfilling their expectations with an angry, aggressive response, surprise them by being personable instead. Do your best to be informative and articulate. When you consistently behave in this manner, you will dispel negative attitudes toward piercees, one person at a time.

A Lifestyle Option: Here to Stay

One great advantage of our modern society is the remarkable array of acceptable ways to customize yourself and your life. Women can opt for careers over children, and men can be stay-at-home dads. You can live a BDSM, vegan, or rave lifestyle—or another alternative of your choice. You can hire a stylist to update your look or a doctor to alter your appearance. If having your fat surgically sucked out and injecting botulism toxin into your face have become standard practices for beautification, it is not a big stretch to understand how a ring or gem in a nose, eyebrow, or navel piercing could gain prevalence.

Body piercing has been a part of our world for millennia, and now that it has earned a place in the grand buffet of personal options, there is no taking it off the table. You have the opportunity to choose for yourself: to pierce or not to pierce. The decision is yours.

The Point

Years ago I read a brief passage written by Jim Ward about a "piercing urge," a passionate yearning for body piercing that cannot be sated by any other means. This book provides the necessary information to help you fulfill it as safely as possible—or perhaps to accept and respect piercing as a valid personal preference, even if you have never fallen under the spell that engulfs some of us. There are numerous variables to consider: piercers and studios, hygiene and sterile environment, piercing placements and techniques, jewelry styles and quality, and aftercare regimens. . . . The details seem endless. But now that you are knowledgeable, you can make educated choices and deal with your piercing in a conscientious way. You have an excellent chance of getting a piercing that heals well and gives you years (or a lifetime) of enjoyment.

Appendix A: A Piercee's Bill of Rights
(Association of Professional Piercers)

Every Person Being Pierced Has the Right:

1. To be pierced in a hygienic environment by a clean, conscientious, sober piercer wearing a fresh pair of disposable medical examination gloves.

2. To be pierced with a brand-new, completely sterilized, single-use needle that is immediately disposed of in a medical sharps container after use on one piercing.

3. To be touched only with freshly sterilized and appropriate implements, properly used and disposed of or resterilized (where appropriate) in an autoclave prior to use on anyone else.

4. To know that piercing guns are never appropriate, and are often dangerous when used on anything—including earlobes.

5. To the peace of mind that comes from knowing that their piercer knows and practices the very highest standards of sterilization and hygiene.

6. To a have a knowledgeable piercer evaluate and discuss appropriate piercings and jewelry for her/his individual anatomy and lifestyle.

7. To be fully informed of all risks and possible complications involved in his/her piercing choice before making any decisions.

8. To seek and receive a second opinion either from another piercer within the studio or from another studio.

9. To have initial piercings fitted with jewelry of appropriate size, material, design, and construction to best promote healing. Gold-plated, gold-filled, or sterling silver jewelry is never appropriate for any new or unhealed piercing.

10. To see pictures, to be given a tour of the piercing studio, and to have all questions fully and politely answered before making or following through on any decision.

11. To be fully informed about proper aftercare, both verbally and in writing, and to have continuing access to the piercer for assistance throughout the healing process.

12. To be treated with respect, sensitivity, and knowledge regardless of gender, sexual orientation, race, religion, ethnicity, ability, health status, or piercing choice.

13. To change her/his mind, halt the procedure, and leave at any point if the situation seems uncomfortable or improper.

Reprinted courtesy of the Association of Professional Piercers.

Appendix B: My Piercings and Jewelry Chart

	Date: _____	Date: _____	Date: _____	Date: _____
Piercing or Stretch				
Placement				
Jewelry Style				
Jewelry Material				
Jewelry Guage				
Jewelry Length or Diameter				
Ball Size				
Piercer/Studio				
Notes				

Appendix C: Gauge Conversion Chart

Brown & Sharpe Gauge	Inches	Decimal Inches	Millimeters (Rounded)	Millimeters
20	1/32	.032	.8	.81
18	5/127	.040	1.0	1.02
16	3/64	.051	1.2	1.29
14	1/16	.064	1.6	1.63
12	5/64	.081	2	2.05
10	3/32	.102	2.5	2.59
8	1/8	.128	3.2	3.26
6	5/52	.162	4	4.12
—	3/16	.178	—	4.76
4	13/64	.204	5	5.19
2	1/4	.258	6	6.54
0	5/16	.325	8	8.25
00	—	.365	9	9.27
—	3/8	.375	10	9.50
000	—	.410	—	10.41
—	7/16	.438	11	11.11
0000	1/2	.460	12	11.86
—	9/16	.563	14	14.29
—	5/8	.625	16	15.90
—	11/16	.688	18	17.46
—	3/4	.750	19	19.00
—	13/16	.813	20	20.64
—	7/8	.875	22	22.20
—	15/16	.938	24	23.81
—	1	1.000	25	25.40

16g
14g
12g
10g
8g
6g
4g
2g
0g
00g
7/16"
1/2"
9/16"
5/8"
11/16"
3/4"
13/16"

Appendix D: Minimum Healing Times Chart

ampallang: 6–9 months

apadravya: 6–9 months

bindi/vertical bridge: 4–6 months

Bridge/Erl: 4-6 months

Christina: 6–9 months

clitoral hood, horizontal (HCH): 6–8 weeks

clitoral hood, vertical (VCH): 4–8 weeks

clitoris: 4–8 weeks

dydoe: 3–4 months

ear cartilage/antitragus: 3–9 months

ear cartilage/conch: 3–9 months

ear cartilage/daith: 3–9 months

ear cartilage/ear head: 3–9 months

ear cartilage/helix: 3–9 months

ear cartilage/rook: 3–9 months

ear cartilage/snug: 3–9 months

ear cartilage/tragus: 3–9 months

earlobe: 4–8 weeks

eyebrow: 6–8 weeks

foreskin: 2–3 months

fourchette: 6–8 weeks

frenum: 3–4 months

guiche: 3–4 months

labia, inner: 4–8 weeks

labia, outer: 3–4months

labret: 6–8weeks

lingual frenulum: 4–8 weeks

lip, side: 6–8 weeks

lip, upper: 2–3 months

lorum: 3–4 months

navel: 6–9 months

nipple, female: 6–9 months

nipple, male: 3–4 months

nostril: 3–4 months

Prince Albert: 4–8 weeks

Princess Diana: 4–8 weeks

pubic: 3–4 months

reverse Prince Albert: 4–6 months

scrotum: 3–4 months

septum: 4–8 weeks

surface: 6–9 months

teardrop: 3–4 months

tongue/tongue tip: 4–8weeks

triangle: 3–4 months

Notes

Introduction

1. MICRA, Inc., condensed from *Webster's Revised Unabridged Dictionary*, "thrilling," Dictionary.com, http://dictionary.reference.com/browse/thrilling (accessed July 23, 2008).

Chapter 1

1. Beth Wilkinson, *Coping with the Dangers of Tattooing, Body Piercing, and Branding* (New York: Rosen Publishing Group, 1998), 77.

Chapter 2

1. Rufus C. Camphausen, *Return of the Tribal: A Celebration of Body Adornment* (Rochester, VT: Park Street Press, 1997), 42; and Wilkinson, *Coping with the Dangers*, 25.

2. Camphausen, *Return of the Tribal*, 6, 13.

3. Global Environment Facility, Biological Diversity, "Russian Federation: Conservation and Sustainable Use of Biodiversity in the Altai-Sayan Montain [sic] Eco-region (UNDP)," Russian Federation, Number 7, Project Document 14, www.gefweb.org/interior.aspx?id=16770&terms=russian+federation+document (accessed June 6, 2008).

4. George M. Gould and Walter L. Pyle, "Anomalies and Curiosities of Medicine: Being an encyclopedic collection of rare and extraordinary cases, and of the most striking instances of abnormality in all branches of medicine and surgery, derived from an exhaustive research of medical literature from its origin to the present day," 1896, The Power Exchange, www.tpe.com/~altarboy/not90726.htm (accessed May 16, 2007).

5. Jody P. Rubin, "Celsus's Decircumcision Operation: Medical and Historical Implications," *Urology* 16, no. 1 (1980): 121–24, The Circumcision Reference Library, www.cirp.org/library/restoration/rubin/ (accessed September 9, 2007).

6. A. Cornelius Celsus, *De Medicina (On Medicine)*, Book VII, Loeb Classical Library edition, Vol. III (1935), 425, http://penelope.uchicago.edu/Thayer/E/Roman/Texts/Celsus/7*.html (accessed September 4, 2007).

7. Donald E. Brown, James W. Edwards, and Ruth P. Moore, "The Penis Inserts of Southeast Asia: An Annotated Bibliography with an Overview and Comparative Perspectives," Occasional Paper No. 15 (Center for South and Southeast Asia Studies, University of California, Berkeley, 1988), 16.

8. Brown, Edwards, and Moore, "The Penis Inserts of Southeast Asia," 6, 13.

9. Blake Andrew Perlingieri, *A Brief History of the Evolution of Body Adornment in Western Culture: Ancient Origins and Today* (Eugene, OR: Tribalife Publications, 2003), 96.

10 "Discover Indonesia Online," http://indahnesia.com/indonesia/KALDEC/decoration.php (accessed September 13, 2008).

11. Joseph Campbell, *The Masks of God*, Vol. 1: *Primitive Mythology* (New York: Penguin Group, 1998), 254–55.

12. Brown, Edwards, and Moore, *"The Penis Inserts of Southeast Asia,"* 14.

13. Jon Reidel, "War of 1812 Dig Yields Surprises for UVM Archaeologists," *The View*, University of Vermont (June 24, 2005), www.uvm.edu/theview/article.php?id=1677 (accessed June 1, 2007).

14. Bernhardt J. Harwood, *The Golden Age of Erotica* (Los Angeles: Sherbourne Press, 1965), 305–6.

15. Perlingieri, *A Brief History of the Evolution of Body Adornment*, 19.

16. Luke Metcalfe, "Horace Ridler," NationMaster.com encyclopedia, www.nationmaster .com/encyclopedia/Horace-Ridler (accessed July 19, 2008).

17. Lois Bibbings and Peter Alldridge, "Sexual Expression, Body Alteration, and the Defence of Consent," *Journal of Law and Society* 20, no. 3 (Autumn 1993): 356–70.

18. Carol Caliendo, Myrna L. Armstrong, and Alden E. Roberts, "Self-Reported Characteristics of Women and Men with Intimate Body Piercings," *Journal of Advanced Nursing* 49, no. 5 (2005): 474–84.

Chapter 3

1. William E. Keene, Amy C. Markum, and Mansour Samadpour, "Outbreak of Pseudomonas aeruginosa Infections Caused by Commercial Piercing of Upper Ear Cartilage," *Journal of the American Medical Association* 291, no. 8 (February 2004): 981–85, http://pubs.ama-assn.org/media/2004j/0224.dtl (accessed July 17, 2007).

2. Janet Yagoda Shagam, "Body Piercing Safety," *University of New Mexico Health Sciences Center Health Smart* (Fall 2006), 1, http://hospitals.unm.edu/AboutUs/ Healthsmart/Fall06.pdf (accessed July 17, 2007).

3. Donna I. Meltzer, "Complications of Body Piercing," *American Family Physician* 72, no. 10 (November 2005), www.aafp.org/afp/20051115/2029.html (accessed July 19, 2007).

4. AIDS project of Southern Vermont, "Learn More about HIV: HIV Transmission," www.aidsprojectsouthernvermont.org/learn/transmission.html (accessed April 8, 2007).

5. Hepatitis Foundation International, "The ABC's of Hepatitis," www.hepfi.org/living /liv_abc.html (accessed April 23, 2007).

6. American Social Health Association, Hepatitis B (HBV) Questions and Answers, www.ashastd.org/learn/learn_hepatitisB.cfm (accessed April 28, 2007).

7. Junaid Hanif et al., "'High' Ear Piercing and the Rising Incidence of Perichondritis of the Pinna," *British Medical Journal* 322 (April 2001): 906–7, http://bmj.bmjjournals. com/cgi/content/full/322/7291/906 (accessed September 25, 2006).

8. Laurance Johnston, "Navel Piercing & Multiple Sclerosis or Chronic Disease?" Alternative and Innovative Therapies for Physical Disability, www.healingtherapies.info/navel_piercing.htm (accessed July 2, 2008).

9. Web MD, "Yeast Infection Overview," eMedicine Health: Practical Guide to Health, www.emedicinehealth.com/articles/16031-1.asp (accessed May 8, 2006).

Chapter 4

1. Dennis Watkins, "Painful Expectations," *Scientific American Mind* 290, no. 1 (January 2004), www.sciam.com/article.cfm?id=painful-expectations (accessed April 4, 2005).

2. Tetsuo Koyama et al., "The Subjective Experience of Pain: Where Expectations Become Reality," *Proceedings of the National Academy of Sciences of the United States of*

America 102, no. 36 (September 2005): 12950–55, www.pnas.org/content/102/ 36/12950.full (accessed July 19, 2008).

3. James G. Hamilton, "Needle Phobia: A Neglected Diagnosis," *Journal of Family Practice* 41, no. 2 (August 1995): 160; BNET Business Network, http://findarticles .com/p/articles/mi_m0689/is_n2_v41/ai_17276569 (accessed May 9, 2006).

Chapter 6

1. Debra Darvick, "Service with a Smile, and Plenty of Metal," *Newsweek*, July 2004, HighBeam Research, www.highbeam.com/doc/1G1-119028355.html (accessed July 20, 2008).

Chapter 7

1. Margot McCaffery and Alexandra Beebe, *Pain: Clinical Manual for Nursing Practice* (St. Louis, MO: CV Mosby–Year Book, 1989), Attachment C, Exercise 1: Slow Rhythmic Breathing for Relaxation.

Chapter 8

1. Johns Hopkins Medicine, "Glove Requirements for Clinical Procedures," *Infection Prevention Guidelines*, 2004 manual, table 4-2; 4-4, www.reproline.jhu.edu/ English/4morerh/4ip/IP_manual/04_Gloves.pdf (accessed December 12, 2006).

2. U.S. Department of Labor Occupational Safety & Health Administration Standard Interpretations, "December 8, 2005, 'Freehand' Piercing without the Use of Forceps or Other Engineering Controls Violates the Bloodborne Pathogens Standards," www.osha.gov/pls/oshaweb/owadisp.show_document?p_table=INTERPRETATIONS &p_id=25338 (accessed April 2, 2008).

3. Karen du Plessis, "Povidone-iodine," *Allergy Advisor*, http://allergyadvisor.com/ Educational/December03.htm (accessed August 8, 2007).

4. Dr. Raymond Mullins, "Seafood Allergy and Adverse Reactions to Seafood," Allergy Capital, www.allergycapital.com.au/Pages/seafood.html (accessed August 8, 2007).

Chapter 9

1. World Gold Council, "The Caratage (Karatage) System for Gold Jewellery," Utilise Gold, www.gold.org/jewellery/technology/caratage/index.html (accessed July 29, 2007).

2. Metal Arts Specialties, "FAQS: Goldplating Primer," www.artisanplating.com/faqs/ goldplatefaqs.html (accessed April 14, 2008).

Chapter 10

1. Mayo Clinic Staff, "Diseases and Conditions of Bones, Joints, and Muscles," MayoClinic.com Tools for Healthier Lives, www.mayoclinic.com/health/ avascular-necrosis/DS00650 (accessed August 10, 2007).

Chapter 11

1. Richard A. Smith et al., "Complications and Implications of Body Piercing in the Head and Neck," *Current Opinion in Otolaryngology & Head & Neck Surgery* 10, no. 3 (June 2002): 199–205.

2. Betsy Reynolds, "Points on Piercing: Oral Health and Home Care Considerations," Lecture presented at the American Dental Assistants Association's 80th annual conference, Anaheim, CA, July 2004.

3. International & American Association for Dental Research, "Lip Piercing Can Lead to Receding Gums," *Science Daily*, www.sciencedaily.com/releases/2005/03/050326010029.htm (accessed January 11, 2007).

Chapter 12

1. David Schlossberg. *Infections of Leisure* (Herndon, VA: ASM Press, 2004), 409.

2. Anne Greenblatt et al., "Piercing FAQ 2D: Body Piercings & Their Suggested Jewelry," rec.arts.bodyart, www.faqs.org/faqs/bodyart/piercing-faq/jewelry/partD/index.html (accessed January 14, 2007).

3. Trisha Macnair, "Protruding Tummy Button," BBC Health, www.bbc.co.uk/health/ask_the_doctor/bellybuttonprotruding.shtml (accessed January 14, 2007).

4. Excerpted from the ASPS/ASAPS (American Society of Plastic Surgeons/American Society for Aesthetic Plastic Surgery) Patient Education Brochures, American Society of Plastic Surgeons, "Tummy Tuck," www.plasticsurgery.org/patients_consumers/procedures/Abdominoplasty.cfm?CFID=80605952&C (accessed January 16, 2007).

5. Elizabeth Quinn, "Sports Injury Cheat Sheet: Quick Tips for Treating Sports Injuries," about.com, http://sportsmedicine.about.com/cs/injuryprevention/a/aa101402a.htm (accessed January 16, 2007).

6. Richard P. Schaedel, "The Karankawa of the Texas Gulf Coast," *Southwestern Journal of Anthropology* 5, no. 2 (Summer 1949): 117–37.

7. Kelly Shanahan, "Risks from Piercing Nipple," Your Total Health, http://yourtotalhealth.ivillage.com/risks-from-piercing-nipple.html (accessed January 14, 2007).

Chapter 13

1. Alyce Schultz, "Efficacy of Cranberry Juice and Ascorbic Acid in Acidifying the Urine in Multiple Sclerosis Subjects," *Journal of Community Health Nursing* 1, no. 3 (September 1984): 159–69.

2. Vaughn S. Millner et al., "First Glimpse of the Functional Benefits of Clitoral Hood Piercings," *American Journal of Obstetrics and Gynecology* 193, no. 3 (September 2005): 675–76.

3. Intellimed, "Female Reproductive System," Innerbody.com Human Anatomy Online, www.innerbody.com/image_repfov/repo20-new.html (accessed July 20, 2008).

4. Natalie Angier, *Woman: An Intimate Geography* (New York: Anchor Books, 1999), 63.

5. Fox Internet Services, "Clitoral & Labial Size," The-Clitoris.com, Dedicated to a Woman's Sexual Pleasure & Health, www.the-clitoris.com/n_html/c_size.htm (accessed August 22, 2007).

6. Mayo Clinic Staff, "Hypospadias," MayoClinic.com Tools for healthier lives, www.mayoclinic.com/health/hypospadias/DS00884 (accessed February 10, 2007).

7. The Gilgal Society, "A Glossary of Terms Related to Circumcision and the Genital Organs," www.circinfo.com/glossary/glossary.html (accessed August 25, 2007).

8. Editors, Deutsche Gesellschaft für Völkerkunde, "Die künstlichen Verunstaltungen des Körpers bei den Batta" (The Artificial Defacements of the Body in the Batta), *Zeitschrift für Ethnologie* 16 (1884): 217–25.

9. Brown, Edwards, and Moore, "The Penis Inserts of Southeast Asia," 4, 33.

10. Circumcision Information and Resource Pages, "Foreskin Restoration for Circumcised Men," www.cirp.org/pages/restore.html (accessed August 25, 2007).

Chapter 14

1. René A. Jackson and Crystal H. Kaczkoski, "Wound Care," *Gale Encyclopedia of Surgery* (2004), http://findarticles.com/p/articles/mi_gx5198/is_2004/ai_n19120083 (accessed August 26, 2007).

2. Tamara D. Fishman, "Phases of Wound Healing," Wound Care Information Network, http://medicaledu.com/phases.htm (accessed August 26, 2007).

3. *The American Heritage Medical Dictionary*, *The Free Dictionary*, http://medical-dictionary. thefreedictionary.com/Sebum (accessed September 19, 2007).

4. Steven D. Ehrlich, "Arnica (Arnica Montana)," University of Maryland Medical Center, www.umm.edu/altmed/articles/arnica-000222.htm (accessed August 9, 2007).

5. Alan Cann, "Bacterial Motility," Microbiology Video Library, www.microbiologybytes .com/video/motility.html (accessed September 19, 2007).

6. State Government of Victoria, "Handwashing—Why It's Important," Department of Human Services Better Health Channel, www.betterhealth.vic.gov.au/bhcv2/ bhcarticles.nsf/pages/Handwashing_why_it's_important?open (accessed September 13, 2007).

7. D. Gould, "TheSignificance of Hand-Drying in the Prevention of Infection," *Nursing Times* 90, no. 47 (November 1994): 33–35, www.ncbi.nlm.nih.gov/sites/entrez?cmd =Retrieve&db=PubMed&list_uids=7800517&dopt=AbstractPlus (accessed August 9, 2007).

8. Ohio State University, "Stress Slows Healing of Dental Wounds by 40 Percent," *ScienceDaily* (June 1998), www.sciencedaily.com/releases/1998/06/980622060800 .htm (accessed September 21, 2007); BBC News, "Stress Slows Healing," April 2000, http://news.bbc.co.uk/2/hi/health/711896.stm (accessed September 21, 2007).

9. Eberhard J. Wormer, "A Taste for Salt in the History of Medicine," *Science Tribune* (March 1999), www.pdwconcepts.com/userfiles/file/CaseStudy.pdf (accessed September 14, 2007).

10. René A. Jackson and Crystal H. Kaczkoski, "Wound Care," *Encyclopedia of Surgery: A Guide for Patients and Caregivers,* www.surgeryencyclopedia.com/St-Wr/ Wound-Care.html (accessed November 11, 2006).

11. Wormer, "A Taste for Salt in the History of Medicine."

12. Pamela A. Brown and Julie Phelps Maloy, *Quick Reference to Wound Care,* Second Edition (Sudbury, MA: Jones and Bartlett Publishers, 2005), 33–39.

13. Jim Swenson, "Skin and Soap pH," Ask a Scientist: General Science Archive www .newton.dep.anl.gov/askasci/gen01/gen01715.htm (accessed November 11, 2006).

14. Aviva Glaser, "The Ubiquitous Triclosan: A Common Antibacterial Agent Exposed," *Pesticides and You* 24, no. 3 (2004): 12–17, www.beyondpesticides.org/pesticides/ factsheets/Triclosan%20cited.pdf (accessed March 14, 2008).

15. Mayo Clinic Staff, "Hand Washing: An Easy Way to Prevent Infection," www .mayoclinic.com/health/hand-washing/HQ00407 (accessed September 25, 2007).

16. Kirsten M. Buck, "Cleaning and Disinfection: The Effects of Germicides on Microorganisms," *Infection Control Today Magazine* (September 2001), www.infectioncontroltoday.com/articles/191clean.html (accessed September 25, 2007).

17. Robert G. Smith, "Wound Care Product Selection," *US Pharmacist*, April 2003, www.uspharmacist.com/index.asp?page=ce/2716/default.htm (accessed July 21, 2008).

18. Bayer HealthCare, "Bactine: Soothing Infection Protection FAQ," www.bactine.com/bactinefaq.htm#usage (accessed November 3, 2007).

19. University Health Services, "Body Piercing: Cleaning and Healing," University of California, Berkeley, Tang Center, www.uhs.berkeley.edu/home/healthtopics/bodypiercing.shtml (accessed September 25, 2007).

20. Buck, "Cleaning and Disinfection."

21. David J. Weber, William A. Rutala, and Emily E. Sickbert-Bennett, "Outbreaks Associated with Contaminated Antiseptics and Disinfectants," *Antimicrobial Agents and Chemotherapy* 51, no. 12 (December 2007): 4217–24; published online October 2007, American Society for Microbiology.

22. Food and Drug Administration, "FDA Issues Final Rule on OTC Drug Products Containing Colloidal Silver," U.S. Department of Health and Human Services, www.fda.gov/bbs/topics/ANSWERS/ANS00971.html (accessed November 3, 2007).

23. Charles P. Gerba, Craig Walis, and Joseph L. Melnick, "Microbiological Hazards of Household Toilets: Droplet Production and the Fate of Residual Organism," *Applied Microbiology* 30, no. 2 (August 1975): 229–37, http://aem.asm.org/cgi/content/abstract/30/2/229 (accessed November 4, 2007).

24. Drugsite Trust, "Emu Oil," Drug Information Online, www.drugs.com/npp/emu-oil.html (accessed October 15, 2007).

25. M. W. Whitehouse et al., "Emu Oil(s): A Source of Non-Toxic Anti-Inflammatory Agents in Aboriginal Medicine," *Inflammopharmacology* 6, no. 1 (March 1998): 1–8, www.springerlink.com/content/38301157u2145526/ (accessed April 9, 2007).

26. Serena DuBois, "Emu Oil: The Undiscovered Secret," *Explore* 8, no. 1 (1997), www.explorepub.com/articles/emu.html (accessed November 4, 2007).

27. Ibid.

Chapter 15

1. Suzanne Morrison, "Inspiring Innovation and Discovery, Study Looks to Find If Soap Best for Cleaning Wounds," McMaster University, www-fhs.mcmaster.ca/main/news/news_2007/soap_wounds.html (accessed November 8, 2007).

2. University of Bonn, "Honey Helps Problem Wounds," *Science Daily* (July 2006), www.sciencedaily.com/releases/2006/07/060727090308.htm (accessed April 9, 2007).

3. Suzie Calne, ed., "Honey as a Topical Antibacterial Agent for Treatment of Infected Wounds," www.worldwidewounds.com/2001/november/Molan/honey-as-topical-agent.html (accessed November 11, 2006).

4. Brown and Maloy, *Quick Reference to Wound Care*, Second Edition, 210.

5. W. Steven Pray, "Caring for Minor Wounds," *US Pharmacist* 31, no. 4 (2006): 16–26, www.uspharmacist.com/index.asp?show=article&page=8_1717.htm (accessed November 12, 2006); Carrie Sussman and Barbara M. Bates-Jensen, *Wound Care: A*

Collaborative Practice Manual (Philadelphia: Lippincott Williams & Wilkins/Wolters Kluwer Health Publishers, 2007), 116.

6. Linda Watts, "Wound Care: It's Not Just Skin Deep," www.diabeteshealth.com/read/1997/11/01/1012.html (accessed October 20, 2007).

7. Brown and Maloy, *Quick Reference to Wound Care*, Second Edition, 33.

Chapter 16

1. Becky Ham, "Pre-Surgery Stress Linked to Signs of Slow Wound Healing," Center for the Advancement of Health, www.hbns.org/news/healing10-23-03.cfm (accessed November 12, 2006).

2. Stephen C. Ross, "Complications of Body Piercing," UCLA Department of Medicine, www.med.ucla.edu/modules/wfsection/article.php?articleid=158 (accessed October 20, 2007).

3 National Education Association, "'Body Art'—A Dangerous Fad," NEA Education Support Professionals, www.nea.org/esphome/jobs/healqual-6.html (accessed December 21, 2006).

4. Myrna L. Armstrong, "Caring for the Patient with Piercings," *RN Magazine* 67, no. 46 (June 2004), http://rn.modernmedicine.com/rnweb/article/articleDetail.jsp?id=110128 (accessed December 21, 2006).

5. Shannon Larratt, "The Alleged Piercing-Related Death of a Teen in Canada," BMEzine.com Press Release, www.bmezine.com/news/pubring/20060313.html (accessed April 16, 2007).

6. Janet Yagoda Shagam, "Body Piercing Safety," *University of New Mexico Health Sciences Center Health Smart,* Fall 2006, 1–4, http://hospitals.unm.edu/AboutUs/Healthsmart/Fall06.pdf (accessed April 20, 2007).

7. Barbara Floria, "Self-Treat? Or See a Doctor?" Wyoming Valley Health Care System, Staywell for Life, www.wvhc.staywellsolutionsonline.com/RelatedItems/1,2971 (accessed April 16, 2007).

8. W. Steven Pray, *Non-Prescription Product Therapeutics* (Philadelphia: Lippincott Williams & Wilkins/Wolters Kluwer Health Publishers, 2007), 530–34.

9. Donna Meltzer, "Complications of Body Piercing," *American Family Physician* 72, no. 10 (November 2005): 2029–34, www.aafp.org/afp/20051115/2029.html (accessed December 21, 2006).

10. V. Jacobs et al., "Mastitis Nonpuerperalis after Nipple Piercing: Time to Act," International Journal of Fertility and Women's Medicine 48, no. 5 (September/October 2003): 226–31, www.medscape.com/medline/abstract/14626379?src=emed_ckb_ref_o (accessed December 22, 2006).

11. Annals of Emergency Medicine Press Releases, "Antibiotics Not Necessary to Treat Most Abscesses, Even in the Presence of MRSA," American College of Emergency Physicians, www.acep.org/pressroom.aspx?id=25880 (accessed September 25, 2007).

12. American Osteopathic College of Dermatology, "Pyogenic Granuloma," Dermatologic Disease Database, www.aocd.org/skin/dermatologic_diseases/pyogenic_granuloma.html (accessed October 22, 2007).

13. Natalie Semchyshyn et al., "Surgical Complications," emedicine WebMD, www.emedicine.com/derm/topic829.htm (accessed July 21, 2008).

14. Sussman and Bates-Jensen, *Wound Care: A Collaborative Practice Manual,* 263.

15. Nancy Tcakz Browne et al., *Nursing Care of the Pediatric Surgical Patient* (Sudbury, MA: Jones and Bartlett, 2006), 93.

16. Maureen Haggerty, "Folliculitis," www.healthatoz.com/healthatoz/Atoz/ency/folliculitis.jsp (accessed December 21, 2006); Maria G. Essig, "Folliculitis-Symptoms," http://health.yahoo.com/topic/skinconditions/symptoms/article/healthwise/hw171649 (accessed July 22, 2008).

17. WebMD, "Follicular Cyst of the Ovary," MedicineNet, www.medterms.com/script/main/art.asp?articlekey=8442 (accessed July 22, 2008).

18. Mayo Clinic Staff, "Folliculitis," MayoClinic.com Tools for Healthier Lives, www.mayoclinic.com/health/folliculitis/DS00512/DSECTION=tests%2Dand%2Ddiagnosis (accessed October 10, 2007).

19. *Encyclopedia Britannica*, "Scar," www.britannica.com/EBchecked/topic/526644/scar (accessed July 22, 2008).

20. Stephen C. Acosta, "Campho-Phenique Overdose," University of Maryland Medical Center, www.umm.edu/ency/article/002606.htm (accessed October 15, 2007).

21. Mayo Clinic Staff, "Nickel Allergy," MayoClinic.com Tools for Healthier Lives, www.mayoclinic.com/health/nickel-allergy/DS00826 (accessed October 10, 2007).

22. Harold S. Nelson, "Contact Dermatitis," Asthma and Allergy Foundation of America, www.aafa.org/display.cfm?id=9&sub=23&cont=329 (accessed June 10, 2007).

23. American Osteopathic College of Dermatology (A.O.C.D.), "Nickel Allergy," www.aocd.org/skin/dermatologic_diseases/nickel_allergy.html (accessed October 15, 2007).

24. Lea Dow, "The Problem-Nickel Allergy, The Solution-Nickel Solution," www.nickelallergyinformation.com (accessed September 16, 2008).

25. Robert F. Diegelmann and Melissa C. Evans, "Wound Healing: An Overview of Acute, Fibrotic, and Delayed Healing," *Frontiers in Bioscience* 9 (January 2004): 283–89.

26. Scott DeBoer and Troy Amundson, "Tongues, Tubes, and Teens: Body Piercing and Airway Management," *Pediatric Emergency Care* 22, no. 10 (October 2006): 755–58.

Chapter 18

1. Erica Skadsen, "Care Instructions and Material Information," Organic Natural Body Jewelry, www.organicjewelry.com/generalinfo.html (accessed May 9, 2007).

2. R. V. Dietrich, "Horn," Central Michigan University College of Science and Technology, www.cst.cmich.edu/users/dietrirv/zoogems/horn.html (accessed May 9, 2007).

3. R. V. Dietrich, "Ivory," Central Michigan University College of Science and Technology, www.cst.cmich.edu/users/dietrirv/zoogems/ivory.html (accessed May 9, 2007).

4. Mark Pellman, "PVD Coatings for Medical Device Applications (Physical Vapor Deposition)," www.allbusiness.com/manufacturing/miscellaneous-manufacturing/589508-1.html (accessed May 9, 2007).

5. BMEzine, "Tissue Resorption," BMEzine.com Encyclopedia, http://wiki.bmezine.com/index.php/Tissue_Resorption (accessed June 22, 2007).

6. BMEzine, "Transdermal Implant," BMEzine.com Encyclopedia, http://wiki.bmezine .com/index.php/Transdermal_implant (accessed June 22, 2007).

7. Deborah Addington, *Play Piercing* (Emeryville, CA: Greenery Press, 2006).

Chapter 19

1. Scott DeBoer et al., "Body Piercing/Tattooing and Trauma Diagnostic Imaging: Medical Myths vs. Realities," *Journal of Trauma Nursing* 14, no. 1 (January–March 2007): 35–38.

2. Association of Professional Piercers, "Oral Piercing Risks & Safety Measures," www .safepiercing.org (accessed June 22, 2007).

3. Transportation Security Administration, "Statement on Alleged Improper Screening at Lubbock, Texas, March 28, 2008," www.tsa.gov/press/happenings/lubbock.shtm (accessed May 8, 2008).

4. Julie Snyder, "Piercings and Tattoos during Pregnancy," www.pregnancy.org/article .php?sid=1861 (accessed June 22, 2007).

5. Jahaan Martin, "Nipple Piercing: Is It Compatible with Breastfeeding?" LEAVEN 35, no. 3 (June–July 1999): 64–65, www.lalecheleague.org/llleaderweb/LV/ LVJunJul99p64.html (accessed July 22, 2008).

Chapter 20

1. U.S. Food and Drug Administration, FDA News, "FDA Mandates New Warning for Nonoxynol 9 OTC Contraceptive Products," December 2007, www.fda.gov/bbs/ topics/NEWS/2007/NEW01758.html (accessed April 16, 2008).

2. Health Services at Columbia University, "Pierced Clit," Go Ask Alice! (questions and answers), www.goaskalice.columbia.edu/0540.html (accessed June 22, 2007).

Chapter 21

1. Kristina Cooke, "Tattoos Still Taboo at Work," www.mindfood.com/at-tattoos-piercings-not-accepted-work.seo (accessed July 22, 2008).

2. Department of the Army, "Wear and Appearance of Army Uniforms and Insignia, Army Regulation 670-1," February 2005, www.usapa.army.mil/pdffiles/r670_1.pdf (accessed June 23, 2007).

3. The National Conference of State Legislature, "Tattoos and Body Piercings for Minors, State Laws on Tattooing and Body Piercing," www.ncsl.org/programs/ health/minorbodyart.htm (accessed June 23, 2007).

4. Associated Press, "Georgia House Bans Genital Piercings For Women," *San Francisco Chronicle,* March 25, 2004, www.sfgate.com/cgi-bin/article.cgi?file=/gate/ archive/2004/03/25/genitalpierce.DTL (accessed January 6, 2007).

Glossary

A

abdominoplasty: cosmetic surgery of the abdomen; also called a tummy tuck

abscess: pus-filled pocket of infection trapped under the skin

acrylic: general term for many varieties of plastic, including those sold under the brand names Plexiglass and Lucite

adipose: containing fat; found in the tissue just below the epidermis and dermis

aerosolize: to become airborne in microscopic particles

aesthetics: physical appearance, especially when considered pleasing

aftercare: wound care; the treatment given healing piercings

alar cartilage: cartilage on the sides of the nose that is pierced in a nostril piercing

allicin: onion or garlic extract, used in scar reduction products

alloy: a mixture of metals and elements combined to create different properties than the materials have individually

American ampallang: horizontal glans penis piercing that does not pass through the urethra

American Society for Testing and Materials Standard (ASTM): now ASTM International; organization that provides technical standards for materials, products, and systems

American Wire Gauge (AWG): standard of measurement for wire gauges used for sizing American body jewelry and piercing needles; also called Brown & Sharpe

ampallang: male genital piercing that passes horizontally through the head of the penis; *See also* American ampallang and European ampallang

anatomy: physical structure; one of the factors in piercing placement

anchor: *See* surface anchor

anchoring: term for procedure to insert a surface anchor

ankyloglossia: Greek for "crooked tongue." *See* tongue-tied

anneal: to heat and cool a metal, alloy, or glass to specific temperatures at certain time intervals to change its properties

anodize: process of altering the way a metal surface refracts light (which appears to change its color) by creating an oxide film

anti-care: *See* dry wound care

anti-eyebrow piercing: *See* teardrop piercing

antihelix: curved elevation of cartilage in front of the helix that runs parallel to it; the mid-antihelix is the site of the snug piercing

antimicrobial: chemical substance that inhibits or destroys microbes such as bacteria, viruses, and fungi

antitragus: small vertical ridge of cartilage above the earlobe (next to the intertragus notch)

apadravya: male genital piercing that passes vertically through the head of the penis; comprised of a Prince Albert piercing on the bottom and a reverse Prince Albert piercing on the top

apex: highest point; in piercing, the deepest anatomical point, such as under the clitoral hood or inside the navel

APP: *See* Association of Professional Piercers

Arnica montana: herb used topically in cream or gel form to diminish bruising

aseptic: free of disease-causing microorganisms

aspirate: to inhale into your lungs

Association of Professional Piercers (APP): international nonprofit membership organization dedicated to the dissemination of vital health and safety information related to body piercing to piercees, piercers, health-care providers, legislators, and the general public

atrophic scar: pit or depression below the surface of the skin, caused by a wound

autoclave: machine used for sterilizing equipment or materials

avascular: not well supplied with fluid and ducts, especially blood circulation of veins, arteries, and capillaries

AWG: *See* American Wire Gauge

B

bacterial endocarditis: See infective endocarditis

bacteriostatic: restricts growth and activity of microorganisms

Bactroban: prescription-only antibiotic effective for topical treatment of localized infections; also mupirocin

banana bell: See curved barbell

barbell: basic body jewelry style; a bar post and two ends that are often spherical in shape

bar-style jewelry: body jewelry with a post portion that functions like a barbell

basal cells: base layer of cells; the first layer of cells formed in wound healing

BCR: ball closure ring. See captive bead ring

BDSM: combined acronym referring to bondage and discipline (BD), domination and submission (DS), and sadomasochism (SM); consensual forms of human sexual behavior

belly button: See navel

benign: not a threat to life or long-term health; noncancerous

bent bar: See curved barbell

Betadine: iodine-based surgical scrub commonly used to clean the skin before piercing

bindi piercing: vertical facial surface piercing between the eyebrows or slightly above them; also vertical bridge

biocompatible: suited for wear in the body without causing irritation, allergy, or infection

biohazard can: waste receptacle used for disposables (other than needles) that may contain blood or blood products

biohazard room: See sterilization room

biological indicator: See spore test

Bioplast: brand name of an inert flexible plastic used for body jewelry

biopsy punch: See dermal punch

bloodborne disease: illness caused by exposure to bloodborne pathogens such as HIV/AIDS or hepatitis B or C

bloodborne pathogen: microorganism that can cause disease when present in blood

blood poisoning: See septicemia

blowout: complication from overstretching; skin pushes out from inside the piercing

BME: largest and longest-running body modification website, www.bmezine.com (Body Modification E-zine) and affiliated sites

body modification: practices that change the body, including piercing, tattooing, branding, and scarification

bridge piercing: horizontal piercing through the tissue between the eyes or a little lower, on the bridge of the nose; also Erl, nasion, or mid-brow

Brown & Sharpe: standard of measurement for wire gauge; also American Wire Gauge

bull ring: See circular barbell

C

caliper: instrument used to measure internal or external dimensions of jewelry and other objects

candidiasis: overgrowth of Candida albicans; called a yeast infection, though not really an infection

cannula: needle covered with a flexible sleeve, commonly used for piercing in Europe; also catheter needle

captive: captive bead ring; also the captive bead or other captive piece

captive bead: spherical closure that fits in the gap of a captive bead ring to secure the jewelry; also captive

captive bead ring: ring with a captive bead or captive piece that can be changed or replaced

captive circular barbell: circular barbell with a captive bead added to the center

captive piece: an alternate shape or design that is worn in a captive bead ring and functions the same way as a captive bead

captive tube: cylindrical captive piece suited to healed piercings

cartilage: dense, avascular tissue that is commonly pierced in the upper ear and nostril

catheter needle: See cannula

CBR: See captive bead ring

cellulitis: inflammation of the cells; spreading infection of tissues beneath the skin

cheese-cutter effect: cutting of tissue caused by jewelry that is too thin in gauge

circular barbell: ring-style jewelry that operates like a barbell: the end or ends screw; also bull ring or horseshoe

cleft of Venus: furrow at the base of the pubic mound where it divides to form the labia majora; also pudendal cleft clitoral glans: external portion of the clitoris usually covered by the clitoral hood; also clitoral head

clitoral head: *See* clitoral glans

clitoral hood: protective fold of tissue that covers the clitoral glans; also prepuce

clitoris: highly sensitive erectile organ visible at the front of the vulva; female counterpart of the male glans

cold abscess: infection of Mycobacterium abscessus (lacks tenderness and inflammation)

cold sterilant: hospital-strength liquid disinfectants that reduce the number of microorganisms; not accepted as a sole sterilization technique for piercing equipment

collagen: fibrous protein that provides strength and resilience to skin

compression technique: application of firm pressure following cartilage piercing to reattach surface tissue to the cartilage underneath to prevent bumps during healing

compression therapy: continuous mechanical pressure used to flatten scars

concave taper: shape at the back end of an insertion taper to fit with a convex jewelry end

conch: *See* concha

concha: deep bowl-shaped central shell of the ear; also conch

conch piercing: piercing of the concha

contact dermatitis: skin rash from contact with an allergen or irritant substance

contaminate: make unclean, especially as a result of contact with something harmful such as disease-causing microorganisms

contraction: step in the second stage of the healing process in which the edges of the wound pull together

C-ring: circular barbell widened to conform to anatomy; same as a U-ring, but not as wide

crus helix: also Crus of helix; *See* helix crus

crusties: nonmedical term for the normal dried discharge around healing piercings

curve: *See* curved barbell

curved barbell: barbell variation that forms approximately one-fourth of a circle; also banana bell, L-bar, bent bar, and curve

cytotoxic: poisonous or harmful to cells

D

daith: piercing of the innermost ridge of cartilage just above the ear canal at the root of the helix crus

dead stretching: expansion of a piercing simply by pushing in a larger object

debridement: removal of dead, contaminated, or adherent tissue or foreign material

deep Prince Albert piercing: Prince Albert piercing placed further down the penis shaft

dental acrylic: biocompatible form of acrylic used for body jewelry

dental dam: sheet of latex used in dental procedures; can shield female genitalia to prevent sharing of bodily fluids during oral sexual contact

dermal anchor: *See* surface anchor

dermal elevator: tool used to lift the tissue to create cavities for pocketing and insertion of subdermal or transdermal implants; also dermal separator

dermal punch: medical tool for tissue biopsies; can be used to create a piercing; also biopsy punch

dermal separator: *See* dermal elevator

dermis: thick layer beneath the epidermis containing blood and lymph vessels, sweat glands, and nerve endings

development: lasting change in the shape, dimensions, and texture of localized tissue following piercing

deviated septum: a displacement from the midline of the tissue that divides the nostrils

Diana piercing: *See* Princess Diana piercing

disinfection: process of reducing the number of microorganisms from a surface or object by applying antimicrobial chemical agents

divot: small depression in the skin left by piercing; also refers to the infranasal depression between mouth and nose

dolphin piercing: deep Prince Albert piercing connected by a single piece of jewelry to a traditional Prince Albert piercing

D-ring: variation of the captive ring; the flat part of the D is worn through a piercing

drool patrol: tissue or paper towel held during an oral piercing to prevent saliva from getting on clothes

dry wound care: no wetting or washing of the area for weeks or months and all care or cleaning products are avoided; also anti-care

dydoe piercing: male genital piercing through the rim of the corona

E

ear cartilage piercing: general term for an ear piercing that is not through the soft tissue of the earlobe; also traditional placement through helix (or through the scapha to frame the helix)

ear head piercing: placed at the root of helix, the juncture of the ear cartilage and the face

earlet: *See* eyelet

ear-piercing gun: device used to insert a pointed earring (not used for body piercings by professional piercers)

edema: buildup of excess fluid in the tissues causing swelling

energy pull: *See* pull

epidermis: thin outermost layer of skin; protects the dermis just beneath it

episiotomy: incision made to enlarge the vaginal opening to facilitate childbirth

epithelial cells: skin cells; cells forming the protective covering on most external and internal surfaces of the body and its organs

epithelialization: process in the growth phase of wound healing involving the formation of skin to completely cover a wound as epithelial cells grow together and thicken

Erl piercing: *See* bridge piercing

essential oils: concentrated liquid plant compounds

European ampallang: horizontal glans penis piercing that passes through the urethra

externally threaded jewelry: style in which the threads are on the part of the jewelry that passes through the body

eyelet: hollow tube-style jewelry worn through the body, usually in stretched piercings; also earlet or grommet

F

female circumcision: *See* female genital cutting (FGC)

female genital cutting (FGC): alteration or partial or entire removal of external genitalia of a girl for cultural or religious reasons; also called female genital mutilation (FGM) and female circumcision

female genital mutilation (FGM): *See* female genital cutting (FGC)

female guiche: *See* fourchette piercing

ferromagnetic: magnetic; attracted by a magnet

fibula: fastening device historically used for infibulation (to insure chastity)

fifth cranial nerve: *See* trigeminal nerve

fishtail labret: L-shaped jewelry for the lower lip; the shorter leg passes through the piercing and the longer end rests in the groove between gum and lip

fistula: flesh tunnel; the channel that forms when a piercing epithelializes with jewelry inside it

flare-up: regression in healing as a piercing secretes and becomes inflamed and/or tender

flash-cycle cassette sterilizer: *See* Statim

flat-back barbell: *See* labret stud

flora: harmless bacteria that inhabit a part of the body

forceps: medical grasping tool used by piercers to secure and support tissue for piercing

foreskin piercing: piercing of the skin covering the glans of the penis

fourchette: "little fork" in French; *See* fourchette piercing

fourchette piercing: vertical piercing of the female perineum

fraenum: *See* frenulum

freehand: piercing method in which the only tool used is a piercing needle (no forceps or needle receiving tubes)

frenulum: a fibrous cord of connecting tissue

frenulum labiorum pudenda: anatomical term for location of the fourchette piercing

frenum ladder: multiple frenum piercings placed in a row

frenum loop: a band worn around the penis shaft secured by a barbell through a healed frenum piercing

frenum piercing: male genital piercing through the pliable tissue on the penis shaft

frowny: piercing of the lower lip frenulum

fungi: microorganisms, including mold and yeast, that feed off other organisms to survive; can cause infection; sing. fungus

fused quartz: *See* quartz glass

G

gauge: numerical standard of measurement for thickness of metal wire; sometimes used as a verb to mean stretching a piercing, or as a noun referring to the jewelry worn in a stretched hole

gauging: colloquial term for stretching

gauging up: term for stretching

genital beading: implant in which round beads are placed within genital tissue to add sensation and/or alter appearance

genital ribs: variation of genital beading in which rod-shaped pieces are used

gentian violet: purple water-based fungicide used as ink in surgical markers and in other methods of marking piercing placements

germicidal: kills microorganisms that cause disease

glabella: anatomical term for tissue between the brows; location of the bridge piercing

glans: head of the penis or tip of the clitoris

Golden Rule of Piercing Hygiene: Do not touch healing piercings with dirty hands.

gold-filled: *See* gold-plated

gold-overlay: *See* gold-plated

gold-plated: base metal coated with a thin layer of gold to create affordable jewelry with the look of gold; also gold-filled, gold-overlay, rolled gold, and vermeil

Gräfenberg spot: *See* G-spot

granulation: phase in the second stage of the healing process; body produces cells, including collagen

granulation tissue: small, grainy tissue particles that grow to cover healing wounds

granuloma: unattractive growth of excess granulation tissue

grommet: *See* eyelet

growth phase: second stage of the wound healing process that includes granulation and contraction; also proliferative phase

G-spot: sexually sensitive area on the front wall of the vagina; also Gräfenberg spot

guiche: a piercing located in the perineum, behind the scrotum and across the perineal raphe

H

hafada piercing: scrotum piercing, especially when placed on one or both sides in the upper portion of the natural fold

half gauges: odd numbered gauge sizes in between the usual even-numbered sizes used for body jewelry and equipment

heat-shrink tubing: thin, inert tubing used by electricians that can be placed over jewelry to facilitate stretching a piercing

helix: curled outer rim of the external ear; location for the traditional ear cartilage piercing

helix crus: anatomical term for daith piercing placement: the innermost ridge of cartilage just above the ear canal that fades out into the shell of the concha; also crus helix and crus of helix

helix root: where the curl of the helix originates at the top of the ear nearest the head; location of the ear head piercing

hemostasis: stoppage of bleeding; part of the first stage of early wound healing

hill: in contrast to valley, an anatomical rise or ridge; female genitals in which the clitoral hood is pronounced and higher than the outer labia

horseshoe: *See* circular barbell

hyperextend: go beyond the normal range of movement for the body or a joint

hypergranulation tissue: excessive growth of granulation tissue; granuloma and pyogenic granuloma are similar conditions

hypertonic: containing more salt than your blood (as opposed to isotonic)

hypertrophic scar: thick, lumpy scar that sits above the surface of the skin

hypospadias: birth defect in which the urinary meatus is not located at the tip of the penis

I

implant: extreme body modification in which a foreign object is placed in the body; includes subdermal and transdermal implants

implant designation: numbered codes that represent a precise standard for the recipe and quality from the American (now International) Society for Testing and Materials Standard (ASTM) and/or the International Standards Organization (ISO)

implant grade: an implant designation for material with biocompatibility levels accepted for medical implant usage

induration: localized hardening of normally soft tissue, often seen in wounds or infections

industrial: *See* industrial piercing

industrial piercing: single barbell through two or more piercings in one ear; also industrial, industrial project, or scaffold piercing

industrial project: *See* industrial piercing

infection: invasion and multiplication of disease-causing microorganisms producing an injurious effect

infective endocarditis: potentially deadly infection of the inner lining of the heart or heart valves (previously referred to as bacterial endocarditis)

inferior crus of the antihelix: small ridge of cartilage that originates near the face in the upper part of the ear; anatomical term for the location of the rook piercing

infibulation: restriction of sexual activity through mechanical means

inflammation: normal, localized protective response to injury that protects the body from infection but is problematic if it becomes chronic

inflammatory phase: first stage in the process of wound healing; includes hemostasis and the laying down of basal cells

infranasal depression: natural midline dip between mouth and the nose; site of philtrum piercing

infused herbal oil: essential oil mixed into an oil base

infusion: tea from flowers, leaves, or roots steeped longer than usual to extract their properties

inner conch: true conch piercing in the concha of the ear

inner labia: delicate hairless folds of flesh situated between the outer labia; also labia minora

innie: concave navel configuration

insertion: to put jewelry into an existing piercing; also jewelry insertion and reinsertion

insertion needle: *See* insertion taper

insertion pin: *See* insertion taper

insertion taper: tool used to facilitate jewelry insertion or reinsertion and for stretching piercings to a thicker gauge; also insertion pin, insertion needle, or taper

interdigital spaces: between the fingers or toes

internally threaded: jewelry with the threads on the ball or end; the portion that passes through the body is tapped with a hole to receive the threads

interstitial fluid: liquid between cells of the body

intertragus notch: groove at the bottom of the opening to the ear canal above the earlobe and below the tragus

iron cross: combination of a horizontal and vertical piercing, usually in a nipple or penis head; also magic cross

isotonic: matches the salinity of human fluids (as in normal saline)

J

J-bar: *See* J-curve

J-curve: J-shaped barbell variation suited to vertical piercings

jewelry insertion: *See* insertion

K

karat: measure of gold purity; 24 karat is pure gold, 18 karat is 18 parts gold out of 24 parts metal in an alloy

keloid: large, dense growth of excessive scar tissue much bigger than the original wound

keratin: fibrous protein that is not water soluble; one of the components of sebum

L

labia: "lip" in Latin; external folds of skin of female genitalia; sing. labium

labia majora: *See* outer labia

labia minora: *See* inner labia

labret piercing: lower lip piercing; from the Latin labrum

labret stud: short barbell with a disc on one side and an ornament (ball, gem, etc.) on the other; also flat-back barbell

ladder: rows of piercings, commonly of frenum, labia, or other genital placement

laparoscopy: medical procedure in which instruments are inserted through small incisions; frequently done in the navel

L-bar: *See* curved barbell

L-bend: L-shaped jewelry worn in a nostril piercing

lingual frenulum: thin web of tissue connecting the tongue to the floor of the mouth

LITHA: minimal aftercare consisting of regular hygiene; acronym for Leave It the Heck Alone

lobule: fleshy portion of the earlobe; the lobe

localized argyria: permanent dark bluish discoloration of skin caused by exposure to silver or silver salts; also tarnish tattoo

lorum piercing: horizontal piercing on the underside of the penis at the juncture of the penis and the scrotum lumen: space inside a tubular structure, such as the hollow interior of a needle receiving tube

lymph: pale fluid of the lymphatic vessels; chiefly plasma and white blood cells

M

magic cross: *See* iron cross

Master Piercer: honorary title earned for expertise, dedication, and contributions to professional piercing bestowed by another Master Piercer

maturation: final stage in the wound healing process in which the collagen becomes more organized and strengthens; also remodeling

Medusa: *See* philtrum piercing

meridian: energy channels in the body (in Chinese medicine)

microbe: microscopic organism such as a bacterium or fungus, especially one that can transmit disease

microbicide: a substance that kills microbes

microdermal: *See* surface anchor

mid-brow: location and alternate name of the bridge piercing

midline: in the center; structure or imaginary line that divides the body into left and right halves

migration: piercing moves from its original position; either settles and heals, or continues to move and rejects

mill certificates: documents to provide evidence of a particular grade of metal; also mill certs or mill test certificates

mill certs: *See* mill certificates

mill test certificates: *See* mill certificates

mini barbell: barbells in small gauges suited to above-the-neck piercings

mirror finish: high-shine, super-smooth surface

mons pubis: *See* pubic mound

mons veneris: *See* pubic mound

motility: ability to move independently (exhibited by some bacteria)

mupirocin: antibiotic in Bactroban

Mycobacterium abscessus: *See* cold abscess

N

nasallang: industrial piercing of the nose through both nostrils and septum

nasion: area between the eyes; location for bridge piercing

naso-labial folds: smile lines around the mouth extending roughly from the corners of the nose to the corners of the mouth

natural materials: materials such as horn, bone, wood, amber, and stone, which can be worn in healed piercings; also organics

navel: place the umbilical cord was tied after being cut following birth; also umbilicus and belly button

necrosis: death of tissue or cells caused by injury or disease

needle receiving tube: hollow tube used in piercing procedures; also receiving tube and NRT

negative space: area between or around; unpierced skin left between holes for aesthetic reasons

nesting: normal tendency of oral jewelry to indent a millimeter or so into the soft tissue

new piercing salute: *See* salute

nipple development: *See* development

non-ferromagnetic: not magnetic; not affected by a magnet

non-iodized: without iodine

normal saline: isotonic sodium chloride solution, having the same concentration as body fluids

nose bone: short post worn in a nostril piercing with a tiny ball that is passed through the tissue to keep the jewelry in place

nostril piercing: piercing through the alar cartilage on the side of the nose

nostril screw: post-style jewelry with a curved tail that rests inside the nostril or on the back of an ear; does not require a backing like a traditional stud earring

NRT: *See* needle receiving tube

O

Occupational Safety and Health Administration (OSHA): U.S. government organization that regulates workplace safety

organics: *See* natural materials

orofacial piercing: piercing from the exterior facial surface through to the interior of the mouth; includes piercings of the upper and lower lips

OSHA: *See* Occupational Safety and Health Administration

outer conch: piercing in the scapha or anti-helix nearer the concha area than the helix

outer labia: thick fleshy folds of the vulva where hair grows; also labia majora

outie: protruding navel configuration

P

PA: *See* Prince Albert piercing

palang: term used by the Dyaks in Borneo for piercing of the penis head and the object ("crossbar") worn in it; apparent origin of the word *ampallang*

palladium: inert elemental metal sometimes alloyed with gold or platinum for jewelry

PA piercing: *See* Prince Albert piercing

parotid duct: conduit for saliva from the parotid gland

parotid gland: largest of the salivary glands

pathogenic: able to cause disease

pathogens: germs such as bacteria or viruses that can cause disease

Pennington forceps: a medical clamp with a triangular jaw commonly used to support and secure tissue for piercing

perineal raphe: faint ridge of tissue that runs from scrotum to anus; location of guiche piercing

perineum: area between the anus and the rear part of the external genitalia; location of guiche piercing in men, and fourchette piercing in women

peritoneum: membrane that lines and protects the abdominal cavity

philtrum piercing: in the center of the natural divot (the infranasal depression) between mouth and nose; also Medusa, divot, and upret

phlebotomy: *See* venipuncture

physical vapor deposition: *See* PVD

pierce and stretch: technique of making a piercing, then immediately stretching it larger using an insertion taper (not recommended)

Piercee's Bill of Rights: list of piercees' rights by the Association of Professional Piercers

piercing needle: super-sharp needle made specifically for performing body piercings

pin-coupling taper: insertion taper style; the back end is a pin shaped to fit inside internally threaded jewelry

plasma: liquid part of blood comprised of serum and clotting factors

platinum: inert, expensive, precious, elemental metal suited for piercing jewelry

play piercing: temporary piercings; insertion of a needle or needles (and occasionally jewelry) for a performance, ritual, or BDSM or erotic scene

plumber's tape: extremely thin inert tape used by plumbers; when wrapped around jewelry can facilitate slowly stretching a piercing

pneumothorax: collapsed lung caused by air in the space between the lung and chest wall

pocketing: body modification in which a post is placed with one end in each side of adjoining pockets formed in the tissue

Polytetrafluoroethylene: *See* PTFE

povidone iodine: *See* Betadine

preauricular pit: tiny natural hole in the skin where an ear head piercing is placed

prepuce: loose fitting fold of tissue; clitoral hood in women and foreskin in men

Prince Albert piercing: male genital piercing on the underside of the penis at the juncture of the head and shaft; jewelry rests inside the urethra and is worn out the tip of the urinary meatus

Princess Albertina: piercing of the female urinary meatus

Princess Diana piercing: female genital piercing placed under the clitoral hood like a VCH piercing, but off to the side(s)

prophylaxis: preventive treatment

PTFE: inert, flexible, autoclavable form of Teflon used as a nonmetallic jewelry alternative; also Polytetrafluoroethylene

pubic mound: soft pad of rounded flesh on the pubic bone present in both genders; also pubis, mons pubis, and mons veneris in women

pubis: *See* pubic mound

pudendal cleft: *See* cleft of Venus

pull: temporary piercing(s) are tethered and pulled in a controlled manner to achieve certain mental or physical states; also energy pull

pus: thick, opaque fluid consisting of white blood cells, dead cells, and bacteria; produced by inflammation and infection

pustule: small round area of inflamed skin with a visible collection of pus; a pimple

PVD: high-tech version of electroplating deposits a durable film of black, copper, and other colors; used on body jewelry and in other industries; also physical vapor deposition

pyogenic granuloma: *See* hypergranulation tissue

Q

quartz glass: biocompatible type of glass made from almost pure silica; also fused quartz

R

receiving tube: *See* needle receiving tube

reinsertion: insertion done on a hole that has been empty or abandoned

rejection: piercing migration in which jewelry is pushed completely out of the body

relaxing: *See* resting

remodeling: *See* maturation

resorption: erosion of bone, cartilage, gum, or other tissue, which is absorbed by the body

resting: practice of removing large-gauge jewelry for a time to relieve tissue of weight and pressure; also relaxing

retiring: removing jewelry to abandon a piercing

reverse PA: *See* reverse Prince Albert piercing

reverse Prince Albert piercing: vertical midline piercing from the upper side of the urethra to the top of the penis glans; also reverse PA

ring expanding pliers: jewelry tool used to widen a ring, usually for inserting a captive bead or to spread the gap of a circular barbell into a C-ring or U-ring; also RXP, snap-ring pliers, ring opening pliers, or ROP

ring opening pliers: *See* ring expanding pliers

ring-style jewelry: jewelry style that functions like a ring, including the circular barbell

rolled gold: *See* gold-plated

rook piercing: placement through the small ridge of cartilage that originates near the face in the upper part of the ear (the inferior crus of the antihelix)

ROP: *See* ring expanding pliers

RXP: *See* ring expanding pliers

S

sadhu piercing: lower conch piercing, especially in a large gauge

salute: ring stands out from the body when jewelry is too small or the tissue of a new piercing is tight; also new piercing salute

scaffold piercing: *See* industrial piercing

scalpelling: using the cutting instrument to create or enlarge a body piercing

scapha: elongated depression of the ear that separates the helix and antihelix

scar: mark left in the skin by the healing of a wound

screw threads: *See* threads

scrumper: *See* smiley

sebum: naturally occurring product of the body that collects in healed piercing channels; contains fat, keratin, and cellular material from oil glands

septicemia: severe total body infection caused by harmful microorganisms throughout the bloodstream; also blood poisoning

septum forceps: specialized clamp with a short piece of needle receiving tube soldered onto each end; sometimes used for septum, conch, and triangle piercings

septum piercing: piercing in the tissue dividing the nostrils

septum retainer: open-ended U-shaped or modified staple-shaped jewelry that conceals a septum piercing by flipping up and hiding inside the nostrils

septum spike: straight jewelry with tapered ends worn in a healed septum piercing

septum stench: the pungent, rotten odor that comes from sebum in a septum piercing

serous: relating to serum

serum: clear liquid part of blood; essentially plasma, without the clotting factor

serous exudates: in piercing, lymph and dead cells

sharps disposal: special container for safely discarding used piercing needles

side lip piercing with ring: self-descriptive type of orofacial piercing

single-point piercing: alternate name for the procedure to insert a surface anchor

slotted forceps: clamp that has a segment of the jaws removed so the tool can be taken off easily, even after jewelry is in place

smiley: piercing of the upper web that attaches the center of the lip to the gums; also scrumper

snake bites: piercing placement on either side of the lips or tongue; also venoms, vipers, or viper bites

snap-ring pliers: *See* ring expanding pliers

snug piercing: horizontal cartilage piercing framing a protrusion between the conch and the helix called the antihelix

spore: form of certain microbes (including pathogenic bacteria and fungi) that often survive harsh environments in a dormant stage; when conditions improve they can germinate and resume their life cycle spore test: validation of autoclave function to determine if all spores were destroyed using strips of heat-resistant spores run through a sterilization cycle then evaluated by a testing laboratory; also biological indicators

Standard Precautions: infection control practices for dealing with blood or other potentially infectious body fluids; formerly Universal Precautions

Statim: autoclave with a fast sterilization cycle suitable for certain situations; also flash-cycle cassette sterilizer

sterile: free of all microorganisms; an object that has passed through the process of sterilization

sterilization: destruction of all microorganisms, including fungi, bacteria, viruses, and bacterial spores

sterilization room: separate room for processing contaminated items; also biohazard room

stretching: practice of gradually enlarging a piercing to a thicker gauge size

stretching crescent: circular insertion taper worn like jewelry; causes damage if used for stretching too quickly

stretch mark: form of scarring; narrow band of discoloration caused by expanding and weakening of the skin

subdermal implant: form of body modification in which an implant is placed under the skin through an incision and the object is enclosed under the surface

supine: lying on the back

supra-alar crease: natural niche on the side of the nose where it flares; common location for nostril piercing

surface anchor: tiny specialized jewelry worn in a single L-shaped opening formed in the tissue (term for jewelry and procedure); also anchor, dermal anchor, and microdermal

surface bar: barbell variation for surface piercings shaped like an open staple, with a longer straight bar post between two shorter upright legs

surface piercing: piercing of a flat area of the body that lacks a defined fold, flap, or protrusion of tissue

suspension: temporary piercing usually for ritual or entertainment in which sterile hooks are inserted through the flesh and used to suspend a piercee by special rigging

sweet spot: anatomical location optimal for piercing placement

T

tandem piercing: pair of piercings simultaneously performed by two piercers

taper: *See* insertion taper

tapping: drilled out hole in threaded jewelry that fits the threads

tarnish tattoo: *See* localized argyria

teardrop piercing: facial surface piercing atop the crest of the cheekbone; also anti-eyebrow

Techni-Care surgical scrub: microbicide commonly used for skin prep before piercings; also used for piercing care

thermoplastic: material that can be shaped somewhat after heating and that will retain its new form once cooled

threaded: having threads for securing removable ends to body jewelry

threaded end: ball or other ornament that has the threads (rather than the tapping)

threaded-pin taper: insertion taper style in which the larger end screws into the tapping on the jewelry

threadless jewelry: alternate jewelry closure style instead of threads; barbell end has a male pin coupling that presses into a female post

threadlocker: product applied to threads to help prevent the jewelry from unscrewing

threads: screw thread pattern cut into the male portion of threaded jewelry; fits into the female tapped portion

thrush: oral yeast infection; candidiasis

tissue manipulation: localized massage of the skin to prepare it for piercing

tongue-tied: having restricted tongue movement due to a tight lingual frenulum; also ankyloglossia

tongue-tip piercing: piercing within the first half-inch of the tongue

tragus: small protrusion of cartilage that juts out from the face over the center of the ear canal

transdermal implant: implant placed under the skin through an incision with an opening made to allow an ornament to show above the surface

transverse: horizontal or crosswise

triangle piercing: female genital piercing behind the nerve bundle of the clitoris

trigeminal nerve: main sensory nerve on each side of the head and face and the motor nerve of muscles used for chewing; also fifth cranial nerve true navel piercing: when the protrusion of an outie navel is pierced (not recommended)

tummy tuck: *See* abdominoplasty

Tygon: flexible autoclavable plastic (silicone) tubing used as a nonmetallic jewelry alternative

U

ultrasonic unit: machine that removes debris using agitation from sonic waves in liquid

umbilicus: *See* navel

underdeveloped: small anatomy that has not grown to its full extent

Universal Precautions: *See* Standard Precautions

upret: *See* philtrum piercing

urethra: tube that delivers urine from the bladder out of the body

urinary meatus: external urethral opening where Prince Albert piercing jewelry is worn

U-ring: custom-bent circular barbell widened out to a U-shape to conform to anatomy; same style as a C-ring, but opened even wider

V

valley: in contrast to hill, an anatomical groove or crevice; female genitals in a very vertical configuration with outer labia higher than the hood

vascularity: supply of fluid and ducts, especially blood circulation of veins, arteries, and capillaries

vasoconstriction: narrowing of blood vessels

VCH: *See* VCH piercing

VCH piercing: female genital piercing through the clitoral hood; also vertical clitoral hood piercing

venipuncture: drawing blood or inserting an intravenous line; also phlebotomy

venoms: *See* snake bites

vermeil: *See* gold-plated

vermillion border: pigmented area of the lips where lipstick or lip balm is applied

vertical bridge piercing: *See* bindi piercing

vertical clitoral hood piercing: *See* VCH piercing

vertical lip piercing: surface piercing through the pigmented part of the lip

viper bites: *See* snake bites

vipers: *See* snake bites

vulva: external female genitalia

W

wound care: promotion of wound healing by minimizing factors that inhibit healing, enhancing the healing process, and reducing risk of infection

wound healing: series of stages in the process of the body regenerating dermal and epidermal tissue following injury

wrecking ball fractures: cracks in teeth caused by jewelry in an oral piercing

Select Bibliography

Armitage, Cecil Hamilton. *The Tribal Markings and Marks of Adornment of the Natives of the Northern Territories of the Gold Coast Colony.* Royal Anthropological Institute of Great Britain and Ireland. London: Harrison and Sons, 1924.

Association of Professional Piercers. *APP Manual*, U.S. Edition. Association of Professional Piercers, 2005.

Bell, David. *An Introduction to Cybercultures.* London and New York: Routledge, 2001.

Brown, Donald E., James W. Edwards, and Ruth P. Moore. "The Penis Inserts of Southeast Asia: An Annotated Bibliography with an Overview and Comparative Perspectives." Occasional Paper No. 15, University of California, Berkeley, 1988.

Califia, Pat. *Public Sex: The Culture of Radical Sex.* 2nd ed. San Francisco: Cleis Press, 2000.

Camphausen, Rufus C. *Return of the Tribal: A Celebration of Body Adornment.* Rochester, VT: Park Street Press, 1997.

Curry-McGhee, Leanne K. *Tattoos and Body Piercing Overview Series.* San Diego, CA: Lucent Books, 2005.

De la Haye, Amy, and Cathie Dingwal. *Surfers, Soulies, Skinheads & Skaters: Subcultural Style from the Forties to the Nineties.* Woodstock, NY: Overlook Press, 1996.

Dunbar, Andrew, and Dean Lahn. *Body Piercing.* New York: St. Martin's Press, 1998.

Featherstone, Mike, ed. *Body Modification.* London: Sage Publications, 2005.

Gay, Kathlyn, and Christine Whittington. *Body Marks: Tattooing, Piercing, and Scarification.* Brookfield, CT: Millbrook Press, 2002.

Hewitt, Kim. *Mutilating the Body: Identity in Blood and Ink.* Bowling Green, OH: Bowling Green State University Popular Press, 1997.

Lloyd, J. D., ed. *Body Piercing and Tattoos: Examining Pop Culture.* Farmington Hills, MI: Greenhaven Press, 2003.

McNab, Nan. *Body Bizarre, Body Beautiful.* Darby, PA: Diane, 1999.

Mercury, Maureen. *Pagan Fleshworks: The Alchemy of Body Modification.* Rochester, VT: Park Street Press, 2000.

Miller, Jean-Chris. *The Body Art Book: A Complete, Illustrated Guide to Tattoos, Piercings, and Other Body Modifications.* New York: Berkeley Book, 2004.

Perlingieri, Blake Andrew. *A Brief History of the Evolution of Body Adornment in Western Culture: Ancient Origins and Today.* Eugene, OR: Tribalife Publications, 2003.

Pitts, Victoria L. *In the Flesh: The Cultural Politics of Body Modification.* New York: Palgrave Macmillan, 2003.

Polhemus, Ted. *Streetstyle: From Sidewalk to Catwalk.* London: Thames and Hudson, 1994.

Robinson, Julian. *The Quest for Human Beauty: An Illustrated History.* New York: W.W. Norton & Company, 1998.

Rubin, Arnold, ed. *Marks of Civilization: Artistic Transformations of the Human Body.* Los Angeles: Museum of Cultural History, University of California, 1988.

Steele, Valerie. *Fetish: Fashion, Sex, and Power.* New York: Oxford University Press, 1997.

Vale, V., and Andrea Juno. *Modern Primitives: An Investigation of Contemporary Adornment & Ritual.* San Francisco: Re/Search Publications, 1999.

Wilkinson, Beth. *Coping with the Dangers of Tattooing, Body Piercing, and Branding.* New York: Rosen Publishing Group, 1998.

About the Author

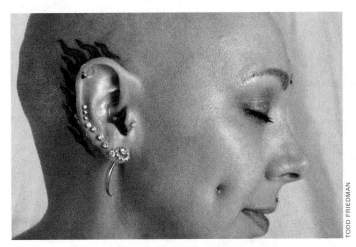

ELAYNE ANGEL has been a professional piercer for more than twenty years and was awarded the President's Lifetime Achievement Award by the Association of Professional Piercers in 2006. A contributing writer for *PAIN Magazine,* she is currently serving her third term on the Board of Directors for the Association of Professional Piercers. She lives in Mérida, Mexico.

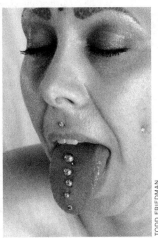

Visit www.piercingbible.com.

Index